Advance Praise for Sky Above Clouds

This book takes us into the inner galactic spheres of creative potential and healing. The fact that Cohen's illness went on for more than 13 years—beating the statistical odds of survival so dramatically that he was told "Medically, you do not exist"—makes this book a miracle story because this is what gave both authors the opportunity to reap such powerful insights. They wrote under the constant threat of his severe metastatic condition, and within the context of raising a child, thriving professionally, and loving one another: The miracle of the life that they weren't supposed to have gave them the opportunity to merge their personal and professional lives, and to flesh out concepts that are not normally underst̶ ̶ ̶ring, illness, and a creative life. This story is amazing to ̶

Sanford Finkel, MD, ge̶ ̶ ̶ ̶sor of
Psychiatr̶ ̶ ̶hool

At various times in one's life and especia̶ ̶ ̶ ̶ ̶tal to be able to creatively assess, interpret, and react t̶ ̶ ̶on. Loss is inevitable, but true strength, power, and hope are found in how we experience and make sense of loss. In *Sky Above Clouds*, there is a sense of continuity despite the chaos of time; there is endurance despite change. Emotional movement that varies from loss, to reflection, to hope, to new futures is a chain that is repeated within smaller sections as well as in the book as a whole. As a reader, I needed to know that people can survive loss, not that they're unchanged by it, but that they are not destroyed. The elements of this book come together into full consciousness, creating this special gift of insight.

Kate de Medeiros, PhD, Blayney Associate Professor of
Sociology and Gerontology, Miami University, author of
Narrative Gerontology in Research and Practice

Sky Above Clouds is a powerful narrative of illness that will reshape current thinking about chronic disease, health care, aging, and the arts. On one level, it is an intensely personal story of Gene Cohen's thirteen-year battle with metastatic prostate cancer and Wendy's insightful observations made throughout the long journey as his wife and caregiver. It chronicles their approach to managing his care when he was deemed a "medical outlier" and the impact of the illness on their relationship, family members, and their professional lives, his as a renowned gero-psychiatrist, researcher, and author and hers as an artist, art therapist, and psychologist. On another level, it portrays how interweaving their unique perspectives as scientist and artist influenced their approach and led to the formulation of an exciting new paradigm about aging and illness, one that emphasizes human potential and the creative spirit to bring new meaning to later life and end of life. Health providers, educators, researchers, and those in the arts and humanities who seek to move beyond entrenched thinking about illness and aging can benefit greatly from this "work of art."

Linda S. Noelker, PhD, Adjunct Professor of Sociology,
Case Western Reserve University

"Tell your numbers in a rhyme if you can," an exercise in imagination associated with the game of cribbage, brought two creative healing souls—artist Wendy Miller and scientist Gene Cohen—together in life and in death. Their book *Sky Above Clouds* reveals the twinkling depths of the unfathomable universe of human compassion and wisdom. This beautiful piece of writing intergeneratively blends the quantum and qualia of life and allows us to experience the swirling galactic energy of their shared relationship. It shows us that one and one are fun and also a few more than two.

Peter Whitehouse, MD, PhD, Professor of Neurology,
Case Western Reserve University,
author of *The Myth of Alzheimer's*

Art therapist Wendy Miller and Gene Cohen, the guru of creative aging, shared a public silence about Gene's terminal cancer for a remarkable 13 years. As the fog of grief surrounding Gene's illness and death has lifted, Wendy has reclaimed her voice and created a poetic reflection of the love affair with art, science, and creativity she shared with Gene. *Sky Above Clouds* is a contemplation on the power of the creative spirit to find sunshine behind and beyond a tempestuous struggle with terminal cancer. It is a story of personal heroism, survival, and recovery with profound lessons for us all.

Michael C. Patterson, CEO of MINDRAMP Consulting,
past manager of AARP's Brain Health Program,
and board member emeritus (with Gene Cohen)
of the National Center for Creative Aging

Sky Above Clouds is the inside story of how science and art come together to create something larger than one plus one equals two. Creativity and the creative imagination are at the heart of this magical transformation. First the father wishes to write a fairytale for his daughter whom he may not see grow up. Then Gene and Wendy come together to bridge, enhance, and illuminate our understanding of "living with loss." With profound gratitude, I thank Gene and Wendy for sharing their unique perspectives on resilience and growth as these creative thinkers integrate theory and life in story. We are our stories. *Sky Above Clouds* is an important tale that shows the power of art and science to uplift and inspire us all in challenging times. In addition, the field of creative aging exists because of the "Creativity and Aging Study" conducted by Dr. Gene Cohen: research, programs, and policy converging into NCCA.

Susan Perlstein, founder, National Center for Creative Aging (NCCA)

Sky Above Clouds

Sky Above Clouds

FINDING OUR WAY THROUGH CREATIVITY, AGING, AND ILLNESS

BY

WENDY L. MILLER, PHD,

and

GENE D. COHEN, MD, PHD

with

TERESA H. BARKER

OXFORD
UNIVERSITY PRESS

OXFORD
UNIVERSITY PRESS

Oxford University Press is a department of the University of Oxford. It furthers
the University's objective of excellence in research, scholarship, and education
by publishing worldwide. Oxford is a registered trade mark of Oxford University
Press in the UK and certain other countries.

Published in the United States of America by Oxford University Press
198 Madison Avenue, New York, NY 10016, United States of America.

Library of Congress Cataloging-in-Publication Data
Names: Miller, Wendy L., 1950- | Cohen, Gene D. | Barker, Teresa.
Title: Sky above clouds : finding our way through creativity, aging, and illness / by Wendy L. Miller and
Gene D. Cohen, with Teresa H. Barker.
Description: Oxford ; New York : Oxford University Press, [2016] | Includes bibliographical references
and index.
Identifiers: LCCN 2015033768 | ISBN 9780199371419 (alk. paper)
Subjects: LCSH: Aging—Psychological aspects. | Older people—Psychology. | Resilience (Personality
trait) | Creative ability. | Mind and body. | Loss (Psychology) in old age. | Art therapy.
Classification: LCC BF724.55.A35 M55 2016 | DDC 155.67—dc23 LC record available at http://lccn.
loc.gov/2015033768

9 8 7 6 5 4 3 2 1
Printed in Canada by Webcom

This is a story of love, a story of loss, a story of care.
It is a love letter, a "heart song," to you, Gene, because that is the only strategy I can choose: a love letter to you and with you.

All stories are illness stories, for all expose the
human condition of mortality.
The care of the sick is a work of art[1].
Rita Charon

Contents

Sky above clouds is a beautiful metaphor that dignifies the process of aging and the process of living, especially in difficult times. Aging can be challenging and often lonely. This can lead to deep spiritual and existential distress as people try to find their inherent meaning and purpose in life. Society moves at a rapid pace, often not giving space to the wisdom of the older person. People can feel useless and cast aside. They can experience deep hopelessness and despair. The other day, at my father's senior living community, I overheard a resident say, "I wish there was someone that could hold my hand and tell me everything will be ok." *Sky Above Clouds* does just that. In the midst of the clouds that at times overshadow our daily lives, there is hope in remembering that there is a sky above these clouds—one that holds the memories of who we were, and the hopes and possibilities of what we are still becoming.

I had the privilege of knowing Gene Cohen at George Washington University. He was a brilliant man who found a new meaning in his own life through his struggle with cancer. I loved his strong will to live with zest and vigor. Even when his body did not have much energy, he continued to learn, teach, and produce amazing works of creativity and scholarship. His experience with illness and his fight to be recognized as a well person, in spite of the label of cancer, inspired him to advocate for a paradigm shift in how we, as a medical community and as a society, view aging and illness. He shattered those images of bodies slumped in wheelchairs, people with vacant stares, and warehouses of the silently suffering ill, with research studies proving that everyone—no matter how ill, how old, how cognitively impaired—has the capacity to grow, learn, and keep living to the very end. And his treatment was creativity—ways to unleash the deep inspiration in all people to help them reconnect with their deep inner selves, their souls, and to find new meaning, new ways of expressing themselves, new ways to hope and to love again. He measured outcomes such as mastery, control, and civic engagement. He also showed how people with dementia improved their quality of life and ability to communicate through creative arts. His passion inspired new clinical models, and transformation of a dreaded ending to life. Instead, he challenged all of us to see possibility to the very end.

Gene clearly impacted many of us in medicine, research, and geriatrics.[1] As his son, Alex Cohen, noted in his eulogy, Dr. Cohen's professional career was "dedicated to the field of aging and geriatrics long before the field even existed. After graduating from Harvard College and Georgetown University School of Medicine, he began shaping the field of geriatrics through his work at the National Institute of Mental Health in the early 1970s. Here he was the first chief of the Center on Aging and Director of the Program on Aging. At that time, this was the first federally supported national center on mental health and aging established internationally. When he arrived only one specialty program in geriatric psychiatry existed, and when he left there were dozens." Dr. Walter Reich, Yitzhak Rabin Memorial Professor of International Affairs, Ethics and Human Behavior, and Professor of Psychiatry and Behavioral Sciences at George Washington University Elliott School of International Affairs, worked with Gene in the Commissioned Corps of the U.S. Public Health Service. In his remarks at the eulogy, Dr. Reich said: "Were we the best and the brightest? I don't know. But I *do* know that the day that I met Gene, I realized I had found someone who, in *any* context, and at *any* time, would be considered among the best and the brightest. I was, in fact, *surrounded* by brilliant researchers and clinicians, whether they'd come *during* the Vietnam War or before. But when I met Gene I realized I'd met someone who wasn't just one of the best and brightest. I'd met someone who was absolutely unique. He had qualities that, even then, set him apart from everyone else, and that exhibited themselves again and again in his long career at the NIMH and the NIH and, later, at George Washington University." Gene's career resulted in so many accomplishments. Dr. Sanford Finkel, Clinical Professor of Psychiatry, University of Chicago Medical School, also worked with Gene from 1977 when they were the only two geriatric psychiatrists in leadership roles for government. He wrote: "Our field was too narrow for him. Whenever he reached a point where the growth curve was slowing a little, he found a new direction that took him and all of us mere mortals to a different level. I don't know what his next direction would have been, but probably something in the intergalactic sphere. He first planted a seed, then a hundred and then thousands, and he stayed to watch them flower and then each would germinate until there was a garden, then a forest of beauty. Only then, knowing that his seminal goals in one area were achieved, would he move to his next areas of exploration and achievement."

It is not often that a book with two co-authors includes one that is dead. Gene Cohen and Wendy Miller were a husband-and-wife team when their preliminary work on this book began nearly a decade ago. Gene's death in 2009 left Wendy to, among other things, write the book and find a publisher. The reader will meet Gene through his writings, which are integral to this book. It was an honor for me to meet Wendy Miller, Gene's wife, several years after his death. Wendy spoke to our GW medical students about her experience of being a wife and of walking the journey of illness with her husband. The medical students were inspired by her stories of courage and deep love and by her commitment to ensure that Gene's life had dignity and his medical team heard what mattered most to him. She gave a voice to his suffering and to his joy in her caring for him. She also challenged the students to remember to treat the whole patient and loved ones—to listen to their stories and not to treat them as diseases but as people with amazing histories and potentials for a fully lived life, even in the midst of chronic and serious illness.

Now, in this book, an act of love and deep respect for Gene, Wendy brings his wisdom to life, gently interwoven with her passion, tenderness, and deep insight into the challenges of people facing serious illness, and some dying, and the struggles of couples facing those challenges together. Both Wendy and Gene clearly believed in a sky above the clouds, living inspired and creative lives—always open to a life full of possibility. This book is born out of those possibilities, and out of the deep love they shared for each other and for the patients and clients they had the privilege to treat.

Christina M. Puchalski,[2] MD
Founder and Director of the
George Washington Institute for Spirituality and Health
Professor of Medicine and Health Sciences at
George Washington University School of Medicine

Preface

This book tells the story of what happens when life's challenges open a new quadrant of existence in our lives. I experience this opening as an existential crack in the personal universe that we have understood up to this point: a crack where both the light and the darkness of vulnerability appear; a crack that reveals the thin veil of another world we may or may not have a desire to enter or even know. Sometimes this crack occurs through a new opportunity; more often, we face it by way of loss or grief, illness, injury, accident, age, or death. At other times we are thrown into this shift in awareness by the pressures of developmental growth or healing, courage or resilience.

When we face challenges of health and age, the light that comes through this crack in the universe can appear reflective or unfamiliar, even as it holds the potential for new discoveries. What pathways of understanding will we discover through this new light? What other qualities accompany the empathy and compassion which so often seem to shine through the light of this existential crack? This book illuminates both the shadowy depths and the safe harbors of this experience.

Both Gene and I loved to study psychological development and the creative arts. With his background in aging, he researched artists in the latter part of their lives. He was always in search of new ways to talk about aging, to translate more vividly the exciting emerging science and clinical stories of aging and insight into new images and metaphors that could represent a truer sense of the potential in our development as we creatively age into wisdom. He was frustrated, as we all should be, by the endless supply of stereotypical images that focus on decline in our older years. All we have to do is search for a birthday card for an older friend or family member to see exactly what these images of aging convey. Even taken as efforts of humor, they are not funny. The stereotypes, as Gene saw them, are damaging, if not immediately to the individual then systemically to our culture, a culture that has historically portrayed and perceived older people as "weird, wicked, and weak"—in a state of decay.[1] He knew that this was a misrepresentation of the truth about aging, growth, and development, and he was committed to changing that image, both literally and metaphorically.

One of our favorite artists was Georgia O'Keefe, who, although she loved to travel, did not fly until later in her life. That new aerial perspective appears to have been especially significant as a visual experience for O'Keefe. In the 1960s she painted first a river series, and later, in her 70s, her cloud series. Each painting in the cloud series was titled "Sky Above Clouds," along with an identifying number, color, or year.[2] These works are dramatic—in size, color, abstraction, and image.

In his talks and presentations on creative aging, Gene frequently referred to O'Keefe's "Sky Above Clouds" paintings as the new metaphor for aging. This was the way we should envision aging, and approach it. As O'Keefe indicated in her paintings, even with her fears of flying, even in spite of her age or any illnesses, there is always sky above clouds.

I have chosen to title our book *Sky Above Clouds* to honor Gene and his vision, to honor O'Keefe and hers, and to honor—in each of us—our own process of creative aging.

The chapters of this book map a journey through life themes common to all of us yet unique to each of us: a philosophical and at the same time practical contemplation of the body, the psyche, the soul, and the family. You will move through different rhythms of time and space, perhaps bringing your own fears, hopes, and dreams into this space with us. Some of our writing is autobiographical, some scientific or psychological; there are other parts that are pure philosophy of living, mixed with the practicality of what this involves. Amidst it, metaphoric reflection. In these pages, as in our work as colleagues and our lives as husband and wife, we share the challenges and joys as we navigate our lives and the urgency of cancer treatment, care for parents with illness and dementia, raise our children and build our careers, and eventually face Gene's own untimely death at just sixty-five years old. Gene and I found the existential and philosophical dialogue within, and with one another, to be of great value in our search for the "sky above clouds," and our desire in writing this book together was to share that with you.

Even as Gene's cancer grew, as did his struggle, his focus was not on his illness but on his career-long push for the paradigm change in our view of aging. One of his final formal "presentations" was as an expert witness in a court battle that was historic in this regard: a fight for the dignity—and fortune—of one of the nation's most celebrated philanthropists of the twentieth century. The elderly matriarch, Brooke Astor, had been dead two years, and the verdict that would decide the fate of her multi-billion dollar estate would rest heavily on Gene's expert testimony about nuances of aging, illness, and mental acuity. In a larger sense, he was there on a mission to protect a vulnerable population—the elderly—from exploitation. What we did not know in those three dramatic days on the witness stand was that his testimony, which represented a culmination of his life's work, would become his closing argument for life as he confronted his own death. On the witness stand, as in his life and work, Gene's intellect, his courage, and his resilience ultimately ruled the day.

Most of all, though, this book is the story of a miracle. Gene's story is in clinical fact a medical miracle—evidenced in the years, the statistics, the prognosis, the outlier status, the going beyond the predicted and the unexpected. Outliers are by definition medical miracles, living outside, beyond the time that the clinical calculations would suggest for a person with a terminal illness.

But that is not the only or most profound miracle to be found here. As I see it, the miracle was to have lived for so long in the shadow of death, yet so fully grounded in our life together. This was—and can be for anyone—the miracle of being together and fully present to one another in the moment, whether these moments are assumed or against all odds. It is a medical miracle that we got the years—the extraordinary gift of time—to experience together a life that we had been told would be cut short soon after the diagnosis.

This miracle put to the test every bit of the theory, research, and science to which we had devoted our careers in the fields of creativity and the brain, adult development, and human potential. In essence, we were granted a unique opportunity to observe, cultivate, and experiment with our own capacity for creativity in meeting adversity, navigating the inner life and outer complexities that illness or loss present: creativity not solely in the conventional sense of making art but creativity in what we make of our circumstances and how we respond to them. Creativity as the catalyst for human resilience is the real miracle story, and it does not have our names alone on it. This way of living into life does not require a medical miracle, but it may contribute to one, as science is beginning to show in the study of the brain and the mind, as well as creativity, illness, and healing.

In the midst of one particularly grueling medical discussion about his poor prognosis, a choice emerged for each of us, as echoed in the biblical passage from Deuteronomy 30:19:

> I call heaven and earth to witness this day. I have put before you life and death, blessing and curse. Choose life, that you and your offspring shall live.

"I choose life," Gene said. "I choose to live it with you," I said. And with that presence, that promise to one another, we lived into our future.

That was the miracle we discovered at the intersection of creativity, illness, and healing, and Gene believed, as do I, that this kind of miracle—a life transformed—is accessible to each and every one of us.

This book was written with the intention of bringing the "sky above clouds" depicted by O'Keefe to life for every reader. As Gene would say, there will always be clouds, thus there will also always be sky above clouds—that space in which life's complexities have the chance to become clear, where we can make the quantum leap into our own potential and our own vision.

The clouds can obscure our view at times. Looking through the clouds, outside in, we may imagine, for instance, that we know what a person confronting a loss or life-threatening illness experiences; or that we know what we ourselves will feel next in adverse circumstances. Yet we do not and cannot know their reality, or even the one that awaits us, with any certainty at all. What we can know is that clear sky above—a *something else*—awaits us, an inner capacity for change and adaptation that is incontrovertible as nature itself. That "something else"—the creative faculty—is what draws us to life, calls forth our love, our resilience, our strength, and our capacity to choose not only life itself but also *what enlivens us*. In that space, we live into the moments of our lives, regardless of what may be in our way—to choose what we must choose, to see what we must see, to hear what we must listen to, to move toward that which we sense within us, to make our way through the clouds, whatever clouds may appear. Sky above clouds opens us not only to potential but to the essential.

A Note to the Reader

Gene's original entries, taken from his notes, drafts, and journals, are presented in italics throughout the book to distinguish them from the main text, written by Wendy.

Gene wrote the fairytale "Phoenix and the Fairy" for our daughter Eliana. It was his way of seeing the family story of challenge and creativity in magical, metaphorical terms that he could share with Eliana from the very—her very—beginning. Short excerpts from his fairy tale, adapted for use here, are placed in the last chapter of the book, reminding us of the universality of fable.

All artwork that appears in this book is Wendy's original work, including drawings, prints, sculpture, and multimedia creations. All photos of her artwork are credited to Joshua Soros or Claire Blatt.

With the exception of professionals and friends, as well as a few others who gave permission to use their names, all names and some personal or identifying characteristics of patients, clients, and others have been changed to protect their privacy. Permission for use of client imagery for educational purposes has been given. Any resulting resemblance to persons living or dead is entirely coincidental and unintentional.

To make reading less cumbersome, when either research or authors are referred to in the text, a full citation or elaboration can be found in Further References, or in Gene's bibliography in the Appendix, both at the back of the book. Wendy's acknowledgements to authors, clinicians, and others who have influenced her thinking and growth in her profession can also be found at the back of the book.

Notes for each chapter and a list of further references are provided for the reader who wishes to further understand concepts discussed and references made.

To provide a chronological sequence of the events and developments treated thematically in the book, a timeline is included the Appendix. These include births, deaths, and other milestones in Wendy and Gene's family and professional lives during the course of Gene's illness. Full text of a summary of Gene's boomer study and an op-ed essay Gene wrote regarding the Brooke Astor case are also included in the Appendix.

Introduction

Saturday, November 7, 2009, 5:15 A.M. EST. Gene has passed quietly tonight. To quote my friend Carol's online tribute that night: "I love you for your passion and courage and the fact that you did 'rage, rage against the dying of the light.' And I love you for knowing, despite Dylan Thomas's advice, that there is a time for many blessings when you do 'go gentle into that good night.'[1] You are surrounded with love."

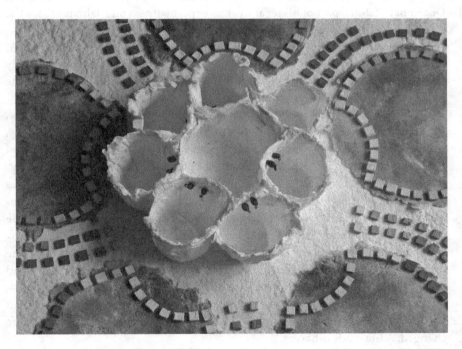

Figure I "A Mother's Plate" (2008), handmade paper pulp with powdered Pearl-Ex pigments and fired clay tiles, 26 × 24 × 6 inches. Artwork by Wendy L. Miller, photo credit: Joshua Soros

Preparing to write this introduction, I find an old leather briefcase folder of Gene's and I decide to write on the legal pad of paper inside. Flipping through the pages to find a blank sheet, I see 1) gauze pads tucked between blank pages; 2) notes on Clara Barton and Harriet Beecher Stowe, some in Gene's handwriting and some in the rapid penciled cursive print of our daughter Eliana, who was in middle school at the time—they had been working on her Humanities homework assignment; 3) Gene's notes from a conversation he had with his oncologist on scans showing nodes and distant disease and his decision to stop a particular medicine and prepare for a clinical trial of combined chemotherapy, and long medical notes in Gene's handwriting, never the words he used to describe to me what the doctor said; 4) a page about two characters in the fairy tale he was writing who were meeting a vet named Dr. Byrd, the kind of play on words that Gene loved; 5) address and directions to a university meeting; 6) an order and result sheet from Sibley Hospital with blood counts and basic panel numbers; 7) notes from listening to an hour and twenty-eight-minute tape about Brooke Astor in December of 2001, part of his legal work as expert witness on Alzheimer's for the soon-to-be-infamous Brooke Astor case in New York City.

And these are just the barest random sample; none of my notes from my work, or our work together on a number of professional fronts, or to-do lists of family responsibilities, the lists that describe a full and fully lived life. Nothing of the week before or the year—or years—before.

This book is about the whole pad of paper: navigating the complexities of life, with stories of creativity, adversity, growth, and development. And that, I can say, is actually less like a pad, one page following the next with an intrinsic order, and more like a cauldron into which one drops the parts: the characters, the episodes, the joys and fears, the details and circumstances of our lives. Our lives themselves are not just one thing; there is our life as a body, as an individual, as part of a couple and of a family, as a professional, as a member of a community. All together the parts get tumbled and shuffled and rearranged in the container, transformed by time, and then one day we wake up, look through all of the parts—the papers, the signs, the awards, the memories, the children as people, the past, the present—and see that we are different. The pieces are different, for they are mere remnants— "artifacts" an anthropologist would call them—and it is our job to try to use them to convey the life lived through them. The history and the substance of a life. A life changed. A life made different.

I can introduce the parts. I can tell you that it is my intention—as was Gene's— that this book share our and others' stories in an attempt to share meaning. And I can tell you that the whole is always greater than the sum of its parts—not only for Gene and me and our family but also in the way these stories resonate for you, the reader, through whatever your experience and however your life is unfolding.

Gene and I met in 1993. He had just "retired" at age forty-nine from a twenty-five year career at National Institutes of Mental Health and National Institutes of Health. But retirement always meant re-hirement for Gene. By 1994, he was directing a new Center on Aging, Health and Humanities at George Washington University,[2] founding a non-profit think tank on aging, called the Washington DC Center on Aging,[3] and launching an entrepreneurial game company, Genco International, Inc.,[4] that specialized in intergenerational board games. Gene had published more than one hundred and fifty academic articles, was the editor of a number of journals in his field, and had ideas for the books he wanted to write. These came to fruition first in *The Brain in Human Aging*, then in *The Creative Age: Awakening Human Potential in the Second Half of Life*, and finally in *The Mature Mind: The Positive Power of the Aging Brain*. Gene was awakening to a mid-life creativity, pulsing with his newfound freedom, direction, and inspiration; a geriatric psychiatrist and physician moving toward creativity and health.

I had lived in the Washington, DC, area for only about six years, having moved there from San Francisco. I was still adjusting to a life so different from my artist/therapist and educator identity back in the Bay Area. I practiced (and still do) as an expressive arts therapist and, in 1994, cofounded Create Therapy Institute, to offer clinical services in arts-based psychotherapy and trainings in the expressive arts, and was very involved in the alternative health movement and mind–body medicine. I also taught as an adjunct instructor at a number of universities in both sculpture and art therapy. This included George Washington University, where, although we hadn't yet met, we shared many colleagues, because my art therapy community was there and Gene was very visible in his program as an advocate for creativity. I also wrote on medical illness and the arts as complementary medicine, on the use of sand tray therapy with internationally adopted children, on experiential approaches to supervision in expressive arts therapy, and on the cultural responsibility of the arts in therapy; I was a creative artist and therapist moving toward medicine.

We met, fell in love, and married within this perfect cauldron of change. We built our lives personally and professionally. Like many couples, our differences softened over time and our similarities became magnets for our common interests and shared perspectives. Of course, this occurred in our family lives, but for Gene and me it also took place in our professional lives. By 2009, the year the metastatic cancer diagnosis reared its ugly head, after an unprecedented thirteen years plus in remission or management or dormancy, he and I were co-presenting and introducing one another at conferences in our fields. We were hatching plans for this book and for a new clinical model, combining our skills to work together with people our own age and older, particularly the boomer generation (born in the baby boom between 1947 and 1966), the sandwich generation (caring for both parents and children), and the sideways generation, (caring for siblings, friends, and colleagues).[5] We wanted to help people who were facing challenges of health, loss, retirement, and re-hirement to tap their inner resources for creativity and new possibilities.

Gene was truly the pioneer of the creativity and aging movement in geriatrics, and I was an expressive arts spokeswoman for mind–body communication in creativity and health. Our last presentation together, which was for the Society for the Arts in Healthcare, was a "he said, she said" format, titled "Developmental Intelligence & Integrative Intelligence—Impact on Creativity, Healing & Cultural Responsibility."[6] Our professional worlds—the world of science and the world of the arts—were speaking to one another, and we felt a responsibility to advance that conversation.

Two Voices, One Vision

So to move forward without him, in life as well as in this book, has reconfigured our plans. On the one hand I am deeply grateful for all that we shared and dared to create. It means that I have a healthy heart and firm ground to stand on to further our ideas and goals. On the other hand, I often feel that I'm half a person trying to recall the full narrative that we intended to create together. Gene speaks for himself in this book, and at times I speak for him and about him.

Thus this book started out as a co-authored book by Gene and me: a husband-and-wife team, made up of a scientist/psychiatrist and an artist/therapist. For five years it held our shared vision of a future working and living together, as it reflected backward on the sixteen years of our life together. We originally thought of it as "The Phoenix and the Fairy, and Other True Stories of Creativity, Challenge and Adversity." As it evolved, it became a holding space for our conversations, our shared hopes, expectations, and goals. That manuscript also included Gene's first venture into fiction writing—an original fairytale he wrote for Eliana to use creative imagery and story, as fairytales do, to capture the heroic life journey in which challenges and setbacks, heroines, heroes, and ogres ultimately illuminate our own fears, creativity, and courage. The entirety of that manuscript combining science, art, autobiography, and fairytale, retitled "Heartsong," was ready for publication when Gene passed away in November 2009, but I wasn't ready to submit it. I couldn't move, much less bring our creation to a publisher.

Our manuscript lay quiet, like me, as grief was rapidly engraving a new story upon our life together. It then took five more years for me as coauthor to become sole author. With the gift of many helpers—friend readers, editors, and writers, *Sky Above Clouds* replaced, rearranged, renewed, and reawakened the original manuscripts. Authoring what had been coauthored required an essential retrieval of what mattered most to each of us as writers and as partners. Even so, that essence changed, too, when the experience of deep loss, grief, and mourning entered the story. A profound shift took place not only inside the book but also inside me. This transformation needed to express itself in the format and storytelling as well. And thus *Sky Above Clouds* was reborn out of the ashes of "The Phoenix and the Fairy" and the early lyrical expression of "Heartsong."

Of his intention for this book, Gene wrote:

> *My goal is not to describe my own special recipe for avoiding or coping with being sick, suffering, and dying. My story is not one of how-to, but of hope and creative possibilities, of tapping into aspects of yourself you may not have known were there for however long you are able to. It is a story of creativity in connection with loss. There is nothing romantic about loss, but it is part of the human condition that when one is struggling to contain or cope with loss, there is also a desire to transcend it. This is a context, however unwanted, for accessing creative potential. So, to provide a series of stories will do justice to the many different ways it can be examined.*

Ultimately, this book came to represent more than the original focus on creativity with aging and illness. While aging is the backdrop for all things as we grow older, often our greatest challenges are not actually about aging itself, they are about health or other life challenges that confront us in adult life.

Our original intention to bring both our voices to the conversation remains a signature aspect of this book. Gene was a scientist, physician, and inventor, and he wrote from those depths of knowledge and sense of the world. I write from an intuitive depth. That's who I am; it's what I do as an artist and art therapist, a mother, and a woman, and it is my way of inviting you into your own intuitive experience to find meaning. This language—my "metaphorical" language as Gene liked to describe it—is juxtaposed against Gene's, which often focuses on the science, the mental processes of creativity, and the positive potential of the maturing brain. My effort here has been to have both of our voices exist on the page, as honestly and creatively as we did in the conversations of our real life.

There is a strong presence throughout the entire book of Chapter 7's theme, being a creative detective: the notion that what we observe may not be what there is to be seen. With this book, I try to bring forward the capacity to see into the complexity through which we lived and through which we all live. One reason for this complexity is that we never know what is going to take place when an illness enters a life; the only certainty is uncertainty. Another reason is that, as the great philosopher Kierkegaard famously said, we live life forward, yet it so often seems that we understand it backward.[7] The book itself is complex, not only in content but also in technique, as I spent five years as a coauthor and then another five years as author of what I thought was the same book. But now I see that the book I was left to do does not "finish up" the one that we started; rather, it tells a unique story of its own. It is no less a piece of Gene's legacy and of my honoring of that legacy. In fact, this book it is all that he envisioned, and more.

That ten-year period of his life between writing his books, *The Creative Age* and *The Mature Mind,* and his death in late 2009 was a time when the fields of healing arts, creative and expressive arts therapy, and creative aging needed his evidence-based research, his policy skills, and his neuroscience of the brain. Yet to ground the work in empirical science, our fields turned themselves away from the "experience" of the image to the "mechanism" of the image, to demonstrate a scientifically valid understanding, and potential for integrative approaches to funding, research, and publishing. Gene was a major voice—some called him the leading voice—in sharing the science that triggered the launch for the paradigm shift across disciplines. In so many ways, my own fields of art therapy and expressive arts therapy have been trying since their inception to do exactly what he was able to do for the field—shift the paradigm away from proving the validity of the arts within the psychological and medical fields to viewing creativity as a resource for accessing potential. But he knew that this shift was not the whole picture either; rather, he felt that my contribution of a deep understanding of integration—the overlay of our developmental and integrative intelligence models, combined with my imagery in story and creative intuition—would take that movement to the next level. He knew that our book would provide the voice I would need to move this next paradigm shift into its complex understanding of creativity and healing. This vision was his gift to me.

Writing this book was part of that process. Finishing this book is still part of it. I just didn't know that I would have to do it without him.

Organizational Structure and Existentialism

Chronology was a very important organizing element when we first began to write together in 2004. Chronology of the illness, chronology of our work lives, chronology of our family lives, chronology of our respective awarenesses. In the next several years and iterations of the manuscript, we juxtaposed these various chronologies with phenomenology: writing about the experiences of hope and expectation, of community support and isolation or fear and acceptance, of truth and denial. Then, after Gene's death, the manuscript draft lay dormant for more than a year, and when I revisited it, our chronological construct no longer made sense to me. The point of the book wasn't that things happened when they did and then in the end Gene died. The point was to use our experience to explore the shared territory of loss and grief, of memory and love, of hope and despair. The book also needed to both honor what we had written—each of us and then both of us together—and honor the truth of my own experience, now so changed by an experience Gene never had: surviving the death of a beloved partner and drawing from these same deep resources to in some way heal and move forward.

Truth be told, for me the illness experience never could have been understood chronologically, but for Gene, the calendar was like a touchstone. It seemed to ground him. Revisiting it chronologically is what helped him write, as it made meaning and gave him the motivation to record such meaning. He remained very motivated, all the way through the last summer of his life, to make sure that even as I rearranged our work, any and all information I might need, he would have written into his master copy of the manuscript, which he labeled "The Entire Book." In reading Gene's sections, he takes us into facets of the workings of the brain and the psyche, through the science of aging. He draws us in very concisely and directly as he describes his own intimate dreams, hopes, and fears. In that sense, his intentions, expressed in his notes and journal entries, continued to inform and guide this book-writing process.

> *Finally, I came to appreciate what so much of my life and professional career have been all about—teaching, sharing information, and helping to improve the quality of life of others. This is what I do as a researcher and as a doctor. It is what excites me, fulfills me, and affords me the chance to make a difference for others. And in my work in the area of Alzheimer's disease, when I shared with others the impact on me personally of my own father developing and dying with Alzheimer's, I discovered how truly powerful personal stories were with audiences. I witnessed how positively affected people were in hearing and learning about the disorder when I added my own personal experience as a professional living with and helping to care for a loved one with this dreaded disease.*
>
> *I certainly did not ever want or welcome the life-threatening crises that came my way, but what I learned from opening up about myself through personal stories in teaching about care for Alzheimer's disease made me aware of how sharing my personal experience could influence the engagement and receptivity of those listening to what I had to say about confronting illness that could affect life and lead to death.*
>
> *Wendy and I then agreed to do this book together, continuing our team effort of working and living with serious conditions that confronted my health, our relationship, and our family. We agreed to continue our team effort, but to make it visible through our writing so that others could witness it and take from it what would be meaningful for them. As Victor Frankl once wrote: "What man actually needs is not a tensionless state but rather the striving and struggling for some goal worthy of him. What he needs is not the discharge of tension at any cost, but the call of a potential meaning waiting to be fulfilled by him."*[8]

My intention is to show facets of our psyches as I write of how we intuitively experience our lives, including our experience of *thinking* about our lives as they unfold. Why do we react the way we do in certain moments? What brings us to impasses and then has us find a way through them? What changes in us day by day, moment by moment, in ways that can either free us or shackle us? Unlike self-help advice or bullets of magic guidance, the stories and conversation shared here are offered as tools to activate the mechanism of seeing into your own life, your own intimate psychological territory. The process of inquiry becomes the mechanism for creative knowledge. Creativity is a generative process that happens within our search for meaning—when we exercise our full capacity for engagement—whether it is in someone else's stories, as you'll read here, or in your own. In this way, creativity is not merely looking at but truly seeing your own experience, by feeling your way as you move through soul stories of experience.

What is most helpful for this creative engagement to take place is that our twin capacities to receive and reflect on experience occur almost simultaneously. We are existential creative beings, and this book aims to reflect our own existential spaces—where you can think about what is happening on the page, and the mirror images in your own experience begin to reveal themselves. True creativity is something that is released, not something named or analyzed, rather something that becomes its own art of knowing. Our stories model a process, slow us down enough to engage in our own experience, and hopefully offer a mirror so that we can see, reflect, and find meaning in our own interpretation. In such a way, looking becomes seeing becomes art.

My hope is that this book will be a companion on such a walk through hard places in life. You do not have to be on that hard path at this time of reading, but only be conscious enough to realize that we will all take these walks. It is not just a walk for ill people or aging people or dying people or grieving people. It is a walk of creativity in the deepest sense, when circumstances (even just reading) slow us down biochemically and psychophysically, and in that slowing down, we have a chance to engage with whatever is present and find meaning in it.

Part One

DISCOVERY

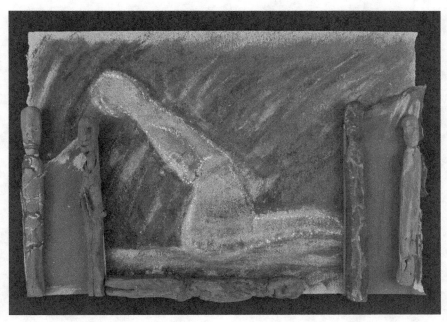

Figure I.i "Waiting" (2004), photo transfer with oil bars on paper and fired quarry tile figures and tiles, 16 × 23 inches. Artwork by Wendy L. Miller, photo credit: Joshua Soros.

1

Heartsong

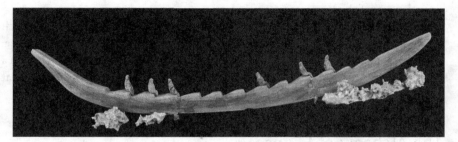

Figure 1.1 "Soul Carrier I" (1996), fired porcelain clay with oxides, 7 × 31 × 3 inches.
Artwork by Wendy L. Miller, photo credit: Joshua Soros

Why did I want to write this book? It was not an easy or immediate deci-
sion, having been decided upon more than a decade after my diagnosis of
metastatic prostate cancer. Part of my hesitation was that expressed by
Norman Cousins, in his classic account of his own life-threatening illness
within Anatomy of an Illness: "I was reluctant to write about it for many
years because I was fearful of creating false hopes in others who were simi-
larly afflicted. Moreover, I knew that a single case has small standing in the
annals of medical research, having little more than 'anecdotal' or 'testimo-
nial' value."[1] However, the longer I beat the odds, the more of an anomaly
I became, the more I saw this less as a purely medical anomaly about ill-
ness, and more of an exploration of life. I felt more and more compelled to
put pen to paper to talk about an extraordinarily trying, challenging, and
continuing time period in my life, one that has taken me on profound and
unexpected new paths.

First, let's dispense with this notion of creating false hopes. This caution about
"not getting people's hopes up" for remarkable remissions or cures is unnecessary,
perhaps even cruel. Gene died in the end. In my thirty-five years as a therapist
for people struggling through illness, and as a daughter, a sister, a mother, and a
friend in the thick of the medical travails of loved ones, I have yet to know anyone
who meets his or her own death, or the death of a loved one, with false hopes. It is
life that has us hold out hope, and looked at squarely, there is nothing false about

that. By that I mean Gene devoted his forty-year career and pioneering energies as a scientist and physician to the proposition that creativity transforms us—in the moment and over time—in sickness and in health, through aging and all manner of life's challenges and passages as we age, and it turns out he was right. That is the life we shared, a reality, and that is the story we share here. Any hope that kindles the idea that the creative spirit uplifts us is not false hope at all; it is honest and true. The most rigorous science in art therapy, guided imagery, psychoneuroimmunology, and mind–body connections shows this to be so, and in my work I witness this transformative power every day.

No, hope doesn't destroy us; silence, however, is another matter. So much around our experience of illness, aging, death, and other loss is marked by silence, held in silence. Not that there isn't conversation, but what is said is so often such a small window into the soul of our experience that the depth and breadth of what remains is left unspoken and held within. Our challenge is to act based on hope & ultimately acceptance of death when it comes – To speak out!

The Alchemy of Silence

The silences of such a story reverberate differently over the years. They reverberate through our hopes and fears, or is that exactly what hopes and fears really are— the "sound" of silence in the register of emotions, the language of our hopes and fears? The silences reverberate through the moments, through the circumstances; they reverberate through the facts. Gene and I, and our kids, lived through the somewhat slow-motion, time-lapse photographic quality of our journey into illness as a tight family, but also each of us alone with our experience. Throughout, the things unspoken or unspeakable shaped our experience at least as much as any clinical measures.

Gene's journey through his illness did not match what the medical profession expected or predicted or really understood. His "numbers" went beyond what the medical profession could validate in its research studies. As he would hear from his own physicians, studies of this disease stopped short of the number of years he had been on his medicines or his treatment regimen.

And yet, even though we eventually came to understand that he was an outlier, it was a knowledge that grew slowly and silently. In the ways in which magical thinking can work on us, we didn't dare say anything out loud. Not to ourselves, not to others; certainly at different times to ourselves and to others, but cautiously. Filtering experience is numbing: we silence how we think about things, how we feel about things, how and to whom we speak about things. Circumstances force us to do so, but then we almost believe the filtered story that gets told. A moment of indecision about what to say, and suddenly indecision becomes something unsaid or cast a certain way, a cryptic version of some truth, and eventually the unsaid thing becomes a secret, and the secret begins to exert its own gravitational pull on disclosure.

Keeping a secret, or simply being less than candid, is hard work. So why do we choose this complicated path? First off, the moment you reveal that you have cancer you have to handle the other person's reaction. Sometimes, it is well worth it to do this, as it provides support and sharing of experience. And we certainly did that, with certain friends and family, and at certain times in our process. But at other times, it can almost be too much, too exhausting to handle someone else's reaction to our new reality and their feelings—assumptions or fears or discomfort—at having to confront this. Not everyone's reaction is caring, ongoing, or helpful. Most close friends, family, and members of the medical team are indeed caring. But it is a risk to reveal a cancer diagnosis, and it is one more thing to brace for and work through when it goes poorly. At one point Gene shared his diagnosis with the parents of one of Eliana's closest nursery school friends, with whom we were sharing more and more time and imagined we would continue to do so. They seemed a part of our extended family and likely to "be there" for Eliana as she went through whatever lay ahead. As the years went by, they distanced themselves from us. Maybe they just decided they didn't like us or they were too busy and invested in other friendships. I never understood it, but Gene always felt that somehow they had written him off, figured that his cancer made us too complicated a family to share a future with, a tragedy waiting to happen. Sometimes people—kids and parents alike—just drift apart. It happens. But when you disclose something this intimate and vulnerable about yourself, you take an emotional risk that the person you've perceived as interested and caring isn't.

As Gene's wife, I felt it was my job to support his decision as to when he wanted to share the diagnosis and with whom. Over time, I began to understand that there could be some refuge in the relationships in which his condition had been silenced out of the conversation. It was not that I was lying or hiding; I was just staying out of the shadow of his diagnosis and the dialog of constant monitoring. I could appreciate some friends as places of respite—loved ones whom I could be with, yet not have them see us through the cancer lens. This gift is seldom spoken of. My friend Joan comes to mind. I chose her to be in this position. She had been on my doctoral committee and has been a mentor to me, as well as a friend, and something of a surrogate mother figure. She had supported me through many challenges in my earlier life, both professional and personal, and I gave myself permission to decide what or when I was ready to bring the topic of Gene's condition into our relationship. I never really knew how much time I would have with him doing so well. She was this refuge for me, a place not where I would hide, but where I could rest. We talked about complexity and art, and it helped me to be able to perceive the moment with her through our mutual passions for art and meaning, a shared lens, rather than through a lens of ill health.

There was no bigger juxtaposition of this complexity than at our wedding, taking place in the intimacy of the living room of Gene's beautiful brownstone in the historic Adam's Morgan neighborhood of Washington, DC. It was filled with this kind of unspoken speech, a mixture of friends and family celebrating with us, some knowing of his diagnosis, some not. (How in the world were they all able to do that?) Everyone knowing we were in love and embarking on our own new chapter. Some holding the bittersweet taste of anticipatory grief, others the sweet taste of anticipatory joy. Joy and grief were just a hairline away from one another as we danced into our uncertain yet available future—a future that went on for almost fourteen years. In some ways, maybe that is true of all futures. We live into them knowing only so much, anticipating or perhaps fearing only that which we can imagine, the rest a mystery. It is an incomplete awareness that invites us to dig in, sink roots, invest wholeheartedly in the reality that is present and fully ours.

The Burden of Silence

The reality is we are not silenced by anyone or necessarily any conscious choice we make. We are silenced by nature because we are protective or confused or worried or exhausted or lost to some parts of our self. Overwhelmed, we are physiologically primed to pull back, or power down. Left to ourselves in that state we may find comfort in our invisibility, or just more pain. I remember a fourteen-year-old boy from my practice. I treated him a year after the sudden and unexpected death of his mother from a medicine she was misprescribed for chicken pox. (She had an allergic reaction to it and very quickly died at the hospital.) He was sad, depressed, and angry. His father brought him in to see me hoping that, as an art therapist using creative methods in addition to talk therapy, I might be able to help his son express himself. The son had so distanced himself from their relationship that the dad felt he could no longer reach him. At fourteen, this boy had no idea that his feelings were rightful aspects of grieving. When I invited him to use art materials to draw—his demeanor made it clear he didn't want to dialog with me directly—he picked a dark oil pastel stick and sketched with angry intensity. He stopped and I looked. He had drawn a stick figure in the middle of the page with dark black strokes of oil pastel, steaming red coming out of the chest. I asked him, "What is happening here in the middle of this body?" In his distant, withdrawn tone, he slowly leaked out the authentic pieces of what he was feeling as he faced his own work: "It's like a burning heart . . . there are flames from everything lost . . . they smoke and burn . . . they really ignite my anger."

I gave him a piece of tracing paper, as I often do so that we can make further marks on the overlay but not change or disrupt an original drawing. It allows us the opportunity to further an image conversation. We placed the clear tracing paper over his drawing and he traced the figure with the same intense blackness, but this time he circled the face with bright blue. I asked him what meaning the blue might bring to the flames. "They are the people who live without such constant pain. They can cool down. They are the people with blue in their heads." Later he made a drawing with both kinds of figures in it—a group of the blue people all together on the left side of the paper, and then short crossed black lines arching over them toward a sole figure with red in his chest in the bottom right corner of the paper. "I feel outside of humanity," he said, "because I am a person who will never belong to the world of the blue people."

Silenced by isolation. Silenced by alienation. Silenced by distance. Silenced by feeling *other than*, not belonging to something as basic as the human race. Yet, in reality, one of the only things certain in life is that each of us will confront illness or other complications in our health or that of our loved ones. We are all in one of two groups: the ill and the not yet ill. Still, we all know this experience of feeling silenced when what we feel does not seem to be accepted or understood by those around us. And it is true: it is not accepted because it is not yet understood. Yet, how can anything we experience in a human life push us to be outside the rest of humanity, as if, shunned by the shame of having our grief or our loss or our encounter, we were being quieted into silence?

It brings to mind another young client, a fifteen-year-old girl who lost her younger sister to suicide—what is called an iatrogenic suicide, resulting from a medically induced delusion when she was given the wrong dosage of a very strong medicine. This older sister, a high school freshman, came in to see me for grief support and art therapy treatment through her high school years as she grieved and learned to manage her post-traumatic stress from her loss. She painted and created poems in her art therapy, calling out through symbols to her lost sister. I remember so vividly the cloth doll figure she worked on to hold everything—all the feelings and thoughts she felt she could not allow to slip out at home or in school. For if she had, she would not be able to survive the hours required to be in those familiar places. She did not want to see a counselor at her school. She needed her inner world and her outer world separated. She painted a cloth doll figure in my office, and on the back of her she wrote, "Eat, Sleep, Dance, Repeat." It might sound coldly regimented or uninspiring to some, but it was her recipe for survival and healing. And a good one at that: it worked for her. She created a ritual that kept her body able to move and gave her being a purpose to stay in school—to be able to dance—and do her school work. By the end of her senior year, she was choreographing dances about her sister's life and speaking at conferences as an advocate for understanding the dangerous side effects of some antidepressant medications. She had found a way to find her voice, something we all do and need to do through time and change.

Gene had his way of doing it. For example, Gene wrote about the impact of each of our prior illness experiences—including the remission or cure we may have experienced—on our experience of a new or recurring illness and the adjustment to the new reality. For him, the diagnosis of metastatic cancer and the grim prognosis were devastating, and yet his earlier experience of a misdiagnosis of ALS (Lou Gehrig's disease) that took two terrifying years to resolve became a source of insight for him in confronting this new diagnosis.[2] He found a way to observe it, and his own deepest feelings, finding the voice and words for that exploration.

> The diagnosis of metastatic cancer was another knockdown blow which I thought would be a knockout, with nobody giving me much time to live. But my experience with the misdiagnosis from my ALS episode two years earlier was that the diagnosis could be wrong. This experience plus my broader knowledge of outliers when it comes to prognoses in general offered me some hope that here, too, my doctors could be wrong. I certainly couldn't count on their being wrong, but I did not have to accept their verdict as my destiny. So I borrowed from another lesson from my experience with ALS, in which I had sought a highly engaging and meaningful diversion in the form of creating a new game to live life the best I could, given the circumstances. With the cancer, I launched a new engaging and challenging diversion in the form of writing the first book entirely focused on creativity and aging: The Creative Age: Awakening Human Potential in the Second Half of Life.
>
> The mistake I did not want to make was to simply stay busy as a form of distraction. Unless that distraction had a sense of purpose and could truly have a positive influence on my state of mind, I felt that I could fall into even greater despair about the meaninglessness of it all. Moreover, I knew from my extensive research on and knowledge about aging that experiences or activities that offered a feeling of sense of control or mastery contributed to a feeling of well-being and enhanced health. In fact, the research of Judith Rodin[3] at Yale (she later became the first female president of an Ivy League university) had shown that while all age groups benefited from experiences that brought about a sense of control, the results were most robust with older adults—a population group I was in the natural process of joining.[4] Furthermore, subsequent biological studies of individuals experiencing a significant new sense of control revealed in effect an immune system boost—enhanced production of T-cells (lymphocytes that attack bacterial infections) and NK cells (natural killer cells that combat cancer cells); the latter certainly would be an added benefit for me.[5] This biological research on "sense of control" experiences contributed to the growth of the mind/body movement and the establishment of the field of psychoneuroimmunology (PNI),[6] reflecting the influence of the mind on the immune system.[7]
>
> The bottom line is that what we ourselves do can alter how we experience illness. Once we move in that direction, we become recalibrated to better cope with the course of illness or new illness episodes, because our prior illness

our perspective ↑
reframe ↑
re constructing ↗

experience influences future illness experiences. If we have discovered better ways to deal with that experience, this new illness wisdom is carried forth. Developmental changes with aging—part of what I have described as the "developmental intelligence" that contributes to wisdom in the second half of life—help us further this process of responding to and altering our illness experience. The change in midlife of the two hemispheres of our brain moving to a kind of all-wheel-drive, working more equally together, provides us with new capacity for understanding our situation in life. Together, the attributes of postformal reasoning become part of the psychological growth process with aging. Together, these positive brain and psychological growth changes with aging create new inner world environments for creativity and creative problem-solving. They don't remove life-threatening challenges, but they enhance our repertoire of life skills for facing them.

our Coping Skills

During the course of my terrifying illness sagas I began to think of myself as living in a parallel universe of the absurd. Every time death and destruction knocked at my door, nobody came to take me away. When each subsequent crisis occurred, I thought back on the experience of the prior one that provided a voice to tell me that however ominous the noise was on the other side of the door, the outcome was never certain.

I was talking to a friend of mine who runs the Smith Center for Healing and the Arts[8] in Washington, DC, a sister program to Commonweal[9] in California, and also organizes wonderful cancer retreats for patients and their families. I had been very involved professionally with the Center and the retreats at their inception, yet I pulled away when Gene's diagnosis arrived, because I was trying to honor the privacy that Gene needed around his cancer. It was not easy for me, as both mind–body medicine and medical art therapy were my professional communities. But I felt that I had to become somewhat invisible—absent myself—the embodied equivalent of silence. After Gene died, I revealed to my Smith Center friend and colleague how I had honored Gene's choice to not share information about his cancer with certain people, and particularly at Smith Center because of the fact that it was located in DC. Gene needed boundaries around his health condition so he could continue his work through the many grants and philanthropic foundations that funded him. She understood, and named it "the burden of silence." It was the name for all that I had kept inside, all that I chose not to share, all that I held in silence for both of us.

Once when Gene was going in for monthly treatments at the hospital, he ran into a colleague from the National Institutes of Health (NIH) with whom he had worked years prior. This colleague was receiving chemotherapy. Gene asked his friend to protect his privacy around his health and to not let others in their profession know of his treatments. This colleague was not able to carry that burden of silence and soon revealed to another colleague that he had talked with Gene when they happened to meet at the hospital; he disclosed Gene's confidential information about the cancer and Gene's treatment. Gene understood, but he felt betrayed and knew that his decision to protect his right of communication and timing had been well founded. The burden of silence is not something that everyone can hold or respect.

There were "the right times" that Gene chose to lift the silence. When he decided to tell the head of our daughter's elementary school, it was a decision to help her understand why we were changing schools before the final sixth-grade year; when he decided to share with Reb David, our friend and rabbi, again it was to clarify the complexity of what he was going through with his broken leg. He made the same choice with some of our other close friends as well.

We each have a right to remain silent. Or to choose how and when to share what we wish. In the medical and healthcare arena there is so little about our clinically diagnosed and scrutinized selves that is only ours to decide. When we step out of that realm and back into our office, our neighborhood, our friendships, and our lives, the option of silence or the time, place, and pace of sharing must belong to us. We must grant ourselves permission to decide when and what we are ready for.

After Gene died, so many in our circle expected me to go into therapy with a professional grief counselor. It is something so often recommended, even urged to those who grieve. But talking to a therapist was an intimacy that I was not ready for. I was not prepared to turn my husband into a clinical story and befriend the counselor or therapist as my confidant. Rather, I stayed close to my already trusted ones, my family and my dearest friends. Yet, every month after Gene's passing, when my hospice counselor called me, my intimacy with her was totally different. And I held that closeness willingly, even though it was concurrent with my not-ready feelings. With her, the rules and contract were not part of a therapy model; they were the hospice model of compassionate reaching out and support. She checked in on me, calling me monthly, and she came to know things that were going on, both with myself, internally, and with my daughter and stepson. Her voice became a beacon of light through the fog of my days, and our conversations were not only life-affirming but life-sustaining. Eventually I became ready and trusted this format for intimacy. I suppose you could call it grief counseling, but the point is that I wasn't ready or willing to name it as that. As time went on, my feelings changed as I grew to appreciate her capacity to comprehend the depths and shapes of loss. In our conversations, I reflected back with her on what it had all been for me. Sharing provided the room for feelings that seemingly had only small spaces in which to breathe. We always have the right to silence in any phase of our health. But when I was ready for this deeply needed opening, what happened was the slow realization of the toll that all that I was experiencing had taken—was still taking—on my own voice and on my intimacy with friends.

Engaging Our Silent Self Opens Inner Dialogue

Learning how to report from inside the experience of our challenges is not an easy or a learned process. I experienced it as what I call heartsong. It was hard to talk about all that we faced at the same time we were living through it. It was as if our hearts were outside of us yet inside of us, singing variations of tone and meaning, sometimes in sound and sometimes in silent pauses between the notes. Challenges seem to pull on our heartstrings. Reporting through the act of writing, laying the notes down on the page, began to feel like a heartsong, singing to us of our own lives, sometimes hoping, sometimes venting, sometimes trying to understand or connect with our own hearts. Hearts that could be hardening and softening at the same time. For any of us, our heartsong may move us toward our own creativity, as well as our own therapeutic needs during challenging times.

Art therapy can combine the two. *Name it, claim it, tame it, aim it.* That's one aphoristic way of framing what we do in therapy as we seek to understand what silences us and how we can begin to hear our inner voice more clearly. It's a way to break down the steps of a complicated process, a way to engage the big feelings, the big struggle, the big blockages into manageable pieces so we can see where they are and what needs to take place. The process goes like this:

You have to name something first, really name it, tell the truth. That step in itself is no easy feat, not because we lie or because we are in denial but because the truth of naming something has to make its way through all the other junk that gets in the way of naming the truth—the labels and other bits of emotional shorthand that deflect the discomfort of deeper reflection. Truly "naming it" means recognizing for yourself what "it" really is that needs to be named. "I have dark dip moods," Gene would say, his name for the cancer shadow that would at times halt his whole being. Naming is step one, and sets up the internal alignment for you to be able to move to step two, when you're ready, which is genuinely claiming your truth as your own. Claiming says, "This is the truth of what is going on for me and it is my issue, it is in my life, it is for me to handle." That is what claiming it means.

Gene's shorthand reference to "dark dip moods" was his way of owning them: "My dark dip moods are the way my own system registers this mortality glitch." Unnamed and untamed, the dark dip moods could prevail in his own mind as the defining truth of his existence. But they weren't the only truth; they were simply part of his larger truth. Only once you have named and claimed the "it"—the dark moods, the loss, the pain, or whatever your "it" is—can you actually do the work of taming your experience, because before it is named or claimed it has unacknowledged and thus unguided power in the psyche. This is why our inner psychological life can wreak havoc in us. We need to learn how to calmly, yet firmly, engage with this part of our personality, to learn to tame our overpowering anger responses or our guilt or our pleasing nature or whatever shape it may take. Gene would close his eyes, sometimes mid-sentence, to allow the movement of the shadows to pass through him. He chose to cultivate a calm, taming response as he moved through feelings and sensations that scared him.

Once we tame it, then we have the potential to aim it. We can decide how and when and what we want to do with this particular trait of ours. We can aim it, like a flashlight, in the direction of what is healthy for us. As Aldous Huxley said: "Experience is not what happens to you. It is what you do with what happens to you."[10] So Gene's deep consideration of science and his own inner life is what he did with what happened to him—how he shined the light in on his experience. He would later write that finding his voice this way was a breakthrough for him. The process focused him.

> It helped me better process my very unsettled feelings, to gain new perspective and get going. I felt a deep and sudden surge of not just hope, but purpose and plans. Dark as these moods may be, they are like a messenger with a sword of regenerative rest I have learned to give myself.

So here I am at the time, naming the truth: my husband's cancer frightens the hell out of me, every day in every way. I try to claim that, but to live in fear is impossible, and so I live by watching—actually super-watching, becoming hyper-vigilant. Perhaps surprisingly, it is a step in the right direction, because it is actually a tamed-down, calming version of my rabid worry. I fear that something will happen to him on my watch, during the night when I am sleeping or taking the necessary alone time for myself—an absolute must these days. I fear that whatever amount of natural patience I have will deplete itself because the necessary renewal of joy that sustains my patience is running low.

To speak of our life without speaking through science would miss the essence of how Gene thought about it. For Gene, science was the language, the medium he used to do all that. Not only medical science, through which he brought his deep understanding of the physical body and brain to bear on an otherwise amorphous threat that grew within him, but also his own and others' pioneering science of creativity and aging gave him a way to understand and thus tame his fears. So often he focused with a sense of marvel at the inner richness and blossoming experience that he attributed, independent of illness, to the positive aspects of aging and creative engagement with day-to-day life. Gene didn't just search for results and explanation and then simply accept what he found; he used science as a sculptor uses material, experimenting with it, shaping it, interpreting it. He loved the distancing power of the process, the stance of reporting, the authority of empirical evidence and insightful interpretation. He loved the sound, the words, the mechanisms of science. He especially loved what it provided for him: a way to see and reframe what he wanted to understand about the intricate forces within us. Science was how Gene spoke from the self that might otherwise have fallen silent.

Creating art was that voice of self-expression for me, and it continues to be. Intuitively arranging and rearranging is the world I live in. I string things together to create patterns, to form shapes of inner landscapes, to move things around until essences magnetize toward one another. I do this physically with materials, poetically with thoughts and feelings, and psychically with therapeutic history. When I cannot do this, I cannot make sense of things. It is the way I work. Everyone has one of these styles. Or would it be better to call them creative capacities? They are our strategies or propensities or temperaments or skills. We each have such a creative trunk, filled with surprising materials and tools, something that is uniquely our way of seeing and interpreting the world, and we use it to make intricacy tangible. We can use it to tame our fears, find our voices, and navigate from quiet to a nourishing connection with others.

Each of us in our own way—Gene through science, I through art—found solace leaning into beauty, and in that experience of beauty, hope. Not false hope. Not denial. But hope that heals the spirit.

Hope and expectation are like siblings; they can work together or be at odds with one another. But their relationship is important, because how it is shaped can affect how each can grow in a positive sense. How their relationship is shaped can also effect a synergy that can influence how we cope with adversity and illness, and how we access our creative potential, regardless of age.

Hope and expectation are two extraordinary human qualities that kindle how we dream when we are awake. The dream becomes a blueprint for action. As Thoreau advised:

If you have built castles in the air, your work need not be lost: that is where they should be. Now, put foundations under them.[11]

And as Martin Luther King, Jr. so passionately and poignantly pointed out,

If you lose hope, somehow you lose the vitality that keeps life moving, you lose that courage to be, that quality that helps you go on in spite of it all. And so today I still have a dream.[12]

What words and concepts connote and denote influences how we perceive and negotiate the world around us and what life deals us. There are those who are uneasy around hope; they view it as denial or clouding reality. These are people who have trouble with nuance, context, and what is relative in the human condition. They have trouble recognizing that reality and hope are not incompatible.

Just as stress can be good or bad, so too with denial. Stress can make you feel bad; it can also <u>motivate you to novel, positive action</u>. Denial can be maladaptive or adaptive. In the latter realm, denial often enables us to go on. If we did not have denial, we would not drive cars, fly in airplanes, climb mountains, or venture into any area that has some risk of accident or adverse outcome. Doctors in particular need to beware: <u>don't drain denial</u> to the extent that you drain <u>hope as well</u>; to paraphrase the old adage, it would be throwing the baby out with the bath water.

One of the most profound things I have experienced about hope is that it does not have to be linked to outcomes, because outcomes and potential outcomes for my illness over time seem to have been undergoing shape-shifting. More important has been how my sense of meaning and possibility within the time for me to live has shaped my feeling of hope. I resonate strongly with what Vaclav Havel has written:

Hope is not the conviction that something will turn out well but the certainty that something makes sense, regardless of how it turns out.[13]

→ being empowered to act.

2

Strategies, Tactics, and Counting

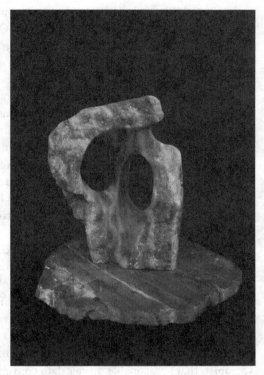

Figure 2.1 "Both/And" (2002), carved alabaster on stone slab, 12 × 9 × 7 inches.
Artwork by Wendy L. Miller, photo credit: Joshua Soros.

Cribbage is a deceptively simple game that dates back to the early 17th century. It has had great appeal as an intergenerational game, typically for 2, 3, or 4 players, fostering play between the young and the old. Cribbage is fast—often over in 15 minutes, but that time is filled with unusual and quite varied scoring combinations that provide depth, breadth, and engagement in playing. The oral scoring that goes on often takes the form of rap-like rhyming, adding a colorful tonal quality to the game. But for me, what always made cribbage very special was that it allowed my father, who worked very long days, 6 days a week, and me to have many quality short

intervals of limited time. I came to appreciate how much fun and meaning-
ful a relationship could be packed into such a brief time period, and that a
quick game for just two people could be so enthralling.

Presently, in thinking about time, which for me is the question of how
much time I have, I find the image of cribbage very grounding. My 14-year-
old daughter Eliana and I are now playing cribbage together.

Our lives together began with cribbage. It was a simple connection amidst a
complicated time in both of our lives. On our first date, I worried about how a
scientist and an artist could truly connect. On our second date, we were casually going over the events of the day when we both became animated with
something we wanted to tell the other. Each of us insisted the other go first, but
I insisted more.

"I applied for a patent for my board game and its scoring system," Gene said.
"It got rejected but I told my lawyer I wanted to appeal it. He told me that
would be a waste of time and money, that patent reviewers never overturn their
decisions, but I decided to present my own case. I could tell by reading the
patent reviewer's report that he was intelligent. His remarks on the application showed insightful observations. I wanted to have a chance to speak with
him directly. I knew I could do a better job having the discussion myself, and
I wanted it. I respected how he had truly studied my application, and my history of cribbage."

"Cribbage?" I said, surprised. "You applied for a patent for cribbage?" I didn't
know which I found more incredible: that this seemingly intelligent man would
apply for a patent on a game that is centuries old, or the coincidence that cribbage
was key in my own story I was waiting to tell him. I didn't know Gene well yet, but
I had come to dinner with him knowing he was a smart, creative type, and that
he was a psychiatrist. Who better to tell about a magical and strangely reassuring
dream I'd had of a close friend from my teenage years? For a psychiatrist and a
therapist, that's reasonable dinner date conversation. But he knew nothing of my
dream yet or the fact that, however improbable it might seem, cribbage had been
part of it.

Gene read the surprise on my face as enthusiasm and he pressed on eagerly,
playing both parts of the lively conversation he'd had with the patent reviewer:

"'So, sir,' I said to the reviewer, 'if I understand your review remarks,
you believe that the changes I am proposing—the double-sided,
double-colored, and double-shaped markers, as well as the return to
the original scoreboard format with the full 60 points—that these
changes are obvious?'

'Yes, Dr. Cohen, that is what I am saying.'

'Well, with all due respect, sir, how many years need to go by before a change is no longer obvious? Three hundred and fifty years have already gone by, and I believe that another 350 years could go by before anyone makes these seemingly obvious changes to this game.' And after a few seconds of silence and a smile, the patent reviewer took out his pen and signed my application for *The Essential Cribbage Board!*"[1]

Gene went on to tell me about how he wanted to show that, through concepts of universal design, one could design an object to meet special needs among the aging without compromising its aesthetic appeal or resulting in prohibitive costs. While his redesign of the game of cribbage made it easier to play for people with motor and visual impairment, his was also a game that looked like a work of art. I later learned that Gene's father loved cribbage, but that in his advancing years, he'd had trouble seeing and moving the pegs. When he initially was hospitalized with Alzheimer's disease and disoriented from pain medicine, Gene had reoriented him back to the present by playing cribbage with him.

As Gene shared his story, something inside me shifted. I listened intently, which is exactly how most people listened to him. He had that effect on you. Some new spark had been magically, unexpectedly awakened. I was also totally astonished. I had no idea about his interest in cribbage.

We toasted his patent victory, and then it was my turn. He turned his attention fully to me, and I felt so comfortable as I began to share my dream story with him.

In my dream, I explained, I see a man—an older-looking man, older meaning late forties or early fifties. He has graying hair and a beard, but he is not an old man. My first impression is that he is my friend Cara's first husband, whose name was also Gene. But then I realize it is not Cara's husband. It is my high school boyfriend Leighton. He looks different because he is now my age, which is confusing because Leighton died when he was in his twenties. But in my dream this is definitely my dear friend older, and he is here to see me. As I move closer to the image, I see he has some sort of knobby protuberance above each of his shoulders—they are wings. Not light and airy like angel images, but wings nonetheless, much like the densely layered shapes I have drawn before in my charcoal drawings; layers superimposed on one another. He appears very sad, his face cast downward. I follow his gaze and see there in his lap is a baby. I had lost a pregnancy a year prior, and somehow in my dream I know it is my baby. I feel vaguely confused and afraid. Is this the baby I lost, or is this some premonition about the baby I hoped to adopt someday?

Gene listened with full attention as I described the questions that had run through my mind in the dream: *Who is this man, this impossibly older Leighton? Is he my guardian angel? Is he watching over me? Why is he so sad? Why does it all feel so sad?* I couldn't tell whether Gene was listening to me as a psychiatrist or as a new friend, but I could certainly feel his capacity for deep empathy and compassion.

In the dream I talked with my old friend Leighton, or at least imagined that I did. This was hardly the playful debate that Gene had just enacted from his day. This dialogue was mystical, and only fragments remained clear in my memory as I retold it to Gene. This older, soulful Leighton of the dream told me that in my previous marriage I hadn't been in the right relationship or in the right space in my life to have a baby, but that that was about to change. "Now, you will have a very healthy child," he said, adding that I was about to find the right man, too. A man who recognized, as I did and held deeply, "that music is the breath of life." Leighton encouraged me to play the piano as I had done when I was younger—as we had done together, sometimes at my house to kick back and relax after school. "Let the notes hold you, strengthen you, provide for you. I will hear you. I will watch over you through thick and thin. I will be with you as I always am," in spirit, he promised. He went on to explain that my life was evolving with meaning beyond my present understanding, but that in time this would become more clear. "It will come to you," he said. "Don't give up. You are stronger than you know." And then he said an odd thing: "Remember cribbage. Play cribbage. Find friends who will just *be* in that way again. Like we were in the ski lodge, with those friends. Remember? I promise you'll find the love you need and deserve. Play cribbage."

Play cribbage? What kind of thing was that to say in a message from the Other Side? On the other hand, it wasn't totally out of the blue. When Leighton and I were sophomores in high school, we played cribbage many nights at Colby's ski slope, where our group of friends gathered after we did our homework. But I contracted pneumonia that year, and my doctor (and my mother) wouldn't let me ski. All my friends skied, so I continued to join them but had to stay behind inside the lodge. Leighton insisted that he had no interest in skiing and stayed inside with me. He made sure I was not alone. We couldn't play piano at the lodge, but he brought a cribbage board and cards, and so we played that. Many times that year, we chose to stay inside the lodge. Foregoing the slopes and enjoying the quieter comforts and special quality of teenage friendships, we sat by the fire and played cribbage.

My relationship with Leighton had been simply that: comfortable and comforting—a dear friendship that was abruptly ended when he was killed in a car accident just after we both graduated from college. That night of the accident I had some strange premonition or psychic vision, something I have never had with anyone else or ever since. And now, twenty years later, here he was, vividly present in my dream, speaking in a familiar quality of tone and all-knowing presence as if he knew more about my life than I did. I remember waking and thinking how odd a dream it was—until my date that night with Gene. Suddenly, the dream and the date felt somehow connected, merged in the present moment with Gene. And here I was, sitting across from someone who could play cribbage, and who had patented, of all the unlikely things, a cribbage board.

As I stared across the table at Gene, who sat with such a compassionate demeanor, I heard the voice from the dream speak to me from within. "Get out of your head," the voice said. "Stop being distracted by the piece of hair that he combs over his balding head. Look at his curls, his smile, his heart. This is a man you could really play cribbage with." I could barely keep from laughing out loud at the fact that in what could only be described as a rare mystical experience, the divine message hinged on: cribbage.

And Gene, what was he thinking? If he was at all surprised by this somber turn in the conversation, he welcomed it with his characteristic curiosity and wonder. He was awed by this piece of synchronicity between us. He could clearly see that I'd found this dream deeply affecting, and he felt moved, too, he said, by what he called "the magic" of my having that dream at the same time as his patent experience. And so, he kissed me.

Cribbage brought us together as a couple and became a metaphor for our experiences just two and a half years later, in 1996, when Gene was first diagnosed with metastatic prostate cancer. In cribbage it goes like this: play the hand, get the cards, add up the number of combinations in your hand, add the numbers, tell your numbers in a rhyme if you can, move your marker to reflect your numbers, then it's the next person's turn. In life after the diagnosis it goes like this: set the time period (a week, a month, a year); count up the clinical numbers (blood cells, prostate-specific antigen [PSA] number, scans, blood pressure, pulse, breathing and oxygen levels, temperature, time elapsed, and so on); add the numbers and set the context, with the emotional response as a rhythm we live in; make your moves; repeat; go on whether you want to or not. Action moves you forward even when you wish it would just stand still. It may sound flippant or just wrong to articulate it like that, as if we could call our own life a game, but I am going to dare to call it that. We do live in rhythm with our lives, and we do notice when something changes it. By nature we seek to move forward, advance through our years, and we develop strategies and coping responses to smooth our way. We feel the vagaries of chance, the roll of the dice, and sometimes the deep grounding of spirit. But from the first diagnosis, Gene and I were always counting, watching the numbers.

When Gene first was diagnosed, in March of 1996, his PSA number, which should have been below 4, was over 300.[2] The diagnosis came as shock.

Gene had come home after several days of presenting at the world's biggest toy fair—Toy Expo—at the Javits Center in New York City, where he had introduced his latest game invention.[3] Despite having had a great day and considerable success at the toy fair pitching his new game to international retail toy buyers, he had returned with an excruciating headache and paralyzing neck pain. On Sunday, he accompanied my sister and me to a crafts fair. He tried to convince us that his neck was some percentage better than the day before. We both told him that he seemed quite miserable and that he should go to a doctor—stop with this self-doctoring and stoic self-diagnosing. The next day, Gene did go to his doctor, who checked his vitals and took some basic blood tests. When the doctor looked at the preliminary results, he said with a startle: "This can't be right!" Gene's blood pressure had soared from normal levels on his last visit not long before to a frightening high reading that foreshadowed a stroke. His doctor said treatment needed to start right away after a few more tests to try to zero in on a more accurate diagnosis. After some additional lab work he instructed Gene to come back the next day.

Gene was concerned but calm when he went back the following day. The promise of a clinical conversation allowed him in a way to step outside his body and observe it in order to understand it. This is often how our psyche responds to upsetting news: *just the facts, please.* This process of giving something startling a chance to "sink in" is the psyche's emergency response; a way of managing the impact of something potentially overwhelming as the facts and implications begin to infiltrate the psyche. The doctor was clearly concerned and he was blunt in his clinical language.

"Please, take a seat," the doctor began. His tone was ominous.

"Now what?" Gene asked.

"I have some very disturbing news."

"More disturbing than yesterday, if that's possible?"

He gave Gene the numbers. "Your last PSA was under 4—within the normal range. Now, a year later, it reads 360—strongly pointing to an aggressive prostate cancer that has likely been metastasizing to other parts of your body. We need to do scans to see what they show."

It was that simple, this swift, clean break between "before" and "after." This marked the beginning of life-by-numbers, in which clinical measures suddenly define your course, your progress, or your setbacks each day. And a new shuffle of information cards is dealt. In Gene's case the scans were done, and the doctor was right: the cancer had already escaped the prostate and metastasized to several different boney areas in his pelvis. The next move: go directly to the oncologist.

Diagnosis established, the oncologist had his own numbers to lay on the table. He advised Gene that he would likely have one good year before the impact of metastatic prostate cancer disease showed itself. The prognosis: Gene might have two to four years to live. Death was certain, and it was that close on the horizon.

We were devastated. Alex had just finished college and had planned to go off adventuring with his girlfriend Kate, but instead he (and weeks later she) came home to be with Gene. Each day, the numbers intensified our awareness and the surreal sense of it all. Here Gene was, soaring in his career, having recently left the NIH after a twenty-five year career there to set up an innovative new research center on creativity and aging, the Center for Aging, Health and Humanities, at George Washington University. On top of that, suddenly his night job as game inventor was meeting some unexpected and satisfying success. And we were not only engaged to be married; we had already adopted our beautiful daughter Eliana at birth. She was now eighteen months old.

So his shocking diagnosis set into motion our new life-game of numbers, just as other life events often do. They become a kind of emotional biofeedback system, telling us what to feel or what to not feel. Gradually, over years, and thanks to daily hormone treatment pills, the PSA numbers that came through our fax machine every month shifted downward and stayed closer and closer to zero. Shock subsided; in its place, vigilance. Our life became defined by tracking the stability of Gene's illness through these PSA numbers. (Low numbers are good, high are bad.)

We lived this numbers ritual through Gene's monthly checkups and lab tests, creating our own quiet ritual of appreciation. One month after another, our monthly ritual extended into years, and then more years, eventually an unprecedented thirteen years. It was a ritual that over time shifted from the tension of fear and worry to an almost routine expectation and trust in a future. Almost, that is.

Life by Numbers: "Medically, You Do Not Exist"

How do any of us get used to a number so powerfully defining our life to us? How do we adjust our internal gauge to respond to the external measurements and the messages they convey? A client of mine undergoing infertility treatments to become pregnant goes in each month for her inseminations, and each month the lab reads her numbers: of follicles, of viable eggs, sperm counts, motility and mobility counts. Then she waits and awaits what is to be, the results of a pregnancy test that either triggers sheer joy in her or drops her as if from the top of a cliff into the valley of despair and discouragement. She has a mere few days to move through this darkness before she has to return to the doctor's office to restart the hormonal pendulum swing and begin to enliven new endometrial cells, new tissue, and new egg formations, and try yet again. The pendulum swings between hope and despair, between winning and losing, between life and death. How do we find our way as it swings between alternate realities? How do we create a strategy and come up with our own tactics to hold ourselves steady?

I think of my mother, who saw her hematologist for years and years, at each visit receiving lab reports stating that although her white blood counts were always very low, her system was just fine. She and my dad would tell us that they had driven to the city to go to lunch or to go shopping. The doctor appointment part of their trip seemed inconsequential—until the day the blood counts marked a shift into multiple myeloma; now the numbers created a very different picture.

The familiar, long-established routine and ritual of reassurance vanished in the mere moments it took for the doctor to announce the new numbers and the new diagnosis that would now become the defining element of their lives. They did what people do: they adjusted to their new circumstances.

Gene saw this capacity to adjust as a developmental gift of aging, supported by neurological scaffolding—how the brain builds on experience. He felt that in our adult lives, we could take advantage of this developmental impetus to energize our creativity as we meet new challenges and, whatever our circumstances, explore new ideas and ways to engage.

> The positive influences of postformal thought, social intelligence, and life experience with aging are well established in terms of how we face adversity. I address these elements in the context of a broader concept that I refer to as developmental intelligence (DI). DI refers to the different qualities of the mind—cognition, social intelligence, emotional intelligence, judgment, and consciousness—with regard to how these qualities mature and interact with one another as we age. Cognition matures as reflected in the development of postformal thought with aging.[4] Social intelligence, influenced by accruing life experience over the course of time with aging, matures.
>
> Emotional intelligence is influenced by changes in the amygdala with aging; the amygdala is the part of the brain integrally involved in processing emotions. Studies on aging find that there is no difference in how the amygdala processes positive emotions with aging. But research reveals that changes in the amygdala with aging reflect the finding that older adults are less affected by negative emotions like fear, range, and envy than younger adults.[5] This discovery helps to explain the counterintuitive studies showing that morale is typically highest in older adults compared to other age groups. High morale is obviously an asset in dealing with adversity as well as the vicissitudes of aging and illness. Good morale in turn also nurtures hope and expectation. I feel very fortunate to have maintained solid morale throughout my ongoing confrontations with illness. Further research on emotions with aging finds that emotional stability, via controlling negative emotions, is also governed by the medial prefrontal cortex, and this capacity of the part of our brain involved in executive function is still improving as we approach our 80th birthday.
>
> Judgment and consciousness (which incorporates how we experience spirituality) also mature with aging. Hence, cognition, social intelligence, life experience, emotional intelligence, judgment, and consciousness all mature with aging. Moreover, in addition to the individual maturing of these critical qualities of the mind, these qualities become better integrated with aging, achieving a higher level of synergy with one another. Developmental intelligence reflects the individual maturing and enhanced

synergy of these qualities and influences on the mind with aging. How DI
shows itself is through wisdom. Wisdom in turn has a positive effect on how
we experience and utilize hope, expectation, and denial with aging.[6]

This was no esoteric theorizing. I could recognize the nuances and gradations of this developmental intelligence as our relationship with this clinical ritual—the anticipation, tests, waiting, and results—and our strategies for maintaining emotional equilibrium evolved. Gene and I got used to the idea that the numbers would show up each month via the fax machine. We waited with worry for so long, then we waited with expectation alongside worry, then with trust alongside worry alongside expectation, then with life alongside distraction alongside lessened worry alongside heightened trust, and on and on it went until it was all just part of how we were living our life. We would kiss. We would celebrate the numbers. We would go to lunch. The numbers said we could have a life. The numbers said we had a whole month to have that life, and then more months. For so long, the moment that fax arrived we got a whole month's reprieve. As soon as the numbers said "your PSA is down" and we knew he wouldn't take that blood test for another month, then we could keep going, have our celebratory lunch, and return to the ordinary.

You might think that you develop a strategy to manage this relentless emotional cycling, but the truth is that the strategy develops you: it takes charge. At some point something shifts inside because you can't let the numbers make you crazy each month; you can't live that way. You adapt and reorganize, recalibrate your emotional "feedback" loop, compartmentalizing the lab reports and doctors' conversations separately from family events and your daughter's basketball games. I use the phrase "emotional biofeedback" to describe the felt sense that most of us know from medical evaluations, even the simplest lab tests: you go into the doctor's office and you feel a certain way, then you get the numbers and the numbers tell you whether to burst into tears or burst into excitement. Nothing has changed inside you, but the numbers on that lab report—the information—become your prompt.

In the case of my client undergoing fertility treatment, a piece of paper says you're either pregnant or not pregnant, and the number throws her into an emotional loop. The feedback loop is predictable: the test, the numbers, the emotional reaction. You breathe and expand as the life of the illness recedes. You never assume that the threat is gone exactly; rather, that the threat is dormant. But only if the numbers give you that chance. If not, then your emotions recalibrate for crisis mode: the dreaded thing isn't dormant, and the life of the illness doesn't recede—it expands. For us, the monthly ritual of reassuring reports gave us hope, kept us believing that all was well, would be well, as the medicine they had told us could hold for a year or two, continued to hold year after year after year, well into its thirteenth year. Gene was surviving, against all odds.

"Medically, you do not exist," one doctor declared about Gene's status as an outlier, an aberration in the annals of medicine. But for us, all that mattered was that medically we were alive; Gene was our case study of one, and his anomaly of survival created a pattern of survival in our minds. Hope and belief became our strategy as we awaited the scores each month.

Gene once noted an uncanny game quality about it. You roll the dice or you pick up your cards and you either get a good hand or you don't, it's lucky or it's not, the game is either fun or it's not. The element of randomness creates suspense, tension.

> Despite hope and positive expectations, the dark side was not ready to retreat. As an inventor of games, I might have anticipated the dark twists and turns inevitable in any realistic strategy game, no matter how optimistic the potential outcome. And our lives at this time had that quality. We had a practical, yet positive attitude, a game strategy. But the unexpected detours, bad cards, and bad rolls came out of nowhere.

The Bad Hand

When bad news comes our way, most of us want to put it out of our mind because our mind cannot comfortably hold it. We each have our own coping strategies, but for some people that first strategic response is not easy. It is mired in the mind—the history and memory and buried associations that envelop us. We get stuck in this internal mud, and trying to assess the situation rationally may not be an option if the internal history is a confusion of past wounds, scars, and tender tissue. It's a fog we can't see through, or even hear or physically move through easily. Mind, body, heart, spirit—everything feels suddenly airless and leaden, or unbound, suspended in time and space. I think of one of my clients, whose obsessive nature spirals her into psychic pandemonium. As if a bully had arisen in the dark, she is flooded with all the ways in which she cannot cope with one more thing. She lashes out at friends and family, venomous when she feels that her competence is being threatened; experiences that overwhelm her competence make her feel she is in a fight for her life. She grows vicious, which pushes people away from her, makes them leave, which only validates for her that she is misunderstood, and so the process repeats itself. The rhythm of the game is torturous rather than melodic, distancing rather than comforting. What a battle, an even harder one, to calm enough to pause, accept, and see through the existential crack in which both faith and mystery move.

Gene and I had such different ways of playing through a bad hand. Fast forward to February 2009, thirteen years from the diagnosis, when the first round of chemotherapy with Taxotere started, as did all the fevers and the sickness and the rushing to the hospital.[7] Months of all of that, each time different, until we learned to control the ups and downs from home. He was his own doctor, working with a team of three other doctors. I wrote in my journal:

> I have to admit, these last six months are the months when our life has been taken from us, bringing us to the chemo days, the procedure days, the side effects days, the cleaning, fixing, arranging and rearranging of places in Gene's body—the bladder, the lungs, the bones, the tests, the infusions, the poisons; the consults, the insults, the results. It is exhausting, depressing, alienating, annoying, frustrating, lonely. Most days no one in the world would know that is what I feel. Most days, we can do it. We have our ways of being both quiet and engaged. Yet now, post the relaxation of a vacation at the lake and the return to our home, to the city life, to the responsibilities of work and caretaking, I must say, *phew*.

I am sitting in a hospital room; Gene is sleeping (as he can do anywhere). I am working to shrug off the annoying voices of a patient outside the door, but I am alone, quiet. Gene's procedure is going to be two hours late, two hours of time from our life. The things we imagine each day that are important to do, our errands or our responsibilities, are just out there, afloat.

How odd it feels to be most content when someone else is responsible for the people I am responsible for. When our daughter Eliana is off somewhere and Gene is off somewhere, I am able to *be*, period. And in that beingness I don't want to do anything anymore. Really. I just want the empty space. The cancer world takes a lot of empty space and fills it up—with cloudy tissue, cloudy thought, cloudy days.

Here we are, once again at the hospital, waiting. This time it is to activate a stent on a tube, a second nephrostomy tube, one of a growing assortment of tubes that have grown commonplace to us now.[8] *Insert. Activate. Adjust. Maintain. Replace.* We come in the doors as ourselves, and then slowly through admissions, the lab, the ward, and eventually radiology, we are stripped of identity. Just coming to the hospital now, I feel it. It used to be a safe place, a place of help. Now I approach it and annoyance is what I feel most. The parking lot is too expensive. The people are too overly kind. The voices are too grating. Even the fountains of water they create to relax people are too loud. My whole system wants to say NO.

We enter the pre-op room. Gene's identity is taken away and he is once again reduced to patient outfit, the gown, the open back, and the bed. The liquid drips into the port, the sound of his breathing sinking quickly into the deep rhythm of sleep. How can he do that, drop so quickly to sleep in this setting, in these kinds of moments? Some might say that his nervous system and its fight-or-flight mechanism were so overwhelmed by stress that this was the extreme version of flight—freeze—and a shutdown into sleep. But I have observed him use this strategy to restore himself so he doesn't get overwhelmed in the first place. I am reminded of something called "capacitance."[9] The word has several meanings in science and math, but also is used in the science of creativity to describe our ability to stretch into places of wholeness even when environments stretch us beyond what we believe we are capable of. Gene did that routinely, and in this case he had simply checked out to regain his energy.

Meanwhile, my confidence in all of this is shaken. My non-confidence grows as a too-talky nurse comes in and goes out of the room. Then comes the nurse who can't seem to find the cap for what she needs, even though she is the one in charge of this procedure. Gene is patient, or at least he taps that talent for survival's sake. I am not, do not; I am impatient, critical, and my fuse is short and ready with sheer annoyance.

I don't like waiting. I am a therapist, and if I am five minutes late for a client, I hear about it for a very long time. "In my profession, we would never get away with that kind of schedule," I say under my breath, "or this response to humanity." It's not audible enough even though I really do want one of these nurses to end up annoyed too, just to even things out. A strange irony of being a therapist, being a person who frames and reframes, who spends hours a day in intimacy with people I grow to love dearly, is that out here in the medical world, there are a lot of people I don't like. I don't like their style, their attitude, or their speed. I know enough to know that it is my anxiety I'm projecting onto them. Many of them are here doing their jobs competently, many doing so extremely well, but my personal annoyance walks in front of me, step by step. Gene's personal kindness walks in front of him. He sees what I see, but he shuts it out. Or transforms it. If not quite spinning gold from straw, he finds just the way to hold an experience to the light and find a thread of value. He was moved to write about this after one particularly insensitive physician decided to lecture him on the hopelessness of his condition. Gene dubbed him "the bludgeoner."

I have witnessed too many cases where the physician's view of the patient needing to know his or diagnosis and prognosis resulted in the physician misinterpreting the patient's expression of hope as reflecting denial that could interfere with following the doctor's treatment plan and interfere with the patient's proper planning for what he or she needs to do in general under the circumstances. Hope, as I said earlier, is not a manifestation of denial, nor a signal that one needs a reality check. It is a wonderful human quality that needs to be properly responded to, in a manner that reflects the art, not the artlessness, of medicine. The "bludgeoner" determined that I needed to hear from him just how limited my days really were, despite my advising him right from the start that I was a physician who thoroughly understood my diagnosis and prognosis. But Doctor/Patient Communication 101 left him on hyper alert for patient denial and for the need to intervene.

> To balance my resulting rage from that travesty of a consultation, in addition to thinking about what else I should have said (will censor myself here), I felt I should be better prepared for what I realized would be similar future encounters with others. I turned to humor, and thought of coining a phrase to capture such outrageous responses that are hurled unsolicited in my direction. I thought about the philosopher Zeno, 20 years Socrates' senior, in ancient Greece. Zeno described a number of paradoxes in thinking. Only 2 or 3 survive today, so I took the liberty of constructing what I refer to as Zeno's 5th Paradox, best expressed in the form of a question: "How can there be more horses' asses in the world than horses?"[10] Then, after every encounter like that with the "bludgeoner" I would sardonically mutter to myself, "Ah, Zeno's 5th Paradox!" I would then also go out and smell the roses. Hardly a day goes by when I don't take time out to simply reflect on the beauty around me—literally, the smell of the roses, the greenness of the grass, the blueness of the sky, the fullness of the moon, the brightness of the stars in the sky (Did I leave out any of the usual suspects of natural beauty?), and the wonderful fleeting beautiful interpersonal reactions that take place—my wife's laugh, my daughter's jokes, my son's pictures of his children (my grandchildren) that he sends. And then I write. I feel that humor and beauty and creative expression restore order to the universe, and to my life.

Gene had amazing coping skills because he was a disciplined person, a patient person, and a kind person, and he approached life like that. He certainly fell into many a dark place, many "dark dips," as he called them, but he used all the aspects of the creative mind that he had written about to find the light. Not as a strategy but in a natural way. He naturally framed things toward potential. He had a capacity to swim through the muck, find the one little gold nugget there in the depths, grab onto it, and bring it up to the surface. He was able to do it when we would go visit his mom in the nursing home, or with his dad, at the end of his time with Alzheimer's. Eliana and I would brace ourselves, emotionally gear up, because this was going to be so hard. Gene would remember that one glimmer in his father's eye when his dad recognized him and he would hold onto that nugget.

Unconscious Competence is the Psyche's Wild Card

The rhythm of this life by numbers, the lull of reprieves and our strategies for managing uncertainty, follow clinical cues, but the body itself doesn't play that game; the body knows with certainty and offers its own clues. But our mind is a complex lens that sometimes obscures what is in plain view and other times allows our fears to magnify benign details into seemingly dangerous ones.

In the fall of 2008, thirteen and a half years after his original diagnosis, Gene developed a stubborn infection that appeared to involve the prostate. His doctors gave him the most aggressive antibiotic, but the infection remained. They gave him another round of the antibiotic, then another, but the infection persisted. The doctors feared the cancer had revived, but his PSA numbers were still so low that we all figured it couldn't be that. The numbers were fluctuating, but nothing dramatic, yet why was it taking so long for the antibiotics to kill the bacterial infection? Gene was walking and moving very slowly, which was not at all typical for him, a man often described as "impish" and tireless by friends and colleagues. But it was not considered indicative of cancer, and we had, after all, had our usual busy year. By December we decided that some sun and a warm, relaxing vacation would be good for all three of us. For Eliana's winter break we decided to break free from the frozen nation's capital and headed for Costa Rica.

Despite the doctors' assurances, I had a frightening intuition that I never spoke of but wrote about before we left Maryland for our trip:

> I have a feeling that my husband is not going to make it. I can't say why. It is just a feeling, a fragility, a quiet between us. A dark feeling. Twelve or thirteen years ago, when the cancer first appeared, I had a feeling that he was going to make it. No reason really. As a matter of fact, it was against reason, but it was a feeling, and it has proved to be true. So this feeling, this dark quiet feeling scares me. I feel myself seeing him fade, walking slower, talking slower, sharing slower, something silent between us. It is not a knowing; as a matter of fact, I think it is an unknowing, a loosening of something inside, a perception based on nothing yet everything.
>
> Now I know something is shifting, something is going, something is leaving. We have no language for this, no symptom, no problem, and no change per se, but something is shifting and I feel it. I don't dare to put this to paper, and yet I wake up in these quiet hours of the night, I can't sleep, I put this to paper. The sands are shifting, gentle, crystalline, sinking, slowly the sands are shifting, and I seem to be the only one noticing. I dare not even say it out loud.

One month later, in January, home from Costa Rica, Gene returned to see his doctors. The cancer was back. The oncologist gave him five months. The internist, only five weeks. He wrote a short but telling email to his friend Sandy: "My cancer has returned. I am devastated."

Looking back, remembering the feeling and reading my journal, it is clear that the unspoken truth was already making itself known to us. At an unconscious level first perhaps, with *unconscious competence*, intuition can discern what is not yet evident or expressed—if we know how to listen.[11] Yet, we can't respond to every worry we have, can't assume every foreboding thought or bad dream is prophetic; we would be overwhelmed with our own anxiety and hopelessly hypersensitive to the ordinary ways our minds process worry and fears. After all, sheer existential terror can frighten or even bully us in our dark places. Worry can wear us down, giving our worst fears all the more traction. We have to find a way to listen to all our senses, to balance everyday worry and even inexplicable foreboding, to hold all that with the thoughts that sustain us—as Gene said, all the "usual suspects of natural beauty." It is all the harder—and more essential—when the numbers come to hold such power over us. All the while, the body knows with accuracy what medical minds and our own minds struggle to discern.

A Gamer's Defensive Strategies: Substitution, Diversions, Projections

displace it

Annoyance over other peoples' actions or assumptions, over perceived slights or slip-ups, or over other routine indignities is another strategy of the psyche under pressure. A strategy of substitution gives us a way to justify being just plain angry. It's a release of tension that makes you feel so much better because you can have the anger and not have the people you love get mad at you—you just aim it elsewhere! After the Costa Rica trip, as the cancer treatment began to take a toll on Gene's body, I moved the dire medical fears aside and replaced them, temporarily at least, with something concrete I could get annoyed over: stereotypes about aging. This was, after all, Gene's life's work, so I was well informed and indignant.

The Costa Rica trip started this process when a desk clerk innocently mentioned in passing, "I haven't seen your father this morning." My father? My father wasn't even here—sadly, he had passed away four years ago. Then it struck me. He was talking about Gene. My husband, whose appearance had wearied practically overnight, who now walked slowly and haltingly, suddenly appeared to strangers as an "old man"—a man old enough to be my father—and just that fast their assumptions about his identity replaced the man.

Gene, the gerontologist, was acutely aware of ageist stereotypes and biases and was quite vocal about them. I thought I understood these on one level, but I had no idea how many buttons that desk clerk's particular question, description and interpretation of who we are and what comprises our relationships would push in me and in Eliana. It was as if a whole separate universe tumbled open.

It made me sad—sad because Gene was visibly slowing down. But my reaction to the clerk's comment and the sadness weren't about age as age; this was about taking Gene out of context. If he were truly my father, I would be proud of my role.

If he truly were her poppy, Eliana would be proud as well. But he was not either. He was her father and my husband. People were seeing him as someone he was not, seeing a family that was not our family. These strangers knew nothing about us, and what they innocently said meant nothing. Yet the world that tumbled open was that of hurtful labels and assumptions: Gene was being labeled. I was being labeled. Our family was being reconfigured by outsiders' assumptions.

At this time Gene was sixty-four, but because of this recent turn in his illness he looked much older, and he moved with the fragile, tentative steps of someone much older. We had been forced into a time period—older age—before our time. In my journal I wrote:

> He moves slower, turns gently, rests on the steps, smells the grass in passing to pace the system, slow passing as the feet don't quite touch the ground with the same confidence of attachment anymore, as the movement between one resting spot and another is one room to the next, one couch to the next, one appointment to the next, one task to the next, one meal to the next, keep the system fueled, keep the eyes on the ball.

The medicines that were intended to manage his cancer had pushed Gene and the rest of us into an unexpected and unwelcomed journey through accelerated time. I had made some kind of peace with the narrower expectations imposed by illness. It is one thing to live in a narrower space, to accept limitations of movement and expectations. It is fine to pace the conversations or exchanges that can occur in a given time frame. It is fine to adjust and tweak and revamp what makes it all possible. We can do this, I thought to myself. Just let us live like this, at least let it stay like this. But the assumptions and labels coming from beyond our protected space moved us into a different conversation, a different context in the eyes of others and, thus, in our own eyes, too.

This is what I was seeing in the present when I would see Gene move through the house during these days. Not so much out in the public world, although I could see it there too, but at home, amidst the daily rituals of showering, dressing, eating, taking care of oneself. The care that has slid into longer time, slower pace, fragile needs is the care of a body that is changing and changing us all.

Here was a man who had devoted his life to confronting ageism. It was such a strange and cruel juxtaposition. Here was the person who had written about it, who had catapulted the field into a focus on potential and toward shifting the stereotypes, assumptions, and myths away from loss; and here it was, coming at us, coming at us when he was giving a presentation, receiving a standing ovation, walking with us to dinner. This wasn't "aging." This was disease. But in the most practical ways it appeared to "age" him, and thus his illness, and others' responses, brought him and his subject together. It was a point, a conversation, we both could hear without exchanging a word. We left it that way. As a couple, our strategy of silence at times was simply merciful.

New Round, New Rules, and Tactics of Tenderness

Just that quickly, the game shifted. Before December 2008, the number coming though the fax machine was a source of joy in that it confirmed our trust that all was well. We awoke each day in generous gratitude for the reprieve. We knew it could change, but we went on hoping for that clean bill of health and that's just what we got. I'd relegated my dark premonition to the silence of my journal, but the Costa Rican hotel clerk had simply voiced what I had already begun to sense. As the medical test results began to catch up to the body's reality, and the doctors' tone and the numbers they shared took a sharp turn for the worse, Gene felt that his last hope had been stolen from him. We could feel the shift; we were in a new game now, more serious than ever, and yet our outlook was still shaped by our past experience—as it is for all of us—and with that came a kind of positivity of last resort. Our experience had been that Gene was an outlier. The original prognosis that gave him just a couple of years at best had been off by more than a decade, we knew now, more than thirteen years later.

Strategies and tactics are coping mechanisms that you base on your past experience; you look at your history. There is never certainty, yet, in our case, the thought was: *you've done this, beat the odds before, so why assume the trajectory of these new facts will be any different?* To call this false hope is a mistake, as I've said. We all live this way, basing our hopes or expectations on experience and history, and sometimes on pure desire. We couldn't do anything in life if we had to wait for certainty. We never know what's going to happen. We can get discouraged or anxious. We can get calm and hopeful.

In moments like this, we don't give up our reality; as a matter of fact, we hold on for dear life. We deepen our mindfulness, expand our compassion to ourselves and others so that we can express our love. These, too, are strategies and tactics. When my friend Carol was taking care of her husband Jerry, she knew that the complementary treatment they had researched and chosen was working. Even when it became apparent that much more time and health would be needed for the treatment to have built up enough momentum in his body to outweigh the fast movement of his disease, this became the ground in which her caregiving became a gardening ritual of love. That blended shake she made, at exactly the same time each day, became their white rose. Gene's soy protein powder drink that he mixed each day for more than thirteen years was his ritual, allowing him an active role in depriving cancer cells of fat, especially meaningful to the scientist struggling for survival.

Cribbage: Rhythms, Counting, and Coping Strategies

I think about my life with Gene before the diagnosis and bleak prognosis hung over our heads. The cancer diagnosis forced a focus to the game of love and marriage that took me right out of so many other concerns. Now, it's as if I can't really go back to the beginning of our story, and I can't push myself into some future that I don't dare to envision, so the present is the only place to stand. Our life has become like the cribbage game Gene and Eliana play. The two of them just sit at the table, open the beautiful board that Gene's game partner Gretchen designed, take out the cards, and play. Maybe they don't even want to play, but they do because for this one short moment, they are in it together, alone together—strategy, tactics and counting: "fifteen two, fifteen four, and the rest don't score." They are calmed and quieted by the game. Gene can't go out onto the basketball court with Eliana anymore or into the lake for a swim. Their communication is not talk as it is with me; it is more kinesthetic play. It is *their* way of being together, their way of finding peace together, father and daughter, in the chaos.

In cribbage and, really, in any game, the play moves forward, however slowly and sometimes with setbacks. But to watch Gene and Eliana play cribbage, with the familiar tactic of connecting both kinesthetically and tenderly as I recall myself at her age in the ski lodge, takes my thoughts back through time to my teenage years, then to my earlier life with Gene, our life before the cancer diagnosis and the turn our lives took soon after. Nothing about our past could have predicted this would be our future, and nothing about the cancer prognosis allows us the luxury of envisioning a future. So we stay riveted on the present; in one sense it holds us in place, in the life together that we love, and yet we also know that it keeps us moving forward, through birthdays, anniversaries, and other milestones and clinical markers that line the way.

Gene struggles in a special way with this pressure to stay in the now but the requirement to plan forward. Previously, his strategy for planning public appearances and other work commitments was a simple matter of scheduling, based on his availability. That has changed.

My sense of time to live completely collapsed. My doctors and all the medical texts informed me that it was limited, and they offered little room for variation. The temporal contrasts I was experiencing were enormous. On the one hand, my doctors were conveying to me that I had no future path, while the rest of the world with no knowledge of my condition was contacting me about program plans down the road. It made me feel like I was in the twilight zone. At the onset of my illness, I became gripped by a strange new sensation whenever contacted to give a future talk. It was a paralyzing, repeating feeling that continued for nearly three years, most pronounced when my invitation was for an event over a year away. My primary oncologist had advised me that I might have only one good year before I became symptomatic from the progression of my cancer. Most likely influenced by this sentence hovering above me, I simply could not fathom a commitment more than twelve months ahead.

Through it all, the effects of the disease and the treatments are dunning, but erratic, adding to the complexity of planning. Gene's strategy is unspoken, intuitive, but I see the pattern emerge. Although his calendar remains full, the projects are almost exclusively sooner or of shorter duration.

There is something about the counting in cribbage, something about the way you move along in the game, the repetition, the path that feels kind of like life, like Gene and me. Cribbage is about strategy, tactics, and counting. What are the tactics I come to count on to navigate the life I now know we've just been thrown into? Listening, waiting, surviving. I need to adapt my strategy for embracing this changing experience as I was able to do in the "old days," when the diagnosis was here, but the life was still our own. "Sticks are nine; go with time. Fifteen two, fifteen four, the rest don't score. Fifteen two, fifteen four a pair is six, move the sticks, I smell a skunk! A double run of three is six and a pair is eight, you're out the gate. I foretell a smell, you're about to be skunked."[12]

3

The Family Body

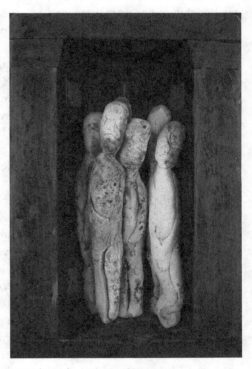

Figure 3.1 "We're All in This Together #3" (1982), raku fired clay figures with oxides and wooden mold, 16 × 10 × 5 inches. Artwork by Wendy L. Miller, photo credit: Joshua Soros.

In everyday language, disease and illness can appear the same, but they are not. The noted psychiatrist, anthropologist, and author Arthur Kleinman distinguishes between them, describing disease as the biological process taking place within the body.[1] Illness goes beyond the biological: it is the lived experience of a process—living with a disease.

Gene's disease became the backdrop for our lives; it took place in his body, not inside mine. But his illness lived in both of us. It lived in our bodies, our hearts, our minds, our spirits, and our social lives. It lived within our family—in *the family body*. It had been with us practically from the beginning of being a family together. We had met and married, both of us having had previous marriages and lives with different people; both of us familiar through our own and other family members' health challenges with illness that redefines life for all. Gene's illness was part of the fabric that created our family, our intimate community, and how we formed our love. It had grown with us, around us, of us.

Illness not only affects a family, it becomes a member of the family. There's a relationship to consider that exists between family members and illness-related needs and requirements, all part of the whole fabric of the family. More than just a condition, illness starts to acquire a life of its own when it requires others to adjust around its impositions or idiosyncrasies. Experience lives through us and the illness experience is no different. Illness lives through us, every day, in every way. That does not mean that we must think about it every minute of every day. But the ways in which illness affects the everyday is the story of our lives—not just Gene's and mine; it is everyone's story. In the fall of 2009, when Gene's cancer was ravaging him physically, he drew strength from other sources and wrote from a deep and loving place of family and relationship.

> Critical illness offers the experience of being taken to the threshold of life, from which you can see where your life could end.[2] From that vantage point you are both forced and allowed to think in new ways about the value of your life. Alive but detached from everyday living, you can finally stop to consider why you live as you have and what future you would like, if any future is possible. Illness takes away parts of your life, but in doing so it gives you the opportunity to choose the life you will lead, as opposed to living out the one you have simply accumulated over the years.
>
> In the terms of the illness author, medical sociologist, cancer and heart attack survivor, Arthur Frank, it was a multilayered opportunity for what I have referred to in my research on creativity as social creativity. The arrangement allowed Alex and me to develop a closeness that for the prior eight years was limited by his living away at boarding school, then college.
>
> At the time of my initial cancer diagnosis in 1996, my son Alex had just moved back for a brief stay after graduating from college. One of the most poignant moments was when I told Alex what I had just learned about my terrible diagnosis and even worse prognosis. We'd put our arms around each other as tears traveled down our cheeks. I flashed back at that moment to a vivid episode in our lives when Alex was two and a half. He had fallen while running and injured a hand and scraped a couple of fingers, causing bleeding. His pride was also hurt. But he got up and we both ran to one another, and as I held him in my arms, he looked wide-eyed at me with a

comforted sense of expectation, asking me, "Daddy, can you fix me?" With his arms now around me, I had the comforting feeling that he would do anything to help fix me. There is something so profoundly moving in deeply sharing love with one's child.

Alex had planned to seek a job in another part of the country, but immediately changed his plans to stay put at our house. Also, his fiancée Kate was going to travel with him, but after they discussed it Kate agreed to move in with him at our house. Fortunately, we had an old four-level 5,500 square foot townhouse, designed by one of Washington's architects in the early 20th century. The house had an interesting history, adapted as a bordello a couple of owners prior to us, and its enormous space offered great privacy. So Alex and Kate moved into the top floor, in effect having their own apartment. We also turned the second-floor wood-paneled library into a nursery for baby Eliana and her crib and toys. To finally have this closeness made me feel so alive again.

Moreover, despite a 21-year age difference between Alex and Eliana, the two bonded with a depth that would likely not have been possible living apart. And as an added bonus, Kate, who later married Alex, became more like a sister to Eliana than a sister-in-law. What more could a father have asked for in the closeness between his children?

Now, with the return of the cancer after a 13-year remission, my relationship with Alex grew yet deeper. Alex was with me when the oncologist gave me only months or weeks to live. Much transpired in our heads after that thunderbolt, but upon leaving the doctor's office Alex gave me the most loving neck message, telling me I could count on him for whatever I needed. And indeed I could count on him. Despite the fact that he was now married with four small children and had a very demanding job, he accompanied me on my out-of-state talks that I had agreed to give before I became ill again. He looked out for me in a most comforting way. There were so many profound experiences of closeness with Alex as the time transpired. One of the talks I gave was among my very best and it was to an audience that was electrified. This was clearly a very moving experience for Alex, even more so with so many at the reception that followed telling him how highly they regarded my work. The pride he showed simply dissolved my heart.

And with my Eliana, at this time of the return, she has watched me month after month. How far does a father's love extend for his daughter Eliana? To the moon and back—as many times as you can possibly imagine. I always wanted a son, and I got a great one. I always wanted a daughter, and got a great one—with wonderful inner warmth and outer beauty. My daughter Eliana, in a word, is lovely. She can always make me smile, especially when she puts her cheek against mine, and softly says from the heart, "I love you daddy."

There are so many things I admire about Eliana—her loyalty, humor, loving nature, musical and artistic talent, persistence, and resilience. Both of my parents wanted me to play piano. I tried, but was not terribly good at it. If my parents were alive, they would beam as I do when I listen to how beautifully Eliana moves her fingers across the piano keys. So, too, with extraordinary photos she takes and with her remarkable graphics.

I'm helping Eliana with her biology homework, which I love to do, especially because when we finish, she moves out of her teenage surliness and gives me a kiss, saying, "I love you daddy!" You can imagine how I melt with that.

We are reading about forest fires as natural events. Nature has its strange and paradoxical ways. The text says that "some ecosystems depend on fires to get rid of debris. A forest fire might change the habitat so drastically that some species no longer can survive, but other species might thrive in the new, charred conditions."[3] My cancer has brought a conflagration to the forest of our family life. Much of the structure we relied upon has been radically changed, but novel and interesting elements have also emerged; there has even been new growth, including this new book by Wendy and me, but written essentially in Wendy's voice. Rather than my being charred, you might say the conflagration set a fire under me to try something new and very different.

This week has been the hardest. I of course keep thinking of my family and my loved ones, my pain of letting any of them down. How would I ever be able to tell Eliana? Decisions moved into grieving as I hoped for renewed energy to return. Then the explanations of my weakness—the need for higher saturation of oxygen, constant oxygen, the complications of nasal dryness with the constant oxygen, the exhaustion of breathing, the appointments, the discussions with the oncologist, and the internist, and now yesterday the cardiologist—our information and caring team. The fifth line of chemo is a long shot by all standards, and the risk is looking so much greater than the potential gain—Wendy and I thought we would have to dream a decision, but in fact, the heavy heart has made the decision for us.

The cardiologist did an EKG (electrocardiogram)[4] and found the cancer has created a hardening of the pericardium sac—the sac that surrounds and holds my heart—and when this layer hardens as it has, probably through the chemotherapies, it becomes more and more difficult to breathe. So between my lungs and my heart and the cancer, yes, breathing is very hard, and it puts me at risk of cardiac arrest. Chemo and surgery (they could cut open my sternum and cut away at the lining—can you imagine choosing that at this point?) both look like on-the-table killers. The cardiologist thinks we need to let nature take its course, as if we aren't in the midst of nature taking its course. The oncologist thinks I have fought as long and as hard as he can imagine. He said if there were even a 3% chance of something working he would carry it to our house daily, but he doesn't have any such thing. And the internist said the surgery is the only life-extender option, and he would follow my lead. But for this, I am clear and it is what I gently have to tell my little loved one, my Eliana: I am not going to make a choice to die on the table. If dying is what is to come, I am going to do it at home.

And so we picked up Eliana at school, who intuitively, somatically seemed to know everything. She had left class midday because she felt too faint to concentrate. When she called Wendy, we were on our way home. We went to pick her up so we could all be together. We came home to the quiet of our intimate words and shared cries. We sat together, all of us on the big comfy chair in the living room. With my slow breathing and my heavy hardened heart, I told her that if the cardiologist operated to fix the hardening of the pericardium, I would die on the table. I don't want to do that. The thing is, darling, do you understand what that means? She said yes, but did she? Could she? She understood in her body that we were in very big trouble, and that her daddy seemed weaker and weaker.

With all this in my head, the three of us, the family body, sat in the chair, quiet.

Each day, I begin my day inside our nuclear family body—Eliana, Gene, and I—waking; moving everyone along to meet the early carpool/school schedule, the daily school/lunch/work needs; making the coffee that awakens us to the process; hearing the mutters of the teenage complaint at something we did or will do: the way we turn the pages of the newspaper, too clumsily, of course, or slurp our orange juice just slightly too loudly for her ever-so-sensitive ears. Work for me entails leaving this part of family life through the back door, walking slowly and carefully down the back steps to the yard, carrying in my arms my food or papers I may need for the day.

I walk along the twenty-four steppingstones that take me to my studio and to Create Therapy Institute, which houses my expressive arts therapy practice that helps people through experiential approaches and the creative arts in therapy.[5] My studio is downstairs—with all my art books, art supplies, sculptures, jewelry, and art works in endless process. The upstairs is my therapy office filled with more art materials, miniature objects for sand tray work, and the furnishings necessary for comfort in the dialog that takes place between me and the people who come to see me. From the studio curtain window, once part of an old carriage house that has since been transformed into my workspace, I look out and observe my home, mindful of the inner workings of this family body we share. From the same vantage point, facing in, I see into the lives of others—children, adults, couples, and families—into the many ways the family body presents in their stories and struggles. The skills I use to listen closely to the discovery process within my clients' imagery are the same ones I use to listen for it within my own family body.

Here, in this space, we take the swift, unsettling changes in their lives and slow them down, to reflect on, examine, and explore them. A brilliant insight or awareness can spark in a second and make so much sense, especially when it is immersed in daily life. The movement is often ever so slight. The steps that transform are slow and sometimes arduous; they are careful undertakings that happen millisecond by millisecond in one's life. Our work is the practice of emotional intimacy and remembrance: psychic history witnessed, recorded, and recalled.

One of my earliest clients was a thirty-three year-old man, a librarian who came to me after five years of surgeries and treatments for melanomas on his upper chest. We worked together for only six months, but during that time his creative quest was based on his very important question: "How can I grow if I don't know what else might be growing inside of me?"

Through a series of drawings and guided imagery (using images to guide attention), deep listening, and moving through the filtered layers of fears and doubts, he came to embrace this inward discovery process of finding out what would "enliven" him. In his mind's eye, he located himself inside a dome inside a pain in his chest where he found a young boy playing with toys beside a closed treasure chest. We worked diligently with this metaphoric chest, drawn as a trunk image, never saying out loud the conscious connection between his own chest as body and the imagistic chest as trunk. His drawings and images evolved through times of protectedness, bumps, and quest for trust and balance, until one day he tied ropes to the chest and drew a man riding on it at fast speed down a steep hill, thrilled to learn to steer and navigate his way. He began to viscerally understand that one day he would know when to open the chest, when he was not traveling upon it, and that everything he had learned from the chest would always be tied to him. He learned to stay anchored to this trust of his own imagistic chest, without ever returning to the conscious description of the physical chest of his past melanomas. I was honored to accompany him in this journey of discernment, and grateful that he affirmed in me the depth of my own faith in following an image, and allowing metaphor and ritual to guide us toward healing.

Gene had his own version of intentional imagery, which he practiced daily. In the shower, for instance, he imagined the prescribed hormones he ingested as being infused with the life-affirming presence of his children, Alex and Eliana, and eventually he was able to expand that infusion to the qualities of his four grandchildren. As the water washed over him, he visualized it—and experienced it, as he described to me—imbued with the healing gifts of love, connection, and belonging. He was very disciplined, so when he chose to add this practice to his repertoire of medicine he could do for himself, he practiced it every single day.

As for me, the image of concentric circles of engagement emerges not so much as chosen therapeutic symbolism but as the de facto sense of my reality. I live in, move through all the circles all the time. I am in dialog with the circles of the individual, the family, and the social body every day. This imagery dialog travels with me, down the steps out of my home and into my studio and office. This is what I do. I listen. I track. I record. I take into my being the presence that is brought ever so delicately to me by people: ill people, healthy people, each of us people, all trying to chart our way through the circumstances that form our lives. The story of living into one's health, whatever that may be, is a story of our belonging to something larger—the community family body—and in that body we are all in this together.

In my concentric circles, within each realm, each circle, are the stories. Gene and Eliana and myself: we are a multitude of stories. Eliana's adoption story—*our* adoption story—is the *Genesis* of our family, and the amazing growth and development of our daughter and ourselves within that story. She is young and moving through middle school, which requires advocacy and tending, tutoring and guiding in the academic arenas; we have our careers that need to run, not on their own, but within the limits of family and community life. We have four grandchildren through Alex and Kate, all under the age of seven at the time Gene died.

It is said that "time heals," but this is not true for me; the way I see it, time passes, and in its time, our time passes into the life it takes to live into our healing. All this requires a great deal of family tending, nourishing, and nurturing, and this life-tending has to run its course, it is its own condition, alongside the illness condition. And in truth it is the whole of it that gets sick, that gets well, that provides the context of what surrounds the life we live. There's the illness part, and you have to take care of that, but there's also all of this family-tending, and you have to take care of that. And what about your self? You need tending too. We cannot separate the strands of illness from the strands of family and individual growth, as if that illness, or that growth, were separate from the condition that shapes our lives.

Gene's guided imagery of being immersed in the family's healing love was not an imagined thing. It was our reality. We do live inside the healing love of the family body. And it is this family body that has emerged, filled with suffering, sorrow, love, opportunity, amazement, and health, and that we grow into as we age and develop. It is an old story, the story as told around the kitchen tables of every generation. It is a love story, a family story, a story of the capacity to endure and to be secure in ourselves. And it becomes our legacy to carry it on, in sickness and in health.

Amid Tension and Transition, a Search for Perspective

At my own father's funeral, in 2005, Eliana, eleven at the time, called to me, "Mom, remember to bring a spoon for Ruby. She's too small to hold the shovel and throw the dirt on top of poppy at the grave. She needs to have something that is smaller, maybe something from your sand tray collection in your studio, so that she'll be able to lift it."

Ruby was two-and-a-half years old at that time. So when Eliana cared about what her niece Ruby would need at the gravesite, I was deeply struck by the juxtapositions of love and panic. We are—I am—raising a child whose family body is already so different than the one I grew up with, surrounded by generations of elders as I was. I feel my love for her, so appreciate that she knows and is able to think of such things as what will matter for little Ruby to be present at the ritual of loss and burial. But that Eliana has the perception and heart to care about how this will be for her young niece sits right beside the part of me that hates that she knows any of this and has to teach a two-and-a-half year old the rituals of death and dying when she herself is only eleven years young.

Four years later, when Gene's treatment had shifted from hormone therapy to chemotherapy and he was six months into that brutal regimen,[6] Eliana and I rested one afternoon on the water trampoline in front of our lakeside camp. We chatted, Eliana, almost fifteen, telling me that it was really hard to see what her daddy had to go through with chemotherapy. On one level, it is such a simple statement. On another level, it is such a complete statement. People ask me all the time, in different tones of caring and worrying, "So, how is Eliana doing?" And I try to answer them, but mostly I sigh. My mother died when I was forty-seven and it took me five years to come out of the anger part of my grief. My dad died when I was fifty-five and although by then I had learned to move through my grief in a different way, not a day goes by when I do not think of them and feel their absence. Not one day.

So, how do I think Eliana is doing? I think she is fifteen—that is how she is doing. She dons indifference, when useful, as a way of being in life. She is naturally and understandably trying to involve herself—in her computer, her TV shows, her friends, her plans, and her desires for independence and freedom. I go back and forth with worry about her and how she is doing, knowing that she is immersing herself in these various other surrogate families, glad that she has the capacity and temperament to do that, and envious that she has the capacity and temperament to do that.

She is watching her so-called normal life completely and profoundly change in a mere eight months. She is watching. At first she didn't know what to watch, but chemotherapy brings it all right home in front of you. We watch the withering, weakening, sleeping, breathing, slowing, sickening, occasional returning of the self that is Gene. Her daddy. My husband. We watch what is happening to love right in front of our eyes. And what is it that is happening? Do any of us know? Are we healing unto life, unto death, unto loss, unto gain? How do we imagine what it is we see?

Gene is quiet. I am quiet. Alex is quiet. Eliana is quiet. We are stunned into our own silences. Fear is a silence of its own.

Eliana wants out.

"It's fun over at his house" or "I like the way her mother laughs" or "the way his grandmother cooks" or whatever her desire is at the moment. "I want to be over there" is what she is saying. She wants OUT and I don't blame her. I want out a lot, too. This summer she never wanted to leave, she wanted IN, so maybe this is a step of some kind of awareness or acceptance. Who knows, but I sometimes have a wish she were more able to share her sensitivity and caring rather than be, well, fifteen: the rolling of the eyes, the turning of the head, the "Whatever!" She is fifteen and that is a hard age regardless of the situation at home. Gene and I cannot imagine what she is making of all this at such a vulnerable age, or how she will make her way through whatever is to come, including the uncertainty of what is to come.

We focus on our daughter's vulnerability, but we are all vulnerable. There is no good age for this. We show feelings and such compassion for one another one moment, and the next our own anger or fear or neediness claws to be heard and tended. Gene, always, is the magnet for our best selves. Eliana has such empathy for her dad, is so watchful of him, but there is not such openness toward me; I am, like the mother of most teenage girls, the one who intrudes on her budding independence with practical questions, requests, and expectations around family duties, homework, and her social life.

How can I imagine that she could step out of herself and see the fear and angst I am living with? If she could see it, I would not be doing my mother job very well, but if she doesn't see it, I am left alone with this familial intimacy, protecting, holding on by the skin of my teeth. The family body is rife with sore spots and inflammations.

My thoughts range from fierce focus on clinical details to the most mundane things to exquisite transcendent moments of mystic dimensions. But all that is a private prelude. In our conversations I choose words very carefully.

To Gene, at the time, I am able to say: "I know how hard this new turn is for you, but I also know how wonderful you have been with it all along as your body and spirit have rallied this long and this far. I see a compass at your core, guiding you in right relationship to your self. When this inner compass gets adjusted, as yours has, it works well forever. It's been working well for so long up to now; we have to remember that, for it has not gone away. I trust you in that adjustment process, hard as it always is to fine-tune."

To Eliana I say something like this: "Everyone's fight is different. Cancer is something that is biological and chemical in the body. The fight for daddy is about being able to tolerate the very strong treatment called chemotherapy, which is what does the hard fight for him. It is not about whether or not you fight well but whether you can tolerate the fight in the body because it makes you look and feel very sick before it makes you better."

She brings up the name of a groundskeeper at her school who died of cancer shortly after he was diagnosed. I explain: "The man at your school who died from cancer didn't find out about his cancer until it was very late in the process. Your daddy has known that the cancer was there for a long time, and his body tolerated the first medicine very well and it lasted a long time—all of your life, as a matter of fact. The doctors are assuming that his body will continue to do well and they are watching him very closely. Because he is a doctor as well, he speaks a similar language to the other doctors' so he understands all those big words. Your daddy also researches and studies what he needs and you know how he is when he is studying! You can be sure he is reading and reading and learning everything he can. We are going to be learning and watching with him so we all will try to know what is happening together; and you have a very open and honest family so if we get to the point where we are worrying, I will tell you so that we can all worry together. That is the way we will do this: together. But we are not worrying now and so you do not have to worry all by yourself either. I promise that I will tell you if a time comes when we have to worry together, but that is not now. OK?"

And I meant it. But eight months later, Gene is looking weaker and weaker to all of us. Eliana, a watcher by nature, a nonintrusive person by nature, a teenager trying to be independent and self-contained, is coming up against her inner full-of-fear child who is her as the watcher, watching the daddy she loves.

This past summer, Eliana watched her brother Alex and sister-in-law Kate worry about him; her aunts and cousin Andy cater to him, worry about his walking, slipping, and climbing the steps; his sleeping and sleeping and sleeping. She is certainly worrying on her own and trying to go places that seem to be more relaxing for her. And no, her mom didn't say it was time to worry. Nor did her brother or her father. She knows she is worrying all on her own. We all do. And when she returns to the house from being with a friend, I see that she has found herself again, and for a short while, she finds her comfort, joy, and pleasantness again. Going out into her world restores her.

She certainly knows something about what she needs. Isn't that what every parent tries to give their children? And me, what about me? What do I need in terms of being that good parent to her. What do I need to restore myself?

Eliana's statement on the water trampoline that day, about the hardships of Gene's chemotherapy, was filled with both the simplicity and the complexity of it all. It is really hard to witness this process, to see the dailyness of it: to watch it, to engage with it, to disengage from it, to pay attention, to worry, to not worry, to act like you are not noticing, yet to notice everything, to know how to play it. It is hard enough for Gene to do it, no less to watch him do it and hold steady with something, anything, inside. To give someone the dignity of their own process, yet to remain in the dignity of your own process. To leave them to do or not to do what they need. And yet, there are so many things he can't do and so many things he needs to do, and knowing which is which, and when to step in and when to leave him alone, and when and what to do is a constant dilemma. When and what and how? To give Gene that, leave Gene that, know when to lean in and when to step back, or just be: every moment is unique in what it calls for, and what it calls forth, in each of us.

And what exactly is going on with him? When is "the time to worry?" If this is not the time to worry, what is that time going to look like? And who am I to say I will know? What does it mean when I say, "My husband doesn't look like my husband anymore?" I don't know whether that's just a passing thing or a clinical sign of an unstoppable downturn. But I can whisper to you that I wake up every single morning and make sure he's alive because the amount of lead weight that I hear walking up the stairs and into the bed at night seems very close to the end of life-force energy. Is she scared? Is he scared? Am I scared?

During the day, I don't feel that way. The me who surrenders to sleep at night is deeply exhausted. Last night, we watched a movie together, just the three of us. That is a big deal because they both love science fiction, horror, and action, and I don't. They always seem to find the tension relaxing. I more often have to get up and leave the room. I mean, how much adrenaline can a person take? Last night, though, even with their choice of action film, I relaxed into our shared time. We were all together and the cat was there and Eliana was not in teen attitude, and he had his head on my lap, and we were our little nucleus of our family together, us, at home. When you have no hair and your head is the cancer head, and you are resting, not dragged into sleep, the vulnerability of the moment is so alive and pulsing. I didn't dare to spend much time looking at him that way this summer. Now as I look at him I see this tender reality of him more and more. I don't know why it's taken me this long to see him this way, to really see him like this.

Everyone says it is a lot on my plate to have a teenage daughter coming into herself at the same time that my husband is dealing with chemo and cancer. Throughout, I've just thought, *this is my life*, and so just truck along. Today, I have woken up to the obvious. I get it. *Yes*, this is *too much on my plate*. I am overwhelmed. I feel like the captain of a ship, trying to keep everything in our life afloat, trying to keep life itself above water, staying focused on the essentials for survival, in a practical sense at least. As Gene left today for an appointment with his urologist he rolled down his car window and asked, "Do you know what the name of my medicine is?" He's referring to the name of this particular chemotherapy cocktail—he can't remember. *What?* My ever-so-detail-oriented, very-focused-on-medicine-and-everything-about-it husband doesn't know the name of his chemotherapy drug? And I blurt out, "Cytoxan."[7] What kind of world is this that I would pull that up into consciousness and he wouldn't? Is it just that his mind is not holding things anymore, the chemo fog, or is it that, in the long run, it no longer seems important enough for him to keep track of, as in *what difference does it make?* Or is it that he is getting worn out, or maybe that his strategy in life of knowing things is not working for this situation. Who knows? The whole picture is so complicated. How do we ever return to the "just-live-your-life mode" when living is so at the edge?

Nine days before he died, Gene wrote in his notes about telling Eliana that things were not good, that there was talk of surgery but he did not want to die on the operating table. He sensed that, in some way, she knew he could be dying in front of her, but she didn't really understand that he would actually die. None of us did at that point.

The Ring of Love: The Past as a Source of Pain, Peace, and Healing

Our family has always grown around challenge—not just Gene's challenge but also mine. That is how we came together. He met me when I was going through infertility treatments, had had a miscarriage, had come out of a divorce years earlier just as he had—we each had had plenty of experience with loss. I wanted to have a child, so I told myself that I couldn't date someone because I was trying to have a child. He was just coming out of a period when he thought he couldn't date someone because he'd had a misdiagnosis of ALS—Lou Gehrig's disease—that took those two terrifying years to resolve.

We met not through some storybook tale of being swept off our feet in love, but with a depth of feeling, love, and respect for one another, built around the recognition of the challenges we each had gone through. It was not just the illness that was a challenge but our pasts as well, including the difficulties and losses of each having been through first marriages that ended. We came to each other with past histories that needed healing. We created, and discovered, a love based on partnership and companionship and a sense of really taking care of one another, not because we couldn't take care of ourselves, but in a deep supportive way, knowing that we were good for one another, and good with one another.

On one level, Gene's condition was the biggest thing in our life. On another level, we could not, under any circumstances, allow it to grow like a cancerous tumor in our family body. If we had, we would have had no hope of living. I don't mean this in some existential sense. I mean you still have to cook and do your laundry. But back then, how could we enjoy Eliana's basketball games? How could we attend to the reverie in our neighborhood walks? How could we keep the everyday alive every day? You have to have the everyday matter, not become something you don't have time for or don't care about.

For a long time I felt that these other story lines, these other people in our lives—my mother, my father, our daughter, our brothers-in law, his parents, and the illnesses that came to our dying family members, eleven over fourteen years of our marriage—these key and important people in our lives were a separate condition, a separate thread of our lives. But I have come to see that all of these threads have been woven into the family body, like a huge hammock within which our conditions rest, rock, and are held. Gene shared this deep sense and appreciation of family.

> *When Wendy and I were living together, we were engaged, not yet married, although we already had adopted Eliana. As the gravity of my situation further sunk in, I began to feel enormously guilty about what it would mean for Wendy to marry a dying person and I strongly recommended that she not do it. These were not at all her thoughts. She said I was ridiculous, that we were deeply bonded—including with Eliana. I pointed out, though, that Eliana was but a baby and that it would probably be easier now than in a couple of years to separate from me. Again, Wendy would hear nothing of it, describing us as a unit. I persisted, and said that she should at least take her time and discuss it with her parents and sisters, and not rush to a decision. She did appease me by doing this, and her extended family's responses were the same as hers. They already saw us embedded in the extended family, and that it was out of the question for me to not be a part of their family. I was so moved then as I am now with their response. It was part of the powerful ring of love that I felt surrounding me.*

Our experience would have been quite different had Gene's deterioration come fast and furious as the doctors imagined initially; if the recurrence had loomed as the most immediate obstacle we faced through the thirteen years that followed, and if our responsibility to it, to its treatment, to its side effects, to its condition, had taken up all the space that it sometimes does in peoples' lives. Instead, we received the unexpected extension of more than a decade of time. But the thought was never far from our minds, in the context of our fuller life: What if he died while his father was in a dementia state? What if there was no one to take care of his mother? What about his brother Franklin; how would he live without all that Gene did daily for him? How about the stability he knew that his brother Joel deserved? How would life be if Gene's life had been the tending of the ill and he had not had the enormous joy and pleasure of being with his daughter, of watching his son grow into maturity and parenthood with a wonderful wife and four gorgeous children?

We couldn't give Gene's condition its full focus; we had so much else to take care of. Gene had described earlier the challenge of both the "sideways" and the "sandwich" generations—those with dependent children and parents or extended family to tend to—and that's precisely where we found ourselves. Beyond his initial concerns for his parents and brothers with his original diagnosis, our worry for him rose alongside that for my own mother, whom I adored, and who was fighting for her life. Then two years later, when she passed away, I struggled through such long and intense grief over her death, while wanting to spend as much time with my father as possible. Five years after she died, my dad developed chronic myeloid leukemia, then a mere few years later came a sudden stroke. One of my sisters developed colon cancer, and both of them faced life-threatening illnesses through their own husbands' declining health. Our family body struggled in the grip of this undertow, taking turns saving and being saved, pulled under then pulled together in the constant waves of illness. Throughout all the years and tears, the family body was being carried as it carried us into the tending that we do together.

By the time she was fifteen, Eliana had been to eleven funerals. Is that a separate story from us? Absolutely not. And through ten of those deaths, her daddy got stronger and stronger. His condition improved. Is that a separate story from our family body? No, it is the family body. But it all happened right in front of our eyes, year after year. We could not come up for air. We were busy. We were living, dying, living, dying. Living.

The night when the three of us watched the movie together comes back to me. That night when we were all together and it didn't matter if the movie triggered an adrenalin rush, and the cat was there, and Eliana was calmly with us, and Gene's head was on my lap, we were our own little nucleus of family at home, together. These are the nights when the simplicity of the family body outshines everything.

Part Two

PARALLEL UNIVERSES OF TIME
AND SPACE

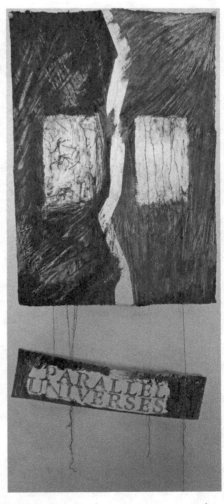

Figure II.i "Parallel Universes" (2007), oil bars, string and encaustic wax on Arches paper, 31 × 15 inches. Artwork by Wendy L. Miller, photo credit: Claire Blatt.

4

The Crucible of Time

Either the well was very deep, or she fell very slowly, for she had
plenty of time as she went down to look about her, and to wonder
what was going to happen next.
–Lewis Carroll, *Alice in Wonderland*[1]

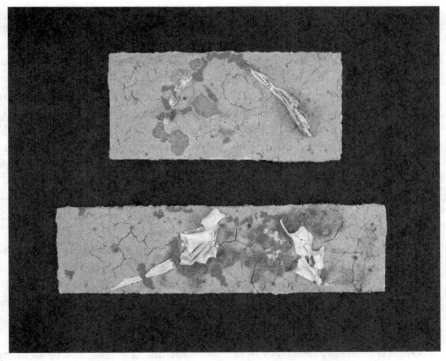

Figure 4.1 "Sandscapes I and II: Encrustment" (2007), cooked sand and mixed media
on canvas with embedded fired porcelain clay fragments and colored paper pulp, 8 ×
16 inches and 7 × 23 inches. Artwork by Wendy L. Miller, photo credit: Joshua Soros

The moment Alice dropped through the rabbit hole and into her famous free-fall,
her sense of time was the first thing to go missing and, with it, any connection to a
familiar reality. As she fell she had dozed, dreamt, ruminated about physics, mar-
malade, kitchen cupboards and her cat, and remarked on the disorienting quality

of time when—*thump!*—she landed on a dirt floor, darkness overhead and a long passage open before her. This was our life, especially and suddenly in the way time itself became otherworldly: compressed, limitless, fast, slow, a clock, an abyss, a mirage, a mystery, an adversary, a gift. All of this we came to call *Illness Time:* not a period of time spent ill, but time itself defined by illness.

Scientists and philosophers have grappled with the idea of time for thousands of years. In a practical sense, it seems that more profoundly than anything else—the earth under our feet, the language or sounds or smells that tell us where we are—time orients us. It organizes us. In the context of time as a linear flow "all things follow one another," the German philosopher Arthur Schopenhauer wrote.[2] Past, present, and future are constructs of time that can lend at least a bare minimum of order to the clutter and chaos of life. Our sense of time, the urgency, or the lack of it, helps us prioritize.

H.G. Wells wrote of time as a fourth dimension, one that represents duration, saying that "there is no difference between Time and any of the three dimensions of Space except that our consciousness moves along it."[3] *Our consciousness moves along it.* True, our everyday consciousness moves along those rails, but the experience is not just one of duration. In this fourth dimension, time also collapses our experience—of moments, days, years, life itself. I stand impatiently waiting for Eliana to get out the door to school, and as I glance and see her so painstakingly brushing on her mascara, I see myself at her age, so completely absorbed in my morning ritual, unfurling my wild curly hair from the jumbo rollers that were supposed to straighten it. I can still feel the pang of hope that the curlers had done their work and my unruly mane would be tame for the day. I see my daughter, feel my past, feel our present, feel Gene's eyes on his daughter he adored. Still, I am no saint: in this moment I am a mother watching the clock, dreading morning rush hour, and I tap my foot, impatient.

In the most practical terms, our everyday relationship with time follows the familiar assumptions we make about the linear nature of life: *Ordinary Time.* We respect their authority and in exchange they provide some sense that things will go as planned, as scheduled. The lunch date. The presentation. The visit from the grandparents. In ordinary time the smallest plan secures our future. Or so we feel.

Ordinary time organizes our lives in so many different ways and by so many different measures that when things are going smoothly and they are all synchronized we barely notice how fluidly we shift between our domains: home, office, friends, family, community, checkups, follow-ups. Somewhere biology imposes its own order—we sleep through an alarm or we miss lunch with a friend who has a cold—but in ordinary time it's manageable. Of course, *Biological Time* is all our cells know; the truest time of all, the one we know most intimately and yet hardly at all, hidden as it is from our conscious knowing.

We think that time is an entity through which we move and we can decide how we're going to move through it and what will happen, when actually it is the other way around: time moves us. The moment you get a diagnosis, everything that you believe you have time for or everything you believe is the way you're going to use time is thrown into chaos, scattered, as Gene once said, "just a big wind."

Illness derails us. It destroys any illusions of certainty, especially about time. Illness lifts the barriers between dimensions and suddenly we are adrift. Our consciousness jumps tracks somewhere between the ordinary here-and-now time that organizes us and illness time, a liminal space between time as we understand it and time that feels mysteriously distorted and which, as it turns out, is not inherently organized at all.

Gene had always wanted to write a science fiction novel. He was fascinated by the complexity of the brain and the mind, how it works in ways we can barely fathom, and what happens when it goes awry. His novel was going to be a thriller, some kind of medical science fiction story in which fluid dimensions of time and a labyrinth of physical, mental, and psychological mysteries stump everyone. As it turned out, he lived it instead.

Illness time is a kind of science fiction, we discover. It is as if we lived in a time machine that takes us backward, then forward, and spins us upside down.

At the Infinity Pool: Reflections on Illness Time

I am stretched out on a lounge chair by an infinity pool overlooking the Caribbean at the edge of the Atlantic Ocean in the Dominican Republic in December 2006. It is a four-hour flight from a cold winter in DC where it seems we spend most of our time in the crisp, sterile, warm climate of our work offices and medical visits. We have decided to take Eliana on winter break for some much-needed time away and fresh air. We have brought Alex and Kate, and their two little girls Ruby and Lucy, their only children at that time, to join us on vacation. We are together as our family. We are also joining the family of one of Eliana's friends, so we make quite a mini-community in and of ourselves. We are not used to this kind of "all-inclusive luxury," as the hotel brochure boasts, but we are delighted to have what we call the "all-of-us-together luxury." Sunbathing, swimming, reading, eating: we are in ecstatic rest-mode—leisure in hyper drive. Correction: everybody else is. Not me.

Everybody else is playing around and having fun. And me? I'm in a totally different universe. Internally, I am critical: this isn't *real* travel, not the kind where a new culture opens itself up to you. This is a club nestled within a tourist enclave designed to let you check your troubles at the door. My mind isn't buying it, consumed instead with the adjustments required to accommodate our here-now-what-next life, and the overlays of clinical and emotional realities, none of which I can check at the door.

Everyone is having a wonderful time together, and finally my mind has the freedom to drift, somewhere else, alone, unmoored from time altogether. How can a moment hold such calm beauty and such fear at the same time, with Gene's condition part of my own? The setting is tranquil enough. If only I could calibrate my inner reflective self to match my outer here-and-now self. Which one is "real"? Which am I supposed to inhabit? I go off on my own to journal a little with paper and pen to the quiet infinity pool on the edge of the spa. It's a start. Mind, body, and spirit feel out of sync. Like Alice tumbling through the rabbit hole, it's hard to tell whether things are moving slowly or we are all just falling a very long way, but whichever it is, there is plenty of time to wonder what's going to happen next. And wonder what "next" means at all.

The Sword of Damocles: The Median Becomes the Message

Gene was fascinated by the interplay of time and age and how they shape our perception of ourselves and our lives.

> Your sense of time varies, depending on whether you are aging, experiencing a life-determining illness, or living with the coexistence of aging and illness. I thought about all of this, a lot, when I was first diagnosed with a life-threatening disease in my second half of life. I was feeling good about my own sense of time with my own aging. But this radically changed when I was diagnosed with a life-threatening disease that acted like the sword of Damocles over my neck.
>
> Dionysius ordered that a shining sword, fastened from the ceiling by a horsehair, be let down so that it hung over the neck of Damocles. It transformed Damocles' sense of time and focus. (Cicero, "The Sword of Damocles")[4]

Gene was gripped by a strange new sensation of time changing for him, and with it, a sense of paralysis now accompanied planning future commitments.

> I suddenly felt overwhelmed and totally exhausted, but I realized I had always been a problem solver, no matter how rough the waters, and following a good night's sleep where my unconscious had a chance to dissect my dilemma, I would awaken with new insights. It did not happen this time. I awoke only to find no exit. Apart from the devastating effects I feared the

cancer would have on my new life with Wendy and baby Eliana, I felt a deep sickness in my stomach at the thought of letting down my frail parents and chronically ill older brother—all who had so relied on my help. It was an almost unbearable feeling. The role of adult children in the sandwich generation has been highlighted in relation to their being sandwiched between responsibilities to parents and their children. But modern life, with extended longevity has also created what I refer to as the sideways and every which way generation, particularly seen with Boomers who are now experiencing the added challenge of siblings in their 60s needing their help as well.[5] I am 15 months older than the oldest Boomer, and had been immersed in sideways responsibilities to my chronically mentally ill, disabled older brother, as well as being sandwiched between frail older parents and my children. I felt I would be letting down so many who were close to me who loved and depended on me. The thickness of the dark clouds increased, and my immediate family was rallied.

It was as if an opaque veil descended in front of my eyes blocking me from having a clear sense of possibilities more than a year away. Though the phenomenon was disturbing, I was also in awe of it. I tried to fit it into a category of mental phenomena I had studied during my training as a psychiatrist. What came into the line-up were phenomena that can accompany momentary or more prolonged periods of anxiety. I figured that my veil was likely a de-realization phenomenon associated with momentary anxiety about whether I'd be around a year from then to deliver on the invitation.

Moreover, it felt like a virtual digital clock was running down the time count right in front of me—not like at New Year's Eve in a celebratory sense to announce the imminence of a new year, but with a starkly ominous, relentless counting down toward my inevitable demise. The sense of prognostic precision and irrevocability was like the horse-hair tenuously holding Damocles' sword. It wasn't just the death sentence draining hope, but the merciless prognosticating that made it hard to focus on anything else—making it hard to focus on life in facing a death sentence. I was being barraged by menacing medians: "The median life expectancy with prostate cancer is low." "The median time to symptoms appearing is this." "The median time that treatment will help is only that." Again, all of the medians were minimal.

When I think of Gene's image of the sword of Damocles over his neck being hung by but thin horsehair, I think about how fragile and thin the threads of life can be for any of us during illness time. In that fragility and tension we nonetheless have to live our lives. How long the thread will hold is not ours to know. This moment is all we know; this is the time we have.

The Hourglass: Time That Adds as It Takes Away

In a public service message Gene did with comedian George Burns during Gene's time as the acting director at the National Institute on Aging, Burns, who was almost ninety-seven at the time, famously replied, when Gene asked how he felt about his age, "It beats the alternative." Gene loved to quote George Burns' humorous, pragmatic views on his own aging—"How can I sit down, when all my life I've been a stand-up comic?"[6] Burns told Gene that he had decided to try it out, and found that sitting down had no adverse impact at all with his audiences. Then he leaned over, grabbed Gene's shoulder, and whispered in his ear, "Dr. Cohen, if necessary, I'll become a lie-down comic!" He was prepared for whatever life would deal him.

A cornerstone of Gene's conceptual theory and personal philosophy of aging was the idea of time, or age, that "adds as it takes away," in the words of the great poet and physician William Carlos Williams.[7] Specifically, Gene was referring to the capacities of the mind and spirit that increase, even as physical capacities may decline. In illness time this aspect of gain amidst loss takes on new meaning and can be a source of resilience and emotional and spiritual healing. All plays out on a larger scale, or with a higher purpose, when we wake up each day aware of the fragility of life. Our appreciation of every moment, every day, can enlarge our sense of time and the richness of it. In illness time, illness adds as it takes away.

I think of my friend Tess, now sixty-two, a three-time cancer survivor over a twenty-year period, who views birthdays as a gift because she is alive to have them. For her, another birthday is the gift of existence. It is a victory that she is here another year. Tess hears others worry or complain about turning fifty or sixty or whatever advancing number, and for a moment she is suddenly made aware of her alien status, one who lives in a different dimension of time, the dimension in which her awareness of death and life is always present and personal for her. For the most part, she says, she experiences time as this positive force—of life accruing. However, on days when concerns about the future of her family or work are pressing, she feels the finiteness of time, the sense of living on borrowed time that's running out.

Marty was in his mid-twenties when he was diagnosed with a small but inoperable brain tumor. Doctors monitored his condition with regular scans a few months apart for several years. At one point, based on the tumor's slow growth and projected rate of growth, the doctors scheduled his next scan for six months later. He was elated. To him, this was a six-month reprieve to focus on living. To his worried family, however, it was a frightening thought "to wait that long" in dread of the ticking biological bomb. Time had different meaning for each of them.

I used to watch the sand run through an hourglass from top to bottom and think only of time running out, time lost.[8] But in illness time, loss is not the only message the hourglass offers. As the sand in the upper chamber slips down and away, the sand in the lower chamber accrues. It gains. The contents shift, but the hourglass never loses a grain of sand; the whole of it shifts and is finite, but in that space is fully present.

Gene and I came to understand that in illness time the two most powerful themes involve this sense of gaining time and losing time. His capacity for deepening time, in essence gaining time, was remarkable. For example: Gene is at the airport and discovers his flight has been cancelled or delayed. He'll have to spend six hours at the airport waiting for his new flight. He does all the necessary negotiations at the counters and on the phone to try for another flight, but there are no other options. He's stuck where he is. Time at the airport is all there is. So he shifts his priorities and sets his anger and frustration to the side. He eats a nice meal, finds a quiet place at the gate, and works on his research or writing and spends that time in a basically good mood. That is, if he is alone and not with me. Unlike Gene, I am always quick to anger over life's snags, especially those that waste time or demand more time from me than I'm prepared to give. So for Gene the time *spent* in this scenario becomes time he *invests*: it gains value. I experience the same time spent as time wasted, an imposition and a loss. For Gene, it is not simply a matter of temperament. It is the way that, in illness time, he has chosen to weigh nuisances and problems like this and decide this is not a big problem. Doing so, he lives in gained time and an experience of positivity that adds to his energy rather than depleting it.

Gene felt that his commitments to others required that he come through responsibly, no matter what. As a devoted family man, he worried about that incessantly, and in his work, he not only was careful to stick to shorter-term commitments but always had colleagues in place whom he felt were superbly able to carry the work forward. The paradox is that as his dependable present evolved into a future he didn't think he could count on, he accomplished more of his ideas—games, books, grants, research—than any one else I knew through that same decade of time.

I Don't Exist, I Exist: The Paradox of Prognosis

I felt that the ramifications of what my doctors were telling me about my prognosis reflected another paradox around time in the two different universes we occupied. On the one hand, the general view of the public and of a great many healthcare providers is that being a ten-year survivor of cancer is a very positive prognostic indication, In my situation, however, where no survivors of metastatic prostate cancer involving bones were reported in the medical literature, did this mean that with time passing I was therefore getting closer and closer to the day of reckoning? Of course, this introduces a further paradox—that with aging, with the passage of time, independent of any disease state, you are getting closer to death. It added even more to my exasperation, as I am sure it does to other persons with cancer who are also what the medical community refers to as outliers.

As a doctor-patient I have a new perspective on why my medical colleagues so often resist talking about hope as a resource for a kind of healing, no matter where a patient may be in a disease process. Now that I'm in it as a patient I experience it differently.

Why is it so hard, I endlessly wonder, for my medical colleagues to simply contemplate, however remotely, the operative word in "continuing remission"—continuing. What it takes to continue, what it takes to go on, physically, emotionally, psychologically—go on in every way? What we are talking about is the art of dealing with hope. If it is so difficult for doctors to encourage—not guarantee—but encourage hope in extreme cases like mine that it really does beg the question: what is it in all the rest of their cases that need and deserve more art and humanity in the encounter? My hope is that my case and others like it, though not in the textbooks, will influence the texts on care of the person, bedside manner, doctor/patient relationships, and the art of medicine. I should point out that I never thought for a minute that I was the only one who lived past 10 years with metastatic prostatic cancer. It was clear that I was an extreme outlier, but I was sure I was not alone. Given: I was a prostate cancer patient reaching an infinite number of "midpoints" in a finite time to my prognosticated demise. Anyone with my condition who was to move from one point to another to end-stage must meet these requirements, and so motion is impossible, and what we perceive as inevitable termination due to metastasized prostate cancer is merely an illusion. Besides, according to all the medical texts, they said I didn't exist anyway.

Illness is certainly not a laughing matter, but lightness is a very good antidote to the heaviness that surrounds devastating disease and disability. And when all my efforts fail at eliciting meaningful responses to personal feelings and troubling thoughts that I share with my healthcare providers, and I get yet further exasperating comments or the lack of any significant comment at all to my serious and sincerely felt concerns, I resort to my made-up Zeno's 5th paradox.

Humor and hope were Gene's antidotes for fear and "dark dips" through this time, as they had been through the years. He would not be reduced, would not have the quality of his time reduced, to a clinical conversation.

Life-threatening illness can be like a culprit opening Pandora's Box where many bad things are released in a short period of time. We then metaphorically struggle with ways to close the box as fast as we can, in a desperate attempt to diminish the damage. When Pandora rushed to close her box, she was able to retain the last of its contents—hope.[9] Hope, in turn, is affected by experience and expectation, about which we have more to say. After a very long remission of thirteen years where my cancer remained dormant, it returned as if Pandora's Box suddenly sprung open. But I still have hope—the same hope that has helped through my string of unfortunate illness events and so far has not let me down.

It was frustrating for him to live into outlier status and at the same time have belief and expectation be constantly questioned, as if he was hoping for all the wrong reasons. As we know, in the end, "cure" was not the "c" word that came to define Gene's final cancer experience. But during his long years of vibrant symptom-free living he had every reason to consider that this indeed might be underway. This is what I meant when I wrote that time does not on its own heal, but having the time to live is truly what is healing. He was living into this outlier status. He wanted to believe it and he wanted his doctors to believe it, but what was happening was he was being told he shouldn't have this "false hope."

There was Gene's oncologist, who had been staring at his scans for years. He had been studying and looking at the biological picture all that time, immersed in biological time. After Gene passed away, I stopped in to see him. I asked if he possibly could have imagined, when he told us it was the time to stop the chemotherapy, that Gene would die in less than two weeks. He pulled up the scans on his computer and showed me what I would call "cloudy tissue" get foggier and foggier. Fair enough: his medical perspective was limited to numbers and images, and so he had collapsed all the dimensions of Gene's reality into *there's no more time for this person.* That is, in fact, precisely what his demeanor had communicated at the time: a distancing. But as we sat now, instead of just informing me that the scans had shown him that the progression of the disease was rapidly permutating, he then chose to tell me that Gene had been "in denial as to how serious his condition had truly become." His words "in denial" shocked me—slapped me, is really what it felt like, for he had collapsed the dimensions of time for his own needs.

It could have been so different, had he simply shared what was his reality, what he was seeing in biological time, without handing down his casual verdict on Gene's state of mind as one of denial. Simply looking at the scans together then I could have said, "Yes, I'm glad you didn't show us these scans that day because we were living in a different dimension, a different experience of the time we were sharing." He had seen the numbers and he knew to tell us when it was time to stop; I am grateful for that expertise. But he had never seen Gene's numbers as anything but indicators of diagnosis and prognosis: disease progression, failing health, and dying. He suffered a kind of medical myopia, a blindness to someone's greater human reality—not just the disease progression but *their* progression through this passage of time, which meant that he never considered the data in the context of what it might suggest about, say, courage or the will to live. That kind of strength of will in the face of mortal danger is something worth studying.

This report was the oncologist's reality, what his understanding of biological time was telling him, and, based on the way he spoke with me, and with Gene in those last few weeks, that was the only way he understood time; the only way he viewed and understood Gene:

Sibley Memorial Hospital Radiology Report: Imaging Services
   Order # X485397-1
   9/11/2009
   Status: FINAL
   Page 1: EXAM: (SMH) CTHOR—Thorax CT W/O Contrast
   HISTORY: Prostate cancer
   The examination was performed without intravenous contrast by request.

The examination of the hilar, mediastinal and chest wall structures shows no evidence for a pleural effusion. There is moderate mediastinal lymphadenopathy. The petracheal node which previously measured 1.4 × 2.0 cm on the study of 7/31/2009 now measures 1.5 × 2.2 cm. A 1.6 × 1.7 cm petracheal node noted on the prior study now measures 1.7 × 1.9 cm. A 2.a cm subcardinal node now measures 2.4 cm. There are minimal sclerotic densities in the thoracic spine and sternum which are unchanged in appearance from the prior study and may be benign.

The examination of the parenchyma shows innumerable confluent pulmonary nodules consistent with metastatic disease. Most of these are somewhat difficult to measure, although there appears to have been significant progression of disease since the study of 7/31/2009. A pleural based mass in the left lower lobe which previously measured 1.3 cm now measures 1.7 cm. A plural based lesion in the right lower lobe which previously measured 8 mm now measures 13 mm. A 1.7 × 1.9 lesion adjacent to the right diaphragm noted on the prior study now measures 2.0 × 2.3 cm.

IMPRESSION: Moderate progression of disease in the pulmonary parenchyma and to a lesser extent the mediastinum.

   Page 2: EXAM (SMH) CAPDPEL—Abdomen & Pelvis W/O Contrast CT
   HISTORY: Metastatic prostate cancer
   The examination was performed without intravenous contrast by request.

The liver, spleen and pancreas are normal. A ureteral stent is present on the left. A nephrostomy tube is present on the right as is a ureteral stent. There is no significant hydronephrosis on the right. There is a moderately prominent extrarenal pelvis on the left which has increased somewhat in size since the prior study. Minimally prominent periaortic lymph nodes are unchanged from the prior study. There is more bulky iliac adenopathy bilaterally. The adenopathy on the left side which previously measured 2.2 × 2.8 cm now measures 2.2 × 2.3 cm. The 2.5 × 2.1 cm node on the right side is virtually unchanged, measuring 2.2 × 2.6 cm. Sclerotic densities are present in the left ischium and right pubic bone consistent with metastases, unchanged from the prior study. Additional sclerotic densities are present in the right ilium. This appears to have progressed very slightly since the prior study. There is also more minimal disease in the left ilium, also somewhat progressed from the prior examination.

IMPRESSION:

1. Persistent periaortic and iliac lymphadenopathy with very little internal change. There may be a slight increase in the size of the nodes on the left since the prior examination.
2. Slight progression of bone metastases.

This was the oncologist's reality, his thorough and intimate yet limited parallel universe, his "time zone." But parallel universes miss something that happens in overlapping universes. Gene and I, and our family, were living each day in the overlapping dimensions of biological time, calendar time, and emotional time—aware of Gene's condition, but fighting cancer in the methodical time frame of chemotherapy appointments, while emotions required their own time to process. I imagine the physicians' daunting multidimensional task: working each hour in "real time," immersed in tracking the disease in biological time, and (for those who do) trying to figure out how to communicate with their patients in emotional time; how to create exchange in the medical narrative we are creating together. No one ever explains—not to the doctors and not to the patients and families—that these dimensions are colliding, confusing everyone: a doctor sees a patient "in denial," the patient feels reduced to a prognosis or invisible to his doctor, and the family is caught in between. It is a slap in the face to the meaning of the word "denial" and a slap to the person labeled as such inside the experience. Who even knows what an *uptake* is or where our *ilium* are? Who knows what they mean—whether "little interval change" or "moderate progression" will turn out to extend life or hasten death? Nocebo - own use of changed neg words.

If he had really been able to not only observe but see, he would have seen that what he labeled "denial" was, in fact, the supply of ingredients, meager as they might be, to sustain the will to live, to breathe each necessary breath that it takes to live into one's dying. Patients don't just die because the numbers show they will die. It is nothing short of awesome to muster what it takes to breathe each breath, knowing there won't be very many more, and to do that with the people one loves the most; to spin gold from straw in the remaining time, never certain of the time they have left until it is gone.

Shared Lives: Shared Parallel, Paradoxical Time

If you're living in an ordinary way, then things just happen. Something is what it is. In illness, a moment could be just a moment. Or it could snag some corner of one's consciousness where past, present, and future commingle, where it registered as a fleeting premonition, already haunted with the meaning. Gene might say how much he loved a visit with the grandkids as they left, and I would hear it in the simple present; or the snag would have me think: *Is this the last time we'll ever talk about this or laugh about this or share moments this way?*

It's not that we transform time; rather, time transforms us, and I am not okay with that. I am railing against the universe because, as a packrat, I thought that I would be able to move through time with all of my people, all my cells, all my loved ones. I didn't yet know that we give up, give over, lose, trade in, all the time, that what I call illness time is the time it takes to come to grips with all that comes your way; that health, illness, healing, and struggle—the whole of it—is what forms the self; that we are all here for one purpose, and that is to help one another through thick and thin no matter what we feel about it. And the rest: weather and dreams.

Perhaps we find illness time so unsettling not only because it is at odds with the familiar linear constructs of time that we have learned practically from birth, but because we are not taught or prepared for it. We are just thrown into it—not as a structure we gain or lose, but as a process of being. Illness time, unlike the others—the clock, the calendar, the biological processes—makes you acutely aware of every minute, every second, every passage of time where the clock can start, stop, slow down, or speed up, unpredictably. Although you feel it, you're helpless to do anything about it besides jump on the good moments, savor them so they don't get away too quickly, even learn to feel deeply during the bad moments—getting irritated, angry at someone, feeling sorry for your situation or yourself, feeling guilty for having these feelings—because who knows how many moments are left. Vulnerability, fear, and gratitude—these are all a part of illness time, and they shape each person's story differently.

People are constantly trying to figure this out. My friend Joanne calls one day and this is her dilemma: she and her two sisters are in fundamentally different dimensions of time regarding how they think and are willing to talk about their ailing 87-year-old mother. Their mother is not doing well. She has already experienced some minor but ever so real strokes. Her being has changed. Joanne can see this, but her two sisters cannot bear to do so. Her older sister has visited their mom only two times this year, even though she lives close by. Her younger sister is determinedly oblivious, and Joanne rails at her about her lack of timely response to their mother, every word a painful reminder to herself: "This is your mother! Would you want to be left there all alone at her age?" They don't want to see their mother or her life reduced to the ticking clock of biological time, so they don't look.

We've been there, many of us. We don't want to see our mom or dad struggle through illness or injury. We don't want to see our loved one deteriorating. So we decide not to look. Joanne's sisters do look at their calendars and schedule their next trip to see their mother, maybe next month, maybe when the weather gets better or when their time opens up. In the meantime, Joanne is confronted with day-to-day decisions about their mother's needs and care. In biological time, the truth is that her mother is aging well, despite her newer needs since the small strokes; no other diagnoses, no other illnesses. And yet, still there is the unspoken family resistance to the reality of aging time.

Time Is the Ultimate Transformer

We don't have to deconstruct time to explain time. Time is a transformer that blends elements of sequential experience together so that they resonate, vibrate, and resound. Time is a container in which we place our experiences and try to understand them in the context of the present. But in truth, our experiences are affected by being in the container of time. So when we experience them again, even milliseconds later, they are different. Time is an expressive filter, expressive in that it is a transformative process—it colors experience, it highlights and low-lights. This lighting affects how we see ourselves as part of a larger story.

Years before Gene's condition had begun its slow but clear decline, yet while the fear of failing health accompanied his internal emotional time, while he was still working as much as he always had, we had decided to write a book together. One afternoon he pressed me for my current notes. I could hear the urgency in his voice. Quietly he told me, "Time is of essence. I need you to write. I need you to work with me. I need to work with you right now."

"Time is of essence," he said, meaning *hurry up*. Later it struck me as a truth in itself, not about the need for speed, but about the nature of time. *Time is of essence.* It is, indeed. Time has substance. It is a dimension that carries meaning, makes meaning, demands our attention. Illness time had etched itself into me. I can't be rushed. I've never been able to be rushed, but I really can't be rushed now.

This was not just something that happened to me alone. It was something that happened between us, between Gene and me. We were really going through his deteriorating condition in two different time zones. There was the real-life/ordinary time zone, with my sisters, with our daughter, with Alex, Kate, and the grandchildren, with the needs of the kitchen or the snowy sidewalks to shovel or my practice or his presentations or whatever needed to be done that day. Then there was the rushed illness time, the time that had said Gene had six months to a year. So at six months, I hear Gene coughing. What does that mean? Are we moving into a new time? I feared this accelerated time, dreaded the shift that Gene was announcing with his sense of urgency about writing.

Maybe we all try to choose a dimension of time that we feel will make things all right; somehow match the rhythm of events and shifts in awareness with our capacity to take in information, respond to questions, plan or even play as the moment allows. Gene, even in the depths of his twilight zone, found hope in the movement of time.

If the initial diagnosis of 1996 made us feel frozen in time, eventually in the 2000's we felt time shift forward again with the momentum of daily life focused on creative living. Things were going well, extremely well by any standard. My cancer hormone treatment was tolerable and seemed to be having a positive effect. My research center was thriving with a series of major studies underway. International commitments kept things lively and interesting, I was publishing, not perishing, and I had a new game in development. At home, despite the knowledge that cancer was out there, in there, somewhere, investing our energies in creative endeavors had helped us find a rhythm in this new but not impossible context. Wendy's creativity took a new form as we moved forward with a home and studio renovation to make our century-old house more livable, and more compatible with Wendy's work as an artist and therapist. For Wendy, the home makeover mirrored a transformation she felt at a deeper level, as her world became more heavily focused on family life, the challenges that aging and illness were bringing home, and her need for a newly evolved professional identity. It was a productive building phase for us all. At last, it seemed, the worst was over. The clock was being reset again—away from illness time.

5

Uncharted Territory

In our sleep
pain that cannot forget
falls drop by drop upon the heart,
and in our despair, against our will,
comes wisdom from the awe-filled grace of God.
—Aeschylus[1]

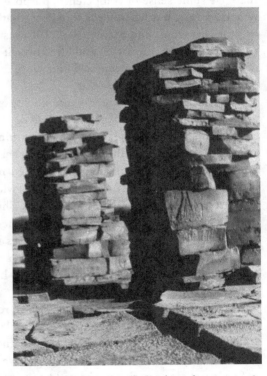

Figure 5.1 "Woman Building: Random Flat Arch Towers" (1982), site-specific installation in the natural clay mudflats of Bodega Bay, California, 2.2 × 5.9 × 10 feet. Artwork and documentation by Wendy L. Miller, photo credit: Joshua Soros.

I enter the house of my friend Antoinette, whom I have known for over forty years. We are exactly the same age, started our young adult life together moving from the east coast to San Francisco where she has stayed, worked, and raised her family through those forty years. I chose to make my home east, and today I have flown out from DC—it has been two years since our last dinner visit in San Francisco. Just six months ago, in December, she got the diagnosis: small cell lung cancer. Two rounds of chemotherapy, one round of radiation to shrink the mass that had metastasized in her brain. She is getting ready to see if she is able to go through another round of chemotherapy. But a close mutual friend called to tell me it was time to come if I wanted to see her. I no longer wait in these moments. I flew west within a few days. Whatever lay ahead, it didn't look promising. Everyone, including Antoinette, knows where this is heading. The past and the future both seem irrelevant just now. All that exists is the precarious present, which seems formless and timeless without the familiar outlines of obligations and responsibilities that give some sense of competence, purpose, and meaning. Antoinette's heart remains strong but her voice is frail, her breath thin. She slowly, determinedly, breathes her words and phrases out. "This was . . . not . . . my plan." She inhales with the same determination and I find myself unconsciously slowing my breath to match hers as she continues. "I like . . . to map out . . . what I do," she says. "I don't . . . know how . . . to do this."

Her words describe the entry into uncharted territory. Not just the sense of not having a plan, but *not knowing how to do this*: the sense that who she is now, her skin, her fragility, her lethargy, her breathing are all new to her. They are not the self that she knows. Those of us around her who have known her can see the same beauty, spirit, and phenomenal magnetism of love that now and always has surrounded her. We surround her because of who she is: her essence, her presence with people. She holds my hands inside hers. She strokes my arm, and as I lean my head on her shoulder, tears streak down our faces. In this moment the decades of our deep friendship don't register as memories across time but as a single, soulful bond that time cannot touch; illness time acts as a kind of transformer in which the energies of a relationship—whatever they have been—become charged with transcendent potential.

Her sister and her partner are in a different room, allowing us to have our own time together. Her medicines fill the coffee table like a centerpiece. The flat screen TV is on Turner Classics, *Wait Until Dark*, with Audrey Hepburn;[2] then Lifetime TV with Perry Mason,[3] a blast from the past we both know and remember.

She is not alone in this uncharted territory. Her sister, her partner, her sons, her parents, her friends: everyone is dropped into a land that must be navigated, with changing markers every day, even each hour of each day. Long-held identities are challenged. The "supermom cook" in the family cannot cure her by feeding her and is grappling for another identity; the "unreliable one" turns out to have the precision and presence of mind to focus on details of Antoinette's care that have overwhelmed others. Antoinette musters all of her energy; at one point she crosses herself, recalling her Catholic upbringing when asking for prayer. She is begging for strength to get out this one big thought, and then slowly pieces together the words that she needs, breathing heavily in between each phrase or word, which I slip together so easily here on the page: "What upsets me . . . is you have this diagnosis . . . there is this big Internet of information . . . and what do you get? . . . Nothing . . . A nurse . . . who walks over to the house . . . two or three times a week . . . and does this," and she motions with her hands the image of the nurse, all business, keying information into her iPad, eyes focused down on the screen. "I feel let down."

Learning to walk in this uncharted territory is an informative and emotional journey of growth. We go through these experiences and slowly, bit by bit, open up not only our knowledge and awareness but our capacity to sustain this deep navigation. With Gene, with Antoinette in San Francisco, with myself and members of my extended family, and, of course, with my clients over the years, I see again, yet always anew, how shocking and disorienting it is for anyone to enter this land and navigate this journey of getting older and facing illness and dying. The new reality is jarring. Illness time and its rhythm feel so unnatural, but of course is entirely natural as a life passage, whether solitary or shared. It's as if a crack has opened in the landscape, exposing strata that have always been there but have never been part of life's landscape on the surface. Deeper territory suddenly presents itself, open to all elements.

I see so clearly in Antoinette's presence how deeply disorienting it is, for my friend who is ill herself and for all of the family and friends rallying to midwife the process of caring for her. I find myself reflecting back to my own home, recalling the conversation at my kitchen counter with my daughter-in law Kate when I explained that the fact that Gene was given no timeline for his course of chemotherapy meant something—and what it meant was not a good sign. She turned to Alex: "Did *you* know that?" as if, in a new light the shades of color in the information we all knew had suddenly and completely changed. Gene's dreams, too, were an indication of how disorienting the whole illness experience was for him. In his dreams, like prey, he was hunted down nightly, forced to come up with more and more clever ways to escape the threat of death.

In one dream, in a classical Italian plaza, he was being chased by a huge ominous monster, nearly ten feet tall, with a head the size of two basketballs. He dashes down alleys and around corners to avoid him and ends up trapped but with an amazing ending:

> *My pursuer sees that I am trapped and a broad sinister sneer covers his grotesque countenance. His oversized hands are now on my throat, and I realize my end is near. Then, suddenly, out of nowhere, a white van appears slowly traveling down the alley. It barely avoids scraping the houses on both*

sides, I flatten myself as tight as I can against the front of one of the houses to avoid being run over, and the monster attempts the same, but his head is too big and as the van passes, his huge head gets caught and crushed.

The Pendulum Swing

We're all familiar with the fight-or-flight response—the adrenalin rush and physical anxiety that a perceived threat triggers in the body. Science has long established the shared pathways of mind–body communication, showing that every thought, every cell, every feeling, every organ is busy listening and responding to this intricate biochemical dialogue. The physical effects of that extreme pendulum swing are well known: our pulse races, our heart pounds, and we begin to sweat. But what I find stunning is that the pendulum swing can yank us so unexpectedly into an emotional state so markedly different from the one we were in just moments before. No less threatening than a predator's attack in primitive times is the power of a piece of information: those numbers on lab reports, the blood counts and bone scans that come through the fax machine can trigger this swing. One moment we're going about the business of our everyday lives, and then there it is, a piece of information—a doctor's comment or news headline about a cancer study—that is either reassuring and calming, or it's a trigger and the fight-or-flight response escalates it in a split second.

Jungian psychology, drawing from the Greek philosopher Heraclitus, uses the term *enantiodromia* to describe the tendency of one pole of an experience to change into its opposite.[4] In 1949, C.G. Jung wrote about enantiodromia in familiar terms, using the example of a pendulum. A pendulum always swings from side to side, fully to one extreme and then back in the opposite direction: that is the intrinsic nature of a pendulum. For Jung, all life and energy are a play of such opposites, and our task is to value both sides of this polarity yet bring ourselves to a calm middle point to engage without being reactive about it. I see enantiodromia and the pendulum as a way to think about our inner balance and especially our emotional regulation. Something throws us off balance and we react instinctively, taking us to the far end of the pendulum swing. Then, as we begin to engage and respond more thoughtfully, the pendulum swings back toward the opposite pole. In the back and forth, we right ourselves, regain our balance, and regulate our emotional state and, with it, our physiological state.

Fight-or-flight has a bad reputation because it is, after all, stressful, and it is, first of all, triggered by a sense of threat. That said, this pendulum swing is generative, actually, creative. In the sway or the swing of the pendulum, for instance, we can experience ourselves being tugged into conscious awareness by an unconscious effort to right an imbalance. This is the way of the unconscious: if our conscious awareness is too one-sided or overwhelming—a sudden recognition that we are helpless in the face of danger, for instance—the unconscious uses its autonomy to bring some of its contents upward to reestablish balance, perhaps through dreams, memories, flashbacks, and sudden insights. Sometimes those same phenomena— dreams, flashbacks, and spontaneous insights—are the equivalent of shock waves reverberating through the unconscious in response to experiences that are deeply affecting. As with any collision of opposite forces, in this case the conscious and unconscious, the energy of that psychic tension is released, sometimes surprising us with something totally new and unexpected—at least partly in our conscious awareness. The frightening sense of helplessness, for instance, gives way as we start to discover sources of support we never realized were there, or find qualities in ourselves that we never knew we had.

The swing slows itself down somewhere toward a neutral place of discernment, a place between the adrenalin surges of fight or flight, where perception, rest, and acceptance might have a chance to take root. I think of this as a float state: not reactive and not shocked into a numb "freeze" state. Sometimes, especially once you're aware of this potential neutral place of discernment, you can feel it in the moment and know it for what it is. A friend who had recently lost his beloved wife described his grief and sense of loss as coming in waves. In the depths, overwhelmed, he would instinctively reach for thoughts or take actions that would, like a lifeline, actively pull him the other way. After several weeks he noted that each time the wave overwhelmed him, then passed, he felt a bit more stable in the trough between the waves. For him, the pendulum swing that had been so extreme upon her death was becoming less extreme; the repeated swing between reaction and recovery was part of a healing process. He felt his loss no less, but his capacity to feel it and yet be less destabilized by it was palpable to him. Or, as he said, "The grieving doesn't change—but you do get better at it."

Medically, *We Do Not Exist Either*

When you are living with a diagnosis such as Gene had, it is hard to imagine this place of rest, acceptance, and having a good life; yet eight years out, here we were: our lives, our careers, our love growing and the cancer apparently not growing. Then, sudden as sudden is, the pendulum swing brought us to the frightening edge again.

It was 2004 and we had come home from our July month in Maine. Gene had had some trouble with his knee that month, some stiffness and discomfort, but not enough to be a concern. Unloading the car from our trip, he started to carry a heavy suitcase up the stairs in the house, and while moving to the first step and swinging the bag to his other hand he fell, and could hear the bone in his leg crack—it was the femur, the largest bone of the body. The ambulance rushed him

to the hospital and just that fast we were all transported back into the scary territory we knew better than to try to predict.

We feared that the fracture was what is called a "pathological fracture," a fracture due to a metastasis of the cancer to the bone, but surprisingly it was not. Tests
would soon disclose that it was due to a hardening of the bones—a side effect of
his cancer treatment. Suddenly, with this startling development came a new turning point, not only in the clinical dimension but in the relational one. This new
complication drew questions and expectations for an explanation that we had not
yet shared openly with everyone. There were people in our life who knew of the
original cancer diagnosis, and others who did not. Now everyone was coming up
with their own ideas about why Gene had broken his leg. He made the choice to
tell some of our friends, and I left those choices to him; but it was a very intimate
time, as suddenly I was explaining to dear friends why I had never told them years
before, and how that choice had been necessary to support Gene's needs at that
time. Whom we told at a particular time was just what happened at that particular
time. Yet, it is very hard to explain to people you love why or how this very important aspect of your life has been kept private.

A metal plate was surgically installed to hold Gene's broken femur together,
followed by weeks of rehabilitation, a hospital bed at home, and physical therapy.
Eliana camped out at the foot of his bed for his first week home. Meanwhile, Gene
jokingly wondered if he would need a lobotomy to cope with the inactivity, and
his thoughts moved to how he could immerse himself in a new creative activity.

As the weeks went by, it appeared that he was making a gradual recovery, but
about two months later he could no longer get around on one crutch and he asked
to go back to using the second one. He tried to rationalize the change with one of
his own authoritative interpretations, but I insisted he let the orthopedic surgeon
make such decisions. Meanwhile, that Saturday, I needed creative space—a break
from my caregiver mode—so while he went off with Eliana for that appointment,
I went across town to attend a workshop in a clay studio. The doctor's office took
an X-ray of Gene's leg, and to everyone's shock and utter dismay, they learned
that the metal plate had broken. The bone had not been healing well, placing such
burden on the metal plate that it had cracked. Eliana and Gene learned together
that he would have to have a new operation, and her reaction said it all: she immediately vomited on the office floor.

After a second procedure, more months of physical therapy, both in a hospital rehabilitation unit and at our home, Gene's leg finally healed for the second
time. But how could a bone, even one as strong as the femur, break a metal plate?
An answer wasn't immediately clear. When Gene came out of surgery that first
time, the orthopedic doctor had told Alex and me that the surgery had taken so
long because his bones were unusually hard. Now, more than six months later,
with Gene again walking, albeit with crutches, we went in search of more information, and that comment from the surgeon reappeared with new significance.

Our internist called a bone specialist at the National Institutes of Health (NIH) Clinical Center, which takes a certain number of cases from the public if they meet NIH research protocols for studies underway. This specialist's research was unusual bone disorders, and his speculation regarding what happened to Gene was the first that anyone heard of this bone hardening as a problem, his various doctors told us.

Dr. M, an endocrinologist who specialized in bone disorders and bone metabolism, studied a childhood disease that looked like osteoporosis but was really a metabolic bone disorder. The treatment for these children was bisphosphonates, the same treatment, Zometa, that Gene had been taking intravenously all of these years as a preventative measure for bone metastasis from prostate cancer.[5] Again, there were no answers regarding the implications of this for Gene.

That day stays so clear in my mind, the impact of the spoken and unspoken, the science and its sudden silence—that snag on the unconscious that says, *this doesn't make sense,* or *this marks a turn.* It was as if we were catapulted into a new geographical landscape, where nothing is familiar and you have everything to learn. I like to believe that there is always a place, a person, book, or even a mystery that can provide some piece of information that can move us closer to understanding. Instead, this day would be our entry into yet another new, stubbornly unknowable part of the uncharted territory into which we were making this illness journey. Beyond the clinical implications, the fact that the medical experts had no answers made Gene—and the rest of us—realize how truly alone we all were now in this journey.

We began to realize that the statement the doctor had made to Gene about his astonishing survival beyond scientific understanding—"Medically, you do not exist"—had now grown to include the rest of us; that "medically, *we* do not exist either." As the family body, we were invisible in the annals of medicine, and invisible to his doctors. As a family searching for advice so we could make a decision around his treatments we embodied this state of not existing: there were no medical facts, which left us with nothing on which to base our decisions. We felt ourselves "put out to pasture," outside medical reach. When a disease process is so rare that it doesn't get funding for research, it's called an "orphan disease." Metastatic prostate cancer is certainly not rare, but surviving it this long, living with it this long, and living into the side effects of treatment that have heretofore been unknown is rare, according to the doctors. In truth, it makes an orphan of patient and family, too, when medical experts don't have a medical answer. In the absence of a medical answer, humanity will do. A companion in the wilderness is not a waste of medical energy. But now, outside the scope of their medical expertise, we could feel the shift in their interest. We had become outsiders to the medical world as well.

The flashes of awareness would come in unexpected moments. One day we made our way through the labyrinth of the NIH Clinical Center, Gene on crutches, to meet for the first time with Dr. M. and his research assistant.[6] They were both so very respectful toward Gene in the sense of the profession's meeting and greeting ritual. The young Dr. M acknowledged the elder Dr. Cohen and praised him. Dr. M. knew Gene's background—that he had headed programs on aging for twenty years, and that he had won the Distinguished Service Medal, the highest honor of the Public Health Service. He knew Gene was an author and a leader in the field of aging. Gene had been a senior official at NIH and a senior official in the Public Health Service Commissioned Corps; he had headed an institute, and that is the highest position at NIH. And Gene was the genial elder statesman, reciprocating with words of appreciation and knowledge of Dr. M's expertise.

I listened as these two men went back and forth, enjoying what I saw as they flapped their scientists' plumage at one another, their chests inflating with the congratulations of recognition that men and mating animals have in common. Then suddenly I felt the seismic tilt of enantiodromia that Jung described: the pendulum shifted. I was tugged right out of this dance of pride and praise and curiosity and swung full force to an extreme otherness, left alone outside of them and outside of myself. I began to digest the strangeness of this brouhaha. How could this ritual save Gene or give us any answers? I wondered how I could turn the attention of these men away from their pluming dance.

The moment came swiftly, as if I had been flung out on a bungee cord. "Doctor, with all due respect," I began, "I, too, love Gene Cohen. He really is an amazing man, and we do want to keep him here. All the praise and pride that you have is lovely, but we are here because we are living in a land where no one goes. No one has been on this medicine as long as Gene has, and therefore the territory that we are entering is not only frightening but very lonely. A treatment that has been used preventatively to strengthen his bones so they would be prepared to face metastasis if they had to has now made them so brittle that they are snapping apart. The medicine has now become the problem, and we are reeling from that. We have been left alone as if we do not exist; and not only do we exist, but we need to know if you can help us."

I know I didn't say exactly that, but all of that got said. The color of the light in the room changed. I am sure I cried. I think the research assistant cried. And the men began to really talk.

Fairies, Phoenixes, and Commonweal: Our Creative Faculty Expands Our Capabilities

To map uncharted territory requires attention to detail, sometimes a diaspora of detail that only slowly comes into view as coordinates start to emerge. No clinical detail was ever lost on Gene. He could, and did, crunch numbers, theorize, and weigh options with the best of his clinicians, sometimes opening new avenues of consideration that proved productive. For instance, at an early point when he went to Commonweal he studied a thread of research about diet and prostate cancer—and when I say "studied," I mean that he examined the research methodology, the outcomes, all possibilities with a scientist's critical eye. He met with Commonweal's founder, Michael Lerner, who had recently received a Macarthur Foundation Genius Award, as well as having published an outstanding state-of-the-art integrative medicine text, titled *Choices in Healing: Integrating the Best of Conventional and Complementary Approaches to Cancer.*[7] Gene learned that there was suggestive evidence that a radical low-fat diet—about 10 percent of normal fat intake—might slow the course of prostate cancer because it would deprive prostate cancer cells of exactly what they love: fat.[8] What Lerner told Gene did not fundamentally surprise him, since while Gene was at the National Institute on Aging, a number of scientists doing research in their laboratories were discovering how very low–fat diets were slowing the course of disease in diverse organ systems throughout the body. But making the choice to do it and sticking to this food regimen for thirteen years was no easy feat, especially, as Gene pointed out, for a lover of chocolate mousse.

Still, Gene decided that it made sense for him to eat this way, and when his physicians, who were not particularly well-versed in the science of nutrition nor interested in it at that point, shrugged it off, he made the choice for himself. Whether it contributed to his remarkable years of survival we cannot know with certainty, but the existing research recommending it would suggest that it did.

More important than the diet itself was the fact that it was one of many choices that emerged from a new willingness to open lines of inquiry, consideration, and deep reflection. These arose, as Gene saw it, from his creative capacity, or creative faculty. With every new level of clinical complexity and concern came a deeper experience of this aspect of his mind, his self. He recognized this and would talk with me about it, his scientist mind fascinated and delighted by observing his own mind in action, actively transforming in this new landscape. This creative faculty expressed itself in surprising and beautiful ways, from imaginative, mythical storylines, to dreams through which the unconscious informed and guided him. During this period of discouraging clinical discovery, as the unexpected side effects of the cancer treatment on his bone density became apparent, Gene's deep love of myth and metaphor emerged to create a narrative that transformed his experience, mine, and especially Eliana's with new meaning. Expert as he was on the subject of creativity and aging, he was himself surprised, even stunned at times, at the power of the unconscious as a trustworthy source of knowing. His dreams were a balancing of that pendulum, weaving storylines so diverse and shockingly drama-filled that his fascination pulled him as if he were a deep-sea fisherman on the waters of his own past experiences. Fishing through time seemed to move chronology backward from the outer world into the timelessness of the inner world. His dreams and reveries became a kind of navigational system to guide through ever-so-new and constantly changing territory. Gene wrote, telling his own story of this period, and our story, through his eyes:

In ancient Greek mythology, the Phoenix is a mythical bird that, across intervals of times, periodically bursts into flames, falls from the sky to the earth, burning into ashes, only to emerge from the ashes renewed to soar again into flight, but destined to repeat the cycle of burning and renewal over and over again.[9] From 1991 to the present I have felt like the Phoenix, three times feeling figuratively as if I were in flames, en route to burning into ashes, only to seemingly miraculously be renewed to spread and lift my wings again in life.

My first flight as a Phoenix was in 1991, when I was misdiagnosed with Lou Gehrig's disease—also known as ALS or amyotrophic lateral sclerosis. ALS is a degenerative neuromuscular disease, characterized by progressive atrophy of the muscles, typically leading to deteriorating function and death within 3 to 5 years of diagnosis. It was only a long 2 years later—after an intense emotional roller coaster ride—that it was determined I had been misdiagnosed. In the process though, I fundamentally reevaluated what I was going to do in my life. I began inventing games as works of art, and with some awards and other success at it, immersed myself in a new direction in my field, setting up a new research center to focus my studies on creativity and aging.

My second flight as a Phoenix came 5 years later, in 1996, when I was diagnosed with prostate cancer that had metastasized to my bones. I chose to use the time to write the first book on creativity and aging—The Creative Age: Awakening Human Potential in the Second Half of Life. Writing the book was a joyous process.

My third flight as a Phoenix came in 2004 when the preventative treatment for my metastasis became the problem. I'd started to carry a suitcase upstairs, and taking the first step I heard my femur crack. It was a severe fracture that was mystifying, and was found not to be due to the cancer but a side effect of one of the drugs used to treat the cancer. Because of my unusual survival rate with the cancer—my doctors knew of nobody on the drug as long as I had been on it—I had become an "N of one" (the only one they knew of) where the drug over this period of time had altered my bones to a state of being very hard and brittle—a very rare condition known as osteopetrosis, the opposite of osteoporosis, or thinning of the bone. The drug had a half-life of 10 years, meaning even after stopping it completely, the level in my body would only have diminished by 50 percent, 10 years later. My doctors were very concerned that with minimal trauma or twisting, many of my bones would break. As it was, the first operation using a metal plate *did not work because the bone was not healing, and due to metal fatigue with the plate not being aided by a healing bone, the plate broke, and the operation had to be repeated. This time, using a long metal rod down the shaft of my femur along with artificial bone grafting, the use of an electromagnetic stimulator to induce more bone growth, plus daily injections of parathyroid hormone, the bone began to heal, and no others broke. It took 10 long months before I was out of a wheel chair and no longer in need of crutches and a cane.*

The lesson of the value of writing a book on a topic I loved during a time of crisis was not lost on me, and this time I used this period of what might be called disability to write my book, The Mature Mind: The Positive Power of the Aging Brain. *And now, with both the cancer and the bone-altering drug presumably still in my body, I began to work with Wendy on this new book you are reading now, imagining myself as a phoenix and Wendy as a fairy.*

The dictionary defines a fairy as a supernatural being with magic powers who could help or harm—usually help—human beings.[10] *In recent legend, fairies have been pictured as very small, and sometimes very lovely and delicate. In medieval stories, however, fairies were often of full human size.*

In our house, fairies are of special interest. Our daughter Eliana from a very young age has been fascinated with fairies, doing beautiful drawings of them and collecting beautiful images, toys, and sculptures of fairies. When Eliana's nanny (Wendy's mother) died, Eliana was three and asked us: "Is Nanny a fairy now? Will she watch us now like fairies watch everything?" Later, when Wendy was planning her 50th-birthday party, and Eliana was almost six, Eliana suggested that Wendy have a dress-up party with her best friends and that Wendy dress up like a fairy. Not long thereafter, when Wendy was caught in the act of placing coins under Eliana's pillow in place of the tooth that was there, Eliana announced her discovery that Wendy Miller was in fact the tooth fairy—not that the tooth fairy did not exist, but that her mother was the tooth fairy. Wendy had achieved the stature of a fairy. Eliana then asked me if I thought her mother was a fairy. I replied, "You are right, she has many qualities of a fairy; she certainly does a remarkable job in looking out for both of us." Eliana nodded her head in agreement.

I reflect now back to those times and think again that Wendy does have many qualities of a fairy. When we met, shortly after it had been determined that my diagnosis of ALS was a misdiagnosis, I was actively engaged in what I have described in my new theory of psychological development as being in the midlife reevaluation phase. Wendy was remarkably in tune with my deliberations, as my ideas were in a similar vein as the work she had researched and written on her developmental phase diagram, and this certainly played a role in the building of our relationship and our love for one another. We could understand each other's intellectual as well as personal and romantic pursuits. One of the more poignant illustrations of the depth of our connection was when we both told our cribbage stories, each a story of healing. It almost seemed magical, like fairies and phoenix seem magical.

Two years later, we were engaged and I was diagnosed with cancer. Wendy, in retrospect, was like a fairy who pointed her wand toward a new path for me to follow, one that on my own I never would have taken. It was a path that I did follow and one that helped shape the perspective on life that I was to adopt. She insisted I apply to become a participant in one of Commonweal's weeklong residential cancer help programs, in Bolinas, California. Commonweal, founded in 1976, having a reputation in the eyes of many medical illness practitioners (traditional and complementary alike) as being the best cancer help program of its nature in the world, made it easier with my traditional training to act on Wendy's recommendation.

Commonweal's stated goal was "To help participants live better and, where possible, longer lives. The Cancer Help Program addresses the unmet needs of people with cancer. These include finding balanced information on choices in healing, mainstream and complementary therapies; exploring emotional and spiritual dimensions of cancer; discovering that illness can sometimes lead to a richer and fuller life; and experiencing genuine community with others facing a cancer diagnosis."[11]

I feel this goal and associated objectives were all met there for me. That so many of the group facilitators were themselves survivors of cancer and other life-threatening diseases made the experience all the more meaningful and poignant for me. Most fundamentally, two major outcomes occurred for me. First, I was enabled to deeply mourn, which then allowed me to move forward. Second, I had an extremely important conversation with Michael Lerner that led to a strategy I would otherwise never have adopted. Since with Michael's recently published book he had comprehensively and meticulously reviewed the state-of-the-art of complementary treatments, beyond traditional ones, I felt he was the one to probe about anything I should consider in the complementary treatment field. I had read an enormous amount about traditional approaches, and had consulted with some of the country's leading experts in this area as well. But the complementary area, which was becoming an area of growing interest for me, was not one where I felt sufficiently knowledgeable.

On the whole, my Commonweal experience allowed me to better process my very unsettled feelings, to gain new perspective, and to get time moving productively again. Hope and expectation became recalibrated.

A further turning point came one afternoon, where I consulted with another leading expert on prostate cancer. After we reviewed my case clinically, he asked me what was I going to do, given my dire circumstances. For a moment I was confused, not understanding the question, but then spontaneously responded, "I choose to live—I plan to live the best I can with whatever time I have." As I said those words, I realized how much I meant them. I felt a deep shift and sudden surge of not just hope, but purpose and plan, a clear intention. There is a place for hope in dark times. More than denial, it can be a catalyst for action, and that can make all the difference. I decided it was time to immerse myself again in my career with whatever time I had left.

Most people feel extremely alone and isolated when they enter uncharted territory. For example, retirement could at first be experienced as uncharted territory because when people retire, all the ways in which they have defined themselves are gone. The same is true with illness. When one faces an illness, the strategies or coping mechanisms so developed through experience and time cannot always save a life or provide the answers. For us, that day at the NIH Clinical Center, to face what we were facing and confront the reality that, as we had been told previously, "Medically, you do not exist," the depth of our aloneness hit hard. Yet, there we were, facing it together. What other choice is there?

Uncharted territory does not mean we do not go there. Uncharted territory means we do go there, or are forced to go there, with uncertainty and the prospect of change. The physician and medical director of Commonweal, Rachel Naomi Remen, writes and teaches medical providers about how our health provides us with a means for evoking wholeness: how our healing relationships develop and strengthen parts of ourselves that we cannot know, or find, or perhaps even think we have; how we discover meaning and value in our life; how we navigate through the often challenging psychological experiences that occur when we age or take care of our loved ones as they age, or when we retire from a career, and certainly, as we face our own and our loved one's serious illnesses; and how our "health is the movement toward wholeness."[12]

I was reminded of my mother's example. In July 1995, eight months before Gene's initial diagnosis, my mom had sat our whole family down at our long dining table at the lake house in Maine. She told us that she had been going to blood doctors for years but now she was going to a hematologist oncologist because her blood profile now showed multiple myeloma.[13] She had never been symptomatic before, but now her blood was changing and they were going to treat her. She and dad had brought home a number of pamphlets from the oncologist's office for each of my sisters and the grandchildren. It was our first entry into cancer world and life-threatening illness. We had lost our nana at age ninety-four; she died of natural causes in her sleep. Next in line to come would be our great uncles, also of natural aging, one at ninety-one, the other at ninety-nine. We knew nothing about facing, treating, or managing life-threatening illness.

Yet, by the time cancer came up in this immediate way, first with my mother's diagnosis, followed so closely by my husband's, I had been primed though my own experience of quality-of-life threatening illnesses. In fact, my education in navigating illness territory had begun years before with my own experience cycling through health and illness. As I saw it, the ground had been seeded, planted, tilled, and harvested through my own experience. I had become a farmer who grew her crops according to the calendar of illness time.

I was the girl with bouts of chickenpox, mononucleosis, Epstein Barr, and shingles. I have tooth discoloration from childhood chickenpox. I got mononucleosis in high school, in college, and then again as a young adult, even though all the doctors told me that you could only have mono once! The last journey through illness time turned into a four-year struggle in the mid-1980s with the addition of chronic fatigue syndrome.[14]

Chronic fatigue syndrome taught me that if my own energy was not going to return to me, then I would have to learn to use my time in a different way. I chose to continue to live in the landscape of my bed, a life of reading and resting. I decided that if this was what it was going to be like, I'd better adapt to it. I enrolled in a university doctoral program that allowed for distance study so I could be guided and accompanied in my study of health and illness. It led me into formal years of training in psychosynthesis, guided imagery and psychoneuroimmunology, the mind–body connections, the use of my field—expressive arts therapy—for healing and studying the alternative health movement.[15] My skills and expertise grew through my life, where health and illness intertwined like the caduceus image of medicine, the serpent around the staff of knowledge forming my health, my profession, and my field. I have spent a lot of time struggling in myself to learn how to cope with the need to change and adapt my pace to my condition. Challenges like this unknowingly accompany any of us and so the past is always with us, informing the present in some way. These earlier experiences become lessons learned, whether cautionary tales or inspiring ones, as they mark the trails for the next time.

The Ultimate Expression of Potential Is Creativity

The illness journey is so often assumed to be only the gradual narrowing and shutting down of life and life force. But Gene often referred to William Carlos Williams' later-life poetry in which he described "an old age that adds as it takes away."[16] In other words, the aging process need not—in fact should not—be defined as an accumulation of losses. Rather, as we struggle with loss, our problems become the catalyst for finding new potential. Williams' work in older age was itself a powerful reminder that our understanding *about* aging usually comes *as* we age, living through our own aging and life experience.

People will sometimes talk about how an illness changed their life for the better, or about "the gift" of the illness, but the listener is often inclined to hear those stories as simply making the best of a bad situation. They may admire it in a person living with cancer or one who has overcome a difficult illness, but they see it as function of attitude, when in fact these stories or testimonials offer a glimpse of the developmentally driven creative faculty that is innate in all of us.

Gene so often insisted, "What has been universally denied is the potential. The ultimate expression of potential is creativity."[17] He referred to creativity as an emotional and intellectual process—a mechanism—that can displace negative feelings with positive feelings of engagement.[18] In the next chapter, when we look at my Phase Diagram, we will also look further at Gene's definition of creativity:

> *Creativity and its effects may be a solo experience in which we develop a new attitude or facet of self understanding, and by doing so, fundamentally alter the way we approach and experience life, relationships and activities. Our creativity may also alter our thinking, our behavior, or our experiences of our community and culture.*[19]

In certain circumstances, change is welcomed. In others, it intrudes on us, maybe even unwelcomed. However unfamiliar or unsettling life's terrain may become, the uncharted territory opens creative, generative space that adds, even as other circumstances may take away. Confronted with the fragility and finiteness of life—our own or others that move us—we may ask the Big Questions with a focus and intensity we did not have before. Gene asked himself always, "What do I really want to be doing? Is that a person or project that I can creatively engage in?" I more often fell into the "Why me?"—more existential questions of why this was happening to us. Yet my why questions also sat right beside the incredible luck I felt as Gene's health kept holding its ground, year after year, and we were able to move forward in our lives, our work, and our love.

Any of us, forced to consider what matters most to us, may be moved to act on intentions that previously were routinely postponed. For Gene and me, it was a particular family vacation we had dreamed of but put off for years; or traveling to Costa Rica and going on a zip-line together. We also discovered, as do so many others in this journey through illness or aging, that we may find our voice to say what has been unsaid; to forgive; to ask; to initiate; to complete; to let go. To say no when needed. To participate in what matters rather than what we are responsible for doing. To stay connected. Creativity allows us to do whatever we came to do. The question only grows stronger: *Have we in fact done what we came here to do?*

The territory that is uncharted is not only the territory of illness or of aging, or even most fundamentally that, although we are thrown into it through these events in our lives. Rather the uncharted territory is most profoundly the territory of our creative faculty—it is what emerges from our life experiences. The familiar ground of our identity undergoes major seismic shifts though illness and aging, through losses and change, and the geography of our landscape—inner and outer—changes. We are changed. Gene became more sensitive to the physical beauty of the world surrounding him. My creative vocabulary became an authentic language of material imagery—I began sculpting. Eliana found the grace and aggressiveness of her basketball body, and used it to save herself. Alex became the best dad he could ever imagine. Kate found ways to bring Gene's presence of unconditional love into their family life. Unanchored, we all still pursued what enlivened our creative faculty.

What uncharted territory really does, then, is allow us to fully engage in the moment with our whole creative self, the capacities that have been there, but so often hidden. It is our resource of deepest knowing. Our lives are filled with raw material, but we don't recognize it as a source of inspiration because in illness time, we are living uncertain and disrupted or painful, making our way through our new experiences. But eventually we begin to search inward for wisdom and ways to develop some control of our experiences and what we do with them. The inner search alone begins to empower us, and our innate creativity becomes our tool for reshaping even the most painful experiences.

Like an earthquake, illness or adversity sends a shock wave through our life: our worlds get shaken up, everything we have defined as ourselves gets shaken up. The emerging landscape is transformed and so unfamiliar—and yet we draw inspiration from it. There can be a brightness that comes through in the upheaval, an unexpected freshness that arises from a deep source. This is the creative faculty, always deeply present, as if a river of poetry runs underground in the life we are living above ground. This, too, is uncharted territory—this creative channel deep within.

Uncharted territory is all of the things that come together or arise out of this earthquake. We walk into this new creative space, out of the disorienting crucible of time, and although the challenge at times only intensifies, we also find that this new space has this brightness to it. Not because it is bright in the conventional sense. As a matter of fact, the emotional part of the experience is dark, but its brightness is that even the darkness becomes grounding. It is generative, intimate, and in the moment. The earthquake as teacher tells us that the ground has to be opened up, and sometimes it happens through acts of nature, in the body as an illness or an injury; in the landscape, an earthquake. But the lesson in it for us is that we should cultivate it, because the hidden potential, the creative faculty, is there anyway in the depths of our being, even when we don't know it. We have a responsibility to cultivate it.

Where Does the "Will" Come From in the Will to Live?

In Chapter 4, I wrote about my experience with Gene's oncologist—how I feel that doctors need to study the so-called will to live. The reason is that "will" is widely misunderstood. We need to study how it manifests individually in us, how it has its own language, how there are inner-world steps we can practice to activate the will, how that practice, that "muscle," helps the immune system and mobilizes healing. And how, in fact, creativity really is an extraordinary medicine, which I got to see in action as Gene, so intimately, so dearly, so courageously, engaged it. We often think of it as determination, or as willpower—some strong force that we have to corral in order to make things happen. In fact, will does require purposeful drive and intention, but it is so much more than that. It is the creative faculty at work. It is not just a determination to live—it is the creative, generative alchemy of living. We all struggle to actually see this territory. I once described it as "orchids growing in skinny places," in the book *Portrait of the Artist as Poet*:

> I have always written. Writing came naturally for a child journal keeper full of private wonderings. Sculpture came later. I was lured into it romantically as a young traveler hiking through the Andes to Machu Picchu.
>
> Almost near the clouds, I saw orchids with only thin air to breathe growing out of stones tightly fit together. When I returned to the States, I knew I had to build. It wasn't that I had an image of myself as an artist, but that I felt the need to express myself in form. Although I got into graduate school through my writing, I kept going to the sculpture studio to build bigger and bigger structures. Writing and sculpting have always gone together for me. My mythopoetic voice speaks in words formed by rhythm and physical relationship, and my sculptures build narratives that tell stories to me. . . .
>
> My words formed recognition, bridged years of silence, grew orchids in skinny places. All of my art is about exploration. I view my poems as word sculptures.[20]

Now, forty years have gone by since I saw those orchids growing out of skinny places. Much has happened. And I know now that my desire to build forms—to sculpt—was my creative faculty speaking to me. I needed to understand a thing in its three-dimensional form: how it is made, how it can stand, how it can piece itself together. As I can see now, this desire to see dimensionality became my professional path as well: as a therapist to see how we are made, how we can stand, and how we piece ourselves together. This creative faculty is not only something that we have as a resource; it is something we can cultivate and strengthen through practice.[21]

We see this in extreme examples, like the famous example of the mathematical savant Jason Padgett, who was hit in the head, and after being released from the hospital with what they called a bruised kidney began to see slow-motion images of mathematical fractals: shapes and colors visually accompanied numbers.[22] He had a profound concussion and brain injury, and what emerged was an entirely new faculty of visual mathematics. Where did this come from? Had it always been there? Was it the neurological earthquake of the concussion that released and awakened it? Did the concussion change his brain this dramatically? I am in no way suggesting that our creative faculty must be traumatically harmed to be released. I am suggesting that our creative faculty exists, and accompanies us. In this accompaniment, we are connected to a large capacity, an unconscious authority and potential within, ready to guide us in our uncharted lands.

A professor of mine, Penny MacElveen-Hoehn, a widow herself, told me after Gene passed away that she saw Gene as a prodigy.[23] I didn't understand what she meant by that. She explained that prodigies are people who appear older than their years, or those, like Gene, who accomplish much despite a shortened life, undeterred (for long) by the obstacles that get in the way for most of us. But prodigy? He certainly wasn't playing concerts at age five or gaining celebrity status with precocious talents on display. Gene accomplished a great deal in a life foreshortened, but he would suggest that the spark that ignited his passion for the science of aging was the same spark that any of us have: the creative spirit. He had begun his scientific research on aging at a mere eleven years old, studying the growth of fish bones, eventually turning that passion for the science of aging into a distinguished career and the founding of a national institute of aging.

In his career, as in life, each time he faced an obstacle or a challenge, he managed to move out of the narrowness of it. He refused to let it define him, or his field, or his lifestyle, or his relationships, or, for that matter, his illness. However notable his accomplishments, in Gene's mind it was all aimed at a singular objective: to have this creative faculty recognized as a source of unlimited potential within each of us. In his mind, the creative faculty fully engaged is what defines a life of meaning, purpose, and accomplishment in every life.

6

Portrait of Healing

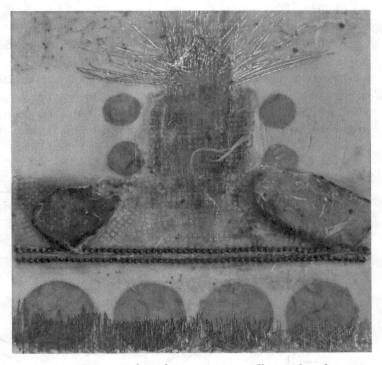

Figure 6.1 "Geography of the Soul" (2011), encaustic wax collage with rock, papers, and chain, 10 × 10 inches. Artwork by Wendy L. Miller, photo credit: Claire Blatt.

As chaotic as life in uncharted territory can feel at times, we are by nature designed to bring coherence to chaos, or at least to try. Even in the chaos of illness, we may find some sense of order in our external world with the schedule of appointments, the routines around medications, or movements that help us navigate the new terrain. When fragilities or the losses of age unsettle us, we make small, practical adjustments to overcome them, then larger ones as they become necessary.

But the uncharted territory within us—the deep psychological terrain that is in disarray in this internal landscape—appears to offer no such markers, no map to orient us and show us a path to move through. In fact, there is an internal process, a healing process, that follows predictable steps—not only a map, but an identifiable process through which we can see an emerging coherence, a portrait of our experience. This healing process through which we integrate the complexities of our experience into a coherent whole has been the focus of my work for more than thirty years. To make the process more accessible—something we can look at and talk about—I developed the Phase Diagram (Fig. 6.2). It is a helpful tool that anyone can use to reflect on their own circumstances and possibilities.

When I first started working with medically ill patients in 1986, it was a conscious choice, not only in how to begin shaping my clinical practice, but also as a way to practice activism. I felt that health was the next political arena for me. I believed that a revolution of consciousness was going to take place in the field of mind–body health. And that has proved to be true, not only in terms of health and healthcare, but also in the various uses of integrative arts medicine. The work grew out of my personal experience with my own immune system illness, chronic

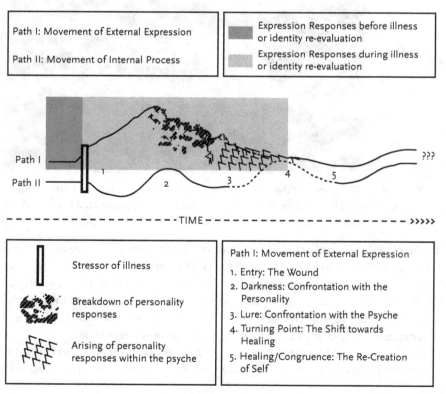

Figure 6.2 The Phase Diagram. Diagram by Wendy L. Miller.

fatigue syndrome, and how that experience intersected with my career, my art, my hopes, my dreams, and my experience of my own "authentic self."

Coming out of this illness and healing period, in 1988, I felt I had learned something very subtle and deep about the intricate process of healing. I knew there were relationships of layering between the emotional (our actions and reactions), biographical (our unconscious responses to internal family dynamics), biochemical (hormonal, neurological, physical responses), and spiritual (values and assessments of meaning) parts of ourselves. I knew that it was important for these parts to come into harmony or congruence with one another, and that imagery was a language subtle and layered enough to capture the signposts for health. Perhaps one day science will be able to "interpret" physical images by better understanding the interactions among the immune system, the brain, the endocrine system, acupuncture points, and all the places in the body that are expressed in imagery.

The extensive literature on illness, which I pored through as I wrote my dissertation on chronic fatigue syndrome, held the great debates and insights of the time about the psychological aspects of living with illness: causes, responses, reactions, personalities, propensities, qualities for healing, and so on. I developed a phase diagram—a visual tool—as a way to help me understand the experience of moving through this inner uncharted territory, as chronic fatigue syndrome was definitely uncharted in the early 1990s.[1] Over the years, I have come to understand that this is not only a diagram of moving through an illness; the Phase Diagram gives us a portrait of what takes place as our inner and outer worlds arrange and rearrange themselves to create integration between them and, in so doing, tap our resources of both creativity and healing.

I have used this diagram in my clinical practice for more than two decades, and it continues to help my clients and me recognize where they are in the midst of a developmental process while they are moving through the uncharted territories of illness, aging and changed identities. The diagram has become a portrait of the healing process of integration.

The nature of healing is the process we go through to bring congruency to these inner and outer levels or paths. It is a seasoned choice, in contrast to the reactivity we initially have entering the experience, when we are pulled and separated from ourselves by these deep levels of the psyche being at odds with one another. Ultimately, this is why healing is both unique and individual to each person, dependent on timing, temperament, biography, biology, and other individual factors. Yet, at the same time, healing has a universal quality in that its direction is toward wholeness and integration. The Phase Diagram is essentially a navigational tool of identity formation. It maps our movement through integration and what some call individuation. More and more of who we are ultimately aligns inside of us so the light of the self comes through all that we are as a whole person: body, mind, emotions, and spirit.

The Phase Diagram provided a touchstone for me, particularly in my role as partner and caregiver, because moving through the illness experience with Gene changed us in so many ways. It created an alternate reality and with it the need for us each to grow and change within it. While that reality continued to shape-shift with changes in the disease and our everyday experiences, we found that we were supported by our capacity to reflect internally. Being both psychological and existential may help intellectually, but the very nature of this unbounded exploration can be something of a psychological free fall; in the upheaval of a major health crisis or loss, you need something more. A map is a better guide.

This next section describes the Phase Diagram, showing the steps and markers to guide you through such an experience. Complex as it may appear at first, imagine the Diagram simply as a map showing the two paths that take us through the textured terrains of change in our inner and outer worlds. Path I shows how our "external expression responses"—or the ways we characteristically respond to challenge—change and develop as we move through experience. Path II shows how our "internal process"—how we think and feel about things—transforms in its own way as we move through the same experience. Two paths, two simultaneous journeys of the self. Now let's look at that textured terrain in terms of phases, or passages, through which these two paths move.

How do you typically respond to challenge? What's your personal style or reaction when faced with a problem in which your physical, mental, emotional, or spiritual health (or that of someone you love) has been impaired or threatened? That's your external expression response style, and we'll look at that first.

The *External Expression Path* (Path I) moves through two phases. Expression responses *before* illness or identity re-evaluation are a starting strategy (first phase). Expression responses *during* illness or identity re-evaluation (second phase) are an attempt to continue this original strategy despite changing circumstances. Together, they show the movement of our external expression responses (see Path I in Figure 6.2) through experience and how it changes us. At the beginning of Path I, in the first phase, a pre-illness history of some kind is accompanied by a starting strategy of choice, meaning that style in which we characteristically meet a challenge in health or in identity. This choice typically reflects a person's personality style. For example, some people may have a natural tendency to engage as problem-solvers (practical, task-oriented researchers), caretakers (looking after the needs of another), overachievers (continuing to accomplish), or avoiders (trying to not notice that the stressor could be changing their life). This first phase simply depicts the continuation of that—our continued reliance on that pre-illness or pre-identity re-evaluation style. The second phase on Path I— expression responses during illness or identity re-evaluation—reflects the type of characteristic responses we have when trying to continue in the style of this strategy. As depicted in the chart in Figure 6.2, these two phases show the movement along the upper *External Expression Path*, which roughly parallels the movement of the other path—the *Internal Process Path*, Path II—which is how we think and feel about things. This internal process path moves through not just two phases (before and during) but five phases in which the complex ways of how we think and feel go through profound changes.

The five phases on Path II are phases of an internal or intrapsychic process of the illness or identity re-evaluation experience. They occur less linearly than they appear in the following list. Rather, they circle through and overlap one another, but as a whole they do create a pattern of movement as internal aspects of our selves become more and more integrated. These five phases are as follows:

1) *Entry* into the experience feels like a "wound" created by illness, physical trauma, or any loss or change. This wound forces us to re-evaluate our physical, emotional, and spiritual being.
2) *Confrontation with the personality* involves how we see ourselves in the context of this new situation and how we assess responsibility for the cause of the ill health or the emotional darkness.
3) *Confrontation with the psyche* occurs when our deepest sense of self, life purpose, and meaning lures us into what feels like an existential crisis in identity.
4) *Turning point* shifts us in the direction of our own healing.
5) *Healing congruence*, or the healing process of congruence between the outer and inner paths, involves a resolution to the confrontations with the personality and the psyche and leads to a re-creation of ourselves.

Healing occurs when both Paths I and II align and move forward in a coherent fashion. Healing is the integration or harmonizing of these *inner and outer paths* and all the phases incorporating pre-illness and illness strategies.

When Something's Gotta Give: Path I Epiphanies

Often our style, our characteristic strategy or approach to life, kicks into high gear under the stress of an illness or an identity re-evaluation, but its effectiveness under these new circumstance varies. Maybe we physically no longer have the same movement independence we used to have, before the illness, which could happen with back injuries or knee replacements; maybe emotionally we don't have the comfort of full, healthy energy because we need to reserve what we have, and it can be hard for family or friends—hard even for ourselves—to recognize this change in us. This is why, in the Phase Diagram, on Path I, we see an initial attempt to continue our personality style under stress as the line aims upward in its trajectory (pre-illness style); then comes a sharp drop, marking the point where our familiar personality style ceases to work any longer. The line breaks and plummets, as if we were falling off a cliff.

Gene's expression responses pre-illness within his personality style were those of a caregiver. He was highly responsible in taking care of others, and his sense of responsibility had served him well in his family, clinical practice, his research, and his career. With the stress of his illness, his response was typical for most of us: work harder and harder in our familiar style to maintain the status quo. In the Phase Diagram, that's the upward climbing line; in real life that's the increasing struggle to hold things together the way we've always held things together. Gene was deeply concerned about the possibility that he wouldn't be here to take care of his parents and brothers; but as he has written, he was able to continue in this role for his family, although as time went on, he also had to take care of and pace his own needs for the stability of his own health. The expression responses of his personality style changed in his outer world during the years of the illness as he was not able to give to others in the same ways as he had, because rather than fulfilling him, it began to take a toll on him and deplete him. To take care of everyone, to be responsible, to research, to plan ahead—it all operated at the expense of his personal self, his health, and he could no longer pay that price.

The breakdown of his pre-illness strategy—the darkened part of Path I— marked the point at which he had to learn how to step back from other people's needs. This was a painful awareness at first. He had to give himself permission to *not* be available to certain people. For example, he didn't work with anyone on his grants and studies if he didn't think they could provide their own passion and creative spark. If he had to provide it for them or convince them, he chose others with whom to collaborate.

Awakening Potential: The Rigorous, Rewarding Inner Journey of Path II

1. ENTRY: THE WOUND

Entry is often experienced as a "fall " or "collapse," beginning with the sudden onset of symptoms or the diagnosis of the illness or the fear, confusion, and isolation that frequently accompany them. The normal routines of life seem to fall apart, and there is often the feeling that the illness is ruining one's familiar sense of being, not only the physical health but also one's sense of self.

For Gene, this entry (Path II on the Phase Diagram) was filled with "dark dip moods," a new accompanying self to his perky, clever temperament. He sometimes wondered if he was becoming bipolar, which was really just a psychiatrist's image for the extremes in his mood and outlook as he entered into this territory, feeling wounded. His extremes were what would be called "situational"—the result of the cancer or side effects of the treatment. The challenge, of course, is that his illness "situation" wasn't going to go away.

2. DARKNESS: CONFRONTATION WITH THE PERSONALITY

To say that the shock of entry into this new adverse circumstance—whatever it is—sets your head spinning is surprisingly accurate in the psychological sense. The personality is thrown for a loop. If your new circumstances mean that you can no longer be the "you" you've always been—not for others and not for yourself—then who are you? Who are you going to be? Who do you need to be—for yourself and for others?

Confrontation with the personality launches an inward search for answers, to bring some sense of coherence to this chaos. Thus the stage is set for this phase of confrontation, a search for explanation, a way to assign responsibility if not blame in the conventional sense. This self-scrutiny often incorporates what might sound like self-blaming—"What is wrong with me? What did I do to bring this on myself? What could I have done differently?"—but more accurately it is an attempt to understand our own participation in the situation, to really understand how this illness came to be.

People often answer these questions by blaming physical factors for their participation in the situation—from a virus to a genetic propensity to an environmental toxin to a missed diagnosis—or sometimes psychological factors: "Well, I have been unhappy since such and such happened," or "Since my husband died, I have not been myself."

Internal reflection and even this sense of blaming or self-blaming, when they arise, are indispensable to the healing process. This inner confrontation is a necessary one in order to move forward; it involves assessing and discerning parts of self, habitual personality strategies that weren't necessarily working very well even before the crisis. The confrontation leads to a deeper, more objective and discerning self-awareness that recognizes there are more parts to the whole of who you are. Art therapy and other forms of creative expression are particularly effective for this listening phase because much of what people first hear from their own symptoms is communicated nonverbally, through strong reactions of feeling and sensations: through pictures, sounds, rhythms, memories, gestures, and actions. One woman moving through the uncharted territory of her illness experience, describing her experience in this phase, drew a candle melted all the way down to the bottom. Beside it was a rose. She felt that her life force was like the candle, almost all the way gone. Yet there was this rose that seemed to want to bloom, clearly inside her as well, but so stifled.

Gene, ever the responsible caregiver, found this confrontation with his highly successful pre-illness personality extremely difficult, a source of considerable inner turmoil. In this confrontation with personality, he had to find ways to manage the conflicting voices of identity within him, had to tap other aspects of himself to find a new and sustainable sense of self. All of this had to come in his own time and in his own way. That is why he told some people of his diagnosis and didn't tell others. If he felt that he would need to take care of their feelings or their reactions or responses, or if their reactions or responses would hinder his work, he chose not to open and share. If sharing supported him or one of his children or one of his projects, he would share the circumstances of his personal life. For him to make this conscious choice, he confronted aspects of himself that had always maintained privacy, kept vulnerability neatly put away as if in a box held for only special loved ones. He was by nature a private person who preferred helping others rather than revealing what he himself might need. He recognized that he had to change—had to open, had to ask, had to consider his needs. He had a recurring daydream mantra:

> In the darkness
> I discovered
> A different light

3. THE LURE: CONFRONTATION WITH THE PSYCHE

Lure is the word I use to describe the feeling when something in us attempts to pull at us, in this case, pulls us out of our usual personality styles. We experience it as a strong yet subtle tug that forces us to confront what is happening. Let's say, for example, that you're someone who, the moment you're told something, you go and research it; you're a problem-solver and you just like more information. So you have this issue come up and your usual strategy is to sit down and learn everything, but the reality is that you're drained and can't think straight and something in you is saying *who cares, it doesn't matter what it is, you need to feel rested, you don't need to be the expert of this.* The pressure continues, and the internal dialogue does, too, and after awhile this other voice that says *stop handling this the way you always handle everything* is getting stronger and stronger. It's not good for your system to be ambivalent in the tension of this pulling, and eventually you say, *okay I used to do it that way but I don't need to do it that way.* That voice gets stronger and stronger. Or if you're normally a person who prefers to keep your head in the sand; this pull the other way may make you want to go research and learn more for a change. The point is that it is a tug—a lure to do the other—because it's not what you would normally do. This confrontation with the psyche is the point where the question changes from "What is the meaning of my illness?" to "What is the meaning of my life?" I worked with a famous orchestral conductor who had Lou Gehrig's disease for five years, from age sixty to sixty-five, and there were many times when we had to circle through this phase so that he could find and re-find his own reasons to stay alive. Confronting his psyche through so many severe physical losses—walking, talking, moving his only one finger or one eye at the computer—made him question his capacity to keep on living.

In my own life with chronic fatigue syndrome, I first tried to fight against my illness with my own personality style of bravado and enthusiasm. In the confrontation with my personality, that strategy began losing its rhythm, intensity, and speed. I could tell, because I didn't have the energy to move at that speed. My communication was quieter, I became more of a listener and watcher instead of the orchestrator of a conversation. In this next phase, the lure into the confrontation with the psyche, a strange sense of faith that I would be OK, began to arise, even though my identity and style were so different. It came to me in many forms—through the color of the light on the lake where I grew up, recognizing beauty during a time when I thought that nothing mattered—slow, slight changes in awareness. This phase pushes in ways that some people describe as a struggle between light and dark, hope and despair; most descriptions are similar to the classic literature on spiritual emergence or on existential crises. The psyche is providing a critical opportunity for moving toward wholeness. A person is drawn (sometimes pulled or pushed) by these transpersonal qualities of self that seem to grow within us—like hope, faith, renewal, acceptance. These qualities are hard to come by within our personalities, but they do arise in and out of us, sometimes in spite of our personalities, and the truth is that we need them. Maybe they are spiritual energy. In Gene's work, he calls this force the "inner push"—in other words, something prompts this energy to sprout up within us, practically pushing us into the next phase.[2] But the process seems to arise or surprise as it emerges from within our unconscious.

For Gene, this is when his own dreams—not the night dreams but the real dreams for his life—came up, and he went for them. To honor his own imagination, he created his games, made notes for his science fiction novel, and wrote his books and editorials.

His confrontation with his psyche I believe arrived through the enormous amount of love and respect that was given to him: he had to learn to receive it—to take it in and own it. Learning to receive was an act of healing for him. He knew well how to give, but receiving was something he had to truly learn. In terms of the developmental map the Phase Diagram offers, as he progressed along Path I, changing his external expression responses, he was changing his relationship to the caregiver within him, the internal process he was on in Path II. This confrontation within his psyche was also releasing this wonderful sense of love and pride he felt—received—from his son's family, his grandchildren. He had grown up to become a caregiver for people who needed him; and now he was raising a loving daughter and enjoying the new life of his son, daughter-in-law, and four beautiful grandchildren, whose love was a beautiful and welcomed gift to him. The caring that he now received himself was a true experience of receptivity for him, and he delighted in his pride and joy. This both opened him up, personally, and released a type of healing love and acceptance.

4. TURNING POINT: THE SHIFT TOWARD HEALING

The shift toward healing is the movement of the personality toward what the psyche is revealing. It seems to come in what could be called transpersonal qualities, perhaps spiritual qualities, such as faith, compassion, surrender, service, purpose, acceptance, wisdom, and love. It is as if these qualities were drawn up from the absolute depths of despair, which is why I don't like to use the terms "positive emotions" or "positive thinking." Maybe some of these qualities do have a "positive" bent, but sometimes so does fierce anger or self-righteousness, and one might not define those as positive. So, I don't like to divide emotions up in that way; rather, to say that something golden grows even when it sprouts covered with the muddy earth from which it has grown. These qualities provide that necessary last bit of energy to shift a person toward this last phase of healing.

For Gene, this meant opening to himself as a creator—all of his books, editorials, and games are an expression of claiming his own creativity, separate from his responsible roles as husband, son, father, psychiatrist, and administrator. The creator was the writer, storyteller, performer, inventor, researcher, and advocate of human dignity. These qualities that infuse the important roles we take in our families interested him: an essential creativity of the whole person, seen with dignity, respect, love, and intimacy; defining and opening the space for the generative, creative faculty to come through as a quiet presence that needed certain conditions to show itself. He knew how much he needed this for his own health and well-being, as this knowledge became stronger and stronger, pushing its way into his psyche; he wouldn't let anything interfere or interrupt it. It became a kind of sacrosanct presence. In fact, he took such delight in real life. He had a quirky but intuitive sense about what he was seeing, and he cultivated these perceptions in new ways. That is what creativity was for him; the more he could think through what he saw, the more he valued it.

5. HEALING/CONGRUENCE: THE RE-CREATION OF SELF

Healing and congruence is the final integration phase wherein the light of the self comes through the whole person—body, mind, emotions, and spirit. As deep spiritual needs that were shunted aside in one's pre-illness life are recognized and met, the self-healing properties of the immune system begin to reassert their power. Our psychological work helps our immune system heal inner wounds that illness can activate around caring, love, meaning, isolation, abandonment, attention, loneliness, and aloneness; and our integrative work brings wholeness to our psyches.

Healing is the congruence between the two paths on the diagram: they move in sync with one another. As Gene allowed himself not to be always responsible for others or available to every request, his creative self strengthened. This creative self became more and more visible both publically and privately as these two paths resonated with each other. His work and his community life became more and more personal, more and more integrated.

Paths I and II represent the outer and inner psychological aspects of our self, and as those become aligned, they create what could be considered a third path, representing the *integrative* self, which we'll explore more fully in Chapter 11.

In his own work, Gene viewed this developmental process through the lens of aging and creativity. In *The Creative Age*, he outlined his "phases of human potential." Each of these stages was, at the core, defined by aging, but equally, and perhaps more importantly, by creativity and the potential that age creates and releases. The natural emergence of creative energy, and the even greater potential for us to cultivate it if we were aware of it within us, drove Gene's work.

My diagram allowed me to navigate in this territory in my work and my life, to follow the internal landscape of what happens when illness causes a huge shock to the system. It was still only a diagram, however. The actual experience with Gene pushed both of us up against the edges of mortality, and for all that any of us might study or read or discuss or believe, for all that we know about that edge, it is all a mere ghost of knowledge. There is no knowledge like direct, lived experience.

Our process of writing together became an intimate expression of so much of this integration and healing process—done together. In our writing our inner lives became exposed to one another, intersected and brought to bear on one another. This held its moments of surprise and tension: we each had become quite accustomed to our own inside view of our collaborative process, and at times, in telling the story on the page, those perceptions conflicted. Gene might be miffed by my interpretation of something he saw differently, or vice versa. I might feel ripped off if I felt he stole my ideas and ran with them. This wasn't really the truth, but sometimes it was the emotional truth. Together we gathered from many angles of our experience, and in sharing them through our writing, we were exposing our selves not only to one another but also to ourselves. It used to be that his medical condition was like a filter, through which he could not see himself into a future. Later, it was if every idea, every encounter, every story was his future and our life was his material. He would be up at 6 A.M. writing; up until 11 P.M. writing, while I, the partner, slowed down, resting, fuming internally from exhaustion, tired from all the responsibilities I was managing in order to keep our household alive and moving. I couldn't find my own voice to create.

It was I whose voice got muffled, and it was my voice that needed to be retrieved to shape our writing and our exchanges. Where was the back and forth? Where did our lives intersect? Where were the entwined voices that shared in their exchange? At times we moved on parallel tracks, as if the separation protected us from something that would happen if we allowed our voices to blend together into the depth of the truth.

Gene's Creativity—A Map for Human Potential

Gene's work on his creativity equation, midlife phases, and developmental intelligence was his unique expression of a view we shared and presented in our work in different ways. For example, his creativity equation, $C = me^2$, arrived for him out of a dream image.[3] His first association, of course, was to Einstein, $E = mc^2$. EMC are also the initials of our daughter Eliana, and that gripped him at a personal level. So he had both the personality level and the psyche level at play, pushing him to interpret and create. His fascination with creativity equaling "me" to a greater power activated the cleverness that Gene loved to access from his personality strategy and his creative skill. M referred to the mass of knowledge or experience one accumulates. As in my Phase Diagram, his interpretation of the two dimensions of experience first included the external life experience path and the internal life experience path. He described one's unique patterns of thinking: looking, interpreting, interacting; one's curiosity, intuition, insight, and inspiration. Then, in the e he saw all of these qualities squared—the ways in which our external and internal lives interact to be able to produce new insights and new energies that fuel our self-expression.

In my diagram, this squaring would be at the place of the shift, the time and space for the confrontations within the personality and the psyche from our inner worlds, interacting with changes that manifest in our outer worlds, preparing the ground for healing, which meant that these levels corresponded and communicated in tandem with one another—an alignment occurring and releasing new energy. He writes:

> Whatever life's variables, $C = me^2$ tells us that you cannot dismiss yourself as a candidate for creative potential. No matter what your age, and especially as you grow older, you do have the capacity for creative expression. The challenge is to recognize it and use it. . . . It is that inner voice that whispers: "Why not?" (The Creative Age, p. 38)

Our understanding of psychic development also overlapped in Gene's perspective on adult development. Developmental psychologist Erik Erikson delineated eight stages of psychological development and then later in life with his wife, Joan Erikson, a ninth stage.[4] Gene expanded on these stages for older adults, and created his four phases of human potential, in which he reiterated that developmental growth cannot be forced. "Wisdom comes to us this way, largely a developmental product of age, smarts, and emotional and practical life experience," he wrote in The Creative Age.[5] Writing extensively on Piaget's "post-formal thought," he described it as a

> thought process that helps integrate the subjective and the objective, feeling and thinking, the heart and the mind, and emerges with aging. It plays a

role in allowing us to understand and express emotions—an asset for any of
us pedestrians along the walk of life. Post-formal reasoning also fosters the
ability to respond to complex situations with more than one right answer.
Post-formal thought transforms our life experience into what we commonly
call "wisdom." (The Creative Age, p. 77)

Gene created his phases, much as I had created mine, because we all need a frame of reference or mirror so we can see ourselves growing and visualize the effects and interactions of our inner resources and our life circumstances. This is what allows us to enliven our lives. My language appears more existential than his, so my diagram focuses on the intrapsychic and spiritual confrontations and exchanges. Yet his goal was exactly the same: "to revive our lives in meaningful, satisfying ways." For me, that is the essence of not only a developmental but also an existential perspective.

If we were to overlay both of our models of developmental phases, we might imagine his *midlife re-evaluation phase,* in which one's creative energy is shaped by a sense of crisis or opportunity, as similar to my first phase, called *entry. Entry* names the reason or event that forces us to re-evaluate. It could take place in either our inner or outer worlds. Gene went on to describe how we are motivated toward more gratifying choices as it is a time that forces reflection.

In his *liberation phase,* he charts more personal freedom and experimentation. He places it into a framework of time and age. I place my two *confrontation phases* that would accompany his *liberation phase* into a framework of circumstances that in many ways match his timeline in age terms. But because I see these phases as occurring over and over again intrapsychically, I don't label them according to age. I see them as spiraling through the relationships of understanding between parts of ourselves, younger ages focusing on taming our personalities, which releases more of our potential as we get older to work with the energies from our creative psyches. These two *confrontation phases* within my diagram are like a spiraling process, returning again and again over time, and certainly they deepen with age and wisdom.

Gene also writes about what he calls "inner drives" in *The Mature Mind.* He believed that our adult development is fueled by the natural impetus for growth and that this natural impetus for growth comes from an *inner push,* in which our brains and our selves are constantly inviting us to create our own paths, choices, and integrations. I see this *inner push* as exactly what emerges from the resources of our psyche, in the third phase on the inner path, *confrontation with the psyche,* when these resources finally have space to breathe, as they have cut through the landscape (with both its hindrances and its openings) of our personality. It has its own force, has its own release, and functions exactly as he describes, like something larger than us that pushes from within and changes our capacity.

In Gene's *summing-up phase*, he describes a time filled with so many creative contributions from one's life. In my phase, *turning point: the shift toward healing*, there is a kind of resolution, a turning toward the resources released through the inner push. Gene's *encore phase* is a time of reflection and celebration, but certainly those words describe the rituals that accompany the process of continuing our developmental growth with this kind of acceptance, comfort, and alignment. It's not that I am equating my final phase, *healing*, with Gene's *encore phase*, but it certainly makes sense that taking care of unfinished business and celebrating the complexity of our lives bring healing. We feel more whole. We feel more wise. We take care of unfinished business and that affirms our lives.

Gene's work on his creativity equation, his midlife phases of human potential, and developmental intelligence reflected an example of his own creative process at work to map the territory for others. Dreams, science, clinical experience, and his own creativity informed his understanding of the interior life and lifelong potential.

The task of integration calls upon us to become creative detectives in this land of creativity, aging, and illness time, and as creative detectives, we are forced to grapple with both darkness and light to make meaning. This is ultimately the primary requirement of creativity: embodied meaning, something we can *feel*, something we *experience*. Many of us may not see ourselves as creative; we may be more familiar with using predominantly intellectual capacities, and yet, we are thrust by circumstances into needing to understand our emotional, spiritual, and physical or kinesthetic faculties. Health requires us to become holistic in our thinking so that we can be both creative and present as we gain greater understanding of our experience and move toward healing. These experiences with illness and aging can offer us images of balance and renewal for the well-being of our whole person. It is our personality, psyche, and spirit that play creative roles in their interactions and movement toward integration. They are our resources for healing, giving both personal and collective meaning crucial to the values of our health and wellness.

Creativity? Healing? They are one and the same, with the same task.

Part Three

NEW LANDSCAPES

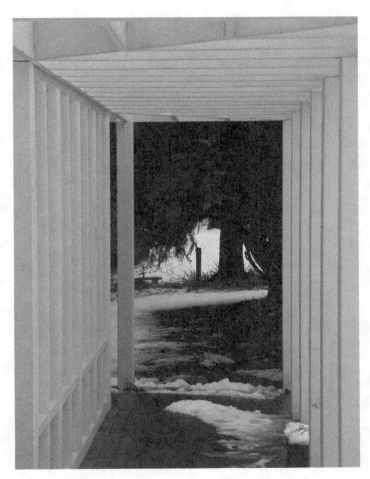

Figure III.i Winter boxwood trees and pergola entry site at Miller's art and expressive arts therapy studio in Kensington, MD. Photography by Wendy L. Miller.

7

Creative Detective

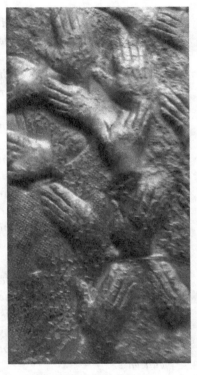

Figure 7.1 "Reaching" (2007), sculpey polymer clay with powdered Pearl-Ex pigments, 8 × 4 × 1 inches. Artwork by Wendy L. Miller, photo credit: Joshua Soros.

In my work as a therapist I often envision myself in the role of a detective, searching for the clues that are buried or stand out as atypical. I am a creative detective, and I need to be one. I spend my days walking and talking with people through their inner landscapes, discovering and uncovering clues. I am always looking for tidbits of information that have been forgotten or left behind. I search for remnants.

As an artist, I have come to understand change in terms of rearrangement of shape and pattern formations. People live under different conditions, including medical illnesses, and the changes in identity that accompany and are accompanied by physical, emotional, and often spiritual challenges.

Gene was fascinated not only by identity development, but also with how we challenge ourselves creatively and what happens to us through such engagement. He was a creative detective who found insight in the overlap of literature and science.

In Nicholas Meyer's novel and screenplay, The Seven Percent Solution, the meeting of the legendary Sherlock Holmes and the eminent Sigmund Freud is described in detail.[1] Meyer advises us that: "This story is true, only the facts have been made up." Both Holmes and Freud are entering midlife and a new stage of cognitive development described as post-formal thought that is apparent when the right and left hemispheres of the brain begin working in better synchrony with one another.

This more mature form of reasoning is characterized by enhanced synthetic thinking and a greater capacity to reconcile seemingly contra-dictory findings—critical in detective work, whether by a sleuth or a psy-choanalyst. Holmes is at a turning point in his life in that his very close friend, Dr. Watson, has arranged for him to see Freud for treatment to recover from his cocaine habit and the adverse consequences it is hav-ing on Holmes' work. Freud, himself, is at a turning point in his career in his rise to fame, and in the interchanges between the psychiatrist and the detective, Freud benefits from criticism he receives from Holmes. One such poignant moment is when Holmes is at first patiently listening to Freud's description of one his cases; then Holmes becomes increasingly impatient with Freud's perceptions, and strongly admonishes the good doctor: "Dr. Freud, you see but you do not observe, a faculty you must cultivate."

Later Freud acknowledges the invaluable contributions that Holmes makes to his observing skills by crediting Holmes: "I have borrowed some of his techniques and have applied them to the mind."

Holmes, in turn, becomes impressed with Freud's improved abilities, now complimenting him: "Your powers of observation and inference could make you a great detective."

What Holmes initially noted about Freud—"You see but you do not observe"—captures how for so long science and society viewed aging. They saw but did not observe. This coupled with the historian Daniel Boorstin's observation that "the greatest obstacle to discovery is not ignorance, but the illusion of knowledge,"[2] reveals the one-two punch that knocked out progress in the field of aging for so long. The interchange between Holmes and Freud also reveals that even the best and the brightest can fail at accurately observing when they are studying an issue. One of the best illustrations of this failure among the best and the brightest is found in the history of views about neurogenesis.

In 1913, Santiago Ramón y Cajal, the great Spanish neuroanatomist who won the Nobel Prize in Physiology or Medicine in 1913, emphasized that "in the adult central nervous system the nerve paths are something fixed, ended, and immutable."[3] Cajal and the leading neuroscientists who followed him throughout most of the 20th century vehemently asserted that nerve cells (neurons) in the brain do not regenerate; neurogenesis was not possible. Their gold standard argument was that nerve cells are not liver cells that can regenerate; they are neurons and neurons do not have the capacity to regenerate—case closed!

A new observation was reported that challenged the view that neurogenesis does not take place in the brain. In the 1980s, Fernando Nottebohm, a bird specialist, became fascinated with the ability of songbirds to sing new songs each season. Upon examining their brains, he made the remarkable discovery that each year, during the season the birds sing most, they generate new brain cells in the part of the brain involved in learning songs.[4] But here is where the illusion of knowledge trumped the observation when the question was raised whether the generation of new brain cells could also be happening in humans. The response again by leading neuroscientists was "no, neurogenesis is not possible in humans!"

But then a truly extraordinary discovery was made at the end of 1998 that revealed how so many of the best and brightest in neuroscience, during even the late 20th century, were unable to look outside the box. The neuroscientists equated neurogenesis—new neuron formation— with regeneration, and continued to assert with a sense of unassailable knowledge that neurons do not and cannot regenerate. What was discovered in a part of the brain known as the dentate gyrus, located in the hippocampus (the part of the brain that processes memories for storage), was a nest of stem cells from which new neuron formation— neurogenesis—happened.[5] The best and the brightest in looking but not observing fixated only on regeneration; they failed to fathom de novo neuron formation independent of regeneration. Their illusion of knowledge, that neurogenesis was not in the genes with aging, interfered with their looking and their observing.

There is more to the story. The bias against growth and development with aging—related to the illusion of knowledge about aging—is so strong that it generates negative knee-jerk reactions to any suggestions of something positive about aging. Hence, when neurogenesis with aging in humans was identified and established, the naysayers took the posture, "Well it's less in the old than the young." But when the discoverers of neurogenesis looked further they found in animal studies that while neurogenesis was less in older animals than younger ones, when the older and younger animals were placed in an enriched, more stimulating environment, the magnitude of neurogenesis was significantly greater in the older animals than in the younger ones. There was a two-fold increase in neurogenesis among the young mice placed in an enriched environment, compared to young mice placed in a standard environment. They then found that there was a three-fold increase in neurogenesis in the old mice placed in an enriched environment, compared to old mice placed in a standard environment.

The ramifications of this research on the value of our challenging our minds—activities that we ourselves can arrange and engage in—are profound.

What about my own life? I feel too close emotionally to observe well as my own creative detective, and yet I need those skills and insights more than ever. This is my husband, not someone else's husband, whom I'm trying to help. What do I need to do, really? A friend of mine once described my work as "holy"—collaborating with someone in service of health. She was referring to the therapist's role with a client, but it is the same for any of us when we become committed partners this way.

I try to hold onto the creative and holy aspects of living through our illness experience, but it is definitely a challenge discerning which internal stirrings need our attention. What does it mean to be a creative detective? This is the point at which language can fall short but images can speak. I painted what I felt, what I sensed that Gene seemed to be feeling, what the family body was experiencing: two shapes on a page, rough scratched, etched colors, one side with dangly chaotic silver thread embedded in wax, the other with vertically laid silver threads—cracked down the middle, separated into their own edges (See Figure 11.1). There was so much going on for Gene, for me, and for our families that no conversation could hold it; there were so many threads left dangling and stuck together.

When I am nervous about changing the chemotherapy, it is because I fear that they have lost hope and are just trying anything to give us something new rather than trying to figure out what truly makes sense, which of course is the real meaning of hope for us. My mind imagines atypical medicines for an atypical person. And I want the doctors to think in that magical way. My mind searches for clues in past experience to learn what is best to do.

With my mom's cancer, I listened and I read about all of what could be in the progression of the illness. The same with my dad. Each of them developed atypical blood cancers: mom, multiple myeloma; dad, chronic myeloid leukemia. But both of them died from something else, or was it really something else? Mom's heart stopped. Dad had a stroke. But now I wonder, did her heart stop because of its own course or because her immune system was so depleted from treatment that there was nothing to fight the bacterial infection she caught that day? I saw something similar with Gene when we first started chemotherapy and his temperature would rise to 104 degrees and we would rush to the emergency room, where his blood pressure was so low and his heart rate so fast. Could his heart die from the stress of that atypical rhythm? Is that what really happened to my mom?

Or my dad's stroke—could it have really been a side effect from the leukemia medications he had taken or the changes made to blood thinner medications, or was it actually that so much had been rearranged in his system that something else went out of whack? Seriously out of whack. What makes me nervous is that chemotherapies or treatments rearrange things in other places in the body and no one is necessarily looking in those other places.

I think about a dream that Gene had:

> *I dreamt it was dark and I was looking out as if I were on a bluff or else on a train that had either stopped at a station or was moving toward its destination. Directly across from me—parallel to my position—I saw an amorphous outline of a form or face that looked to be in a rage as in pain, and was yelling or screaming at me, but in silence. It had some dark red or bloodlike coloring, appearing ominous.*
>
> *Suddenly, I felt the other form was myself either in my inner psychological or physical life or even in a parallel universe. I felt it was trying to get me. Overall, it elicited a feeling of terror and angst that if it reached me, terrible things would happen.*
>
> *At the same time, there was a faint, vague feeling of empathy and sadness that it elicited, as if it were trapped and in misery, trying to escape. But I felt it would be a very serious mistake to have contact, and if such happened, a bad outcome for me would follow.*
>
> *I thought of the image of Woody Allen looking from a train window, seeing himself in a different state across the tracks in another train going in the opposite direction.[6] But this parallel form was stationary or moving at exactly the same speed and in the same direction as I was, staying opposite to me, parallel all the time. Its activity and agitation were increasing, though it still could not reach me, and in a growing state of uneasiness, I awoke.*

Gene's dreams, clinical reflections, forebodings, and spontaneous flashes of insight, along with my own, might as well have been a continuous tickertape of news and clues. We were surrounded by evidence but never sure what to make of it, wary of premature conclusions.

Together our dreams were like vivid novels not being written by someone else but by our own inner selves. Dreams awakened Gene to a hidden potential to write thrillers. If he could dream them, why couldn't he write them? And for me, the inner knowing and description of emotional landscapes brought forth the writer in me who had been recording dreams since a child, listening and playing with dreams at work all day long; now they became a partner in my own voice.

Dreams: Threat or Beauty?

Gene's dreams "knew something," as if there were an authority to the unconscious—the unconscious competence I mentioned earlier.[7] That doesn't necessarily mean that we knew in any complete sense what they were expressing, but they did speak to something inside of us that was deeply connected to a psychophysical process. His dreams pumped adrenalin—adrenalin that he had to keep in check during the day and yet refilled itself each night. Like the Sorcerer's Apprentice,[8] the harder and faster he bailed, the more swiftly the dark dreams arrived to flood his sleep and spill over into his days. He read the cryptic biochemical message embedded in his dreams: his body knew, the adrenalin knew that he had to use every ounce of his system to escape the cleverness of cancer; that the cancer could get you in any way, any day, that it would come in from left field. And of course it was, in fact, already always *there*: a constant presence biologically as well as in the unconscious. For more than thirteen years these dreams came up with different scenarios, activating the adrenalin, injecting a maintenance dose of fear on a nightly basis. What kind of knowing is that? Is it part of our creative faculty?[9]

> But then again, the conscious world of purposeful thought and reflection can hide what we can't allow ourselves to bring to the surface. Shortly after my diagnosis, I began to have recurring nightmares characterized by a repeating theme—one I never before had experienced in my dreams. For the first year, more nights than not, the nightmares would occur, gradually tapering, but not at all disappearing in the second year. Even now, I will occasionally have one of these nightmares, usually following a day when prostate cancer was very active in my consciousness or if something unsettling happened in relation to my illness or treatment.
>
> These nightmares have been unusual in that each one has had the same terrifying theme of my being chased or attacked by ominous figures

or creatures with the goal of killing me. Though the theme is always the same, the content is always different. While I dread having these dreams, I marvel at the unvarying consistency of their theme but constantly changing content—like whodunits that always have different stories, or a "Perils of Pauline" format.[10] They are like a very long running (with no reruns) TV horror series that I cannot shut off. Yet, each dream had striking visual elements, often suggesting natural beauty, art, Americana, or movie-like sets—such as images from great paintings, historic architecture, wondrous natural vistas, classic cars, and theatrical street scenes, as well as extraordinary lighting and colors. But in each dream the terror overrides the beauty. In describing them, they at times have comic book violence qualities, but in the dream they all feel too real. Each dream portrays my life being in severe jeopardy, with me escaping only in the final moment and in the most unlikely manner. At the moment of my escape, I typically awaken somewhat out of breath and sweating.

1997, ONE YEAR POST INITIAL DIAGNOSIS

In my dream, I am standing in a striking sunlit field of towering golden grass, moving lyrically in the gentle breeze, with the sunlight shimmering off them. It is an unusually bright and beautiful day, with the field flowing into a fertile valley at the foot of majestic mountains rising into a deep blue sky with soft patchy very white clouds. I am standing there savoring the extraordinary beauty, when suddenly the whole environment becomes blurry in the midst of a powerful tremor, stirring unsettling and ominous feelings. The tremor ceases and the blurriness fades away, as gradually two exotic birds appear in the distance. As they approach, it becomes apparent they are not exotic, but prehistoric. They are pterodactyls—flying dinosaurs.

They were huge, with wingspans of about 40 feet, and terrifying lance like beaks, at least six feet in length. The birds pause and peer at me. Then one starts flying full speed toward me with its beak aimed at my eyes. I quickly scan my surroundings and can see no hiding places, no way for an escape. The pterodactyl is practically upon me, and I feel it's about to be my demise, when unexpectedly I spot out of the corner of my eye a 50 pound bail of hay just a few feet from where I am standing. I rush to it and with a tremendous effort lift it and throw it at the pterodactyl just as it is about to lance me between the eyes. The bail hits is beak and the creature is knocked abruptly to the ground, stunned, dazed. It wobbles upright and flies off to join its mate. Then the two of them focus once more on me, at which point I lift the bail again. They choose instead to fly off, and I awaken from my state of terror, panting.

5/24/98

I dreamt I died. In my dream, I was going to the funeral, wondering whether in some way my death could be reversed. I recalled a movie where Superman's girlfriend died, but Superman figured out how to fly at the speed of light such that time could be reversed and he could intervene for his girlfriend.[11] But I was not Superman, nor could I fly. Then I realized that in traveling to the funeral I didn't have my bag with me. I must have left it at the airport. I started to go back for it, but was told it would interfere with the funeral. At first, I hesitated, then thought, "I need that bag." So I left to go get it. The next thing I knew, I realized that in so doing, my death was cancelled.

6/21/98

It is Father's Day. In my dream, it was like there was a seal, a large rectangular thin flat lid that kept out what wasn't good for me and kept in—holding together—my essence. The seal then seemed to be separating at the edges, with some of my essence beginning to ooze out. It was as if I myself was in a tall narrow rectangular container—like Houdini[12]— the lid being above my head. At this point, at a slight distance away, a second intact seal appeared. I had a hopeful feeling about it, but the turmoil and deeply unsettling feeling surrounding the seal in jeopardy awoke me in a sweat.

8/1998

I am in a classical Italian plaza. The plaza is nearly deserted. It looks like a de Chirico surrealistic painting.[13] It is late in the day with the sun about to set. There is a sharp distinction between the part of the plaza with its deep muted colors of orange, brown, and green lit by dim light and the part filled with very dark shadows. Classical statues and small isolated figures in the plaza are overpowered by their own shadows. The architecture is that of oppressive arcades with stark white facades in the lit part of the plaza and nearly black ones in the shadowy part where I am hiding. I am being chased by a huge ominous man, nearly 10 feet tall with the largest head I have ever seen—the size of two basketballs. His face is contorted. He is wearing a black heavy wool suit that looks like it was purchased very cheaply at a second-hand store. His hat is the size of a small umbrella. I move down narrow alleys off the plaza. They are lined by narrow historic row houses, all in dark shadows.

Just as I think I have evaded the monstrous man, by sneaking down another alley, he reappears around a corner behind me. He is now getting closer with his arms outstretched to grab my neck and strangle me. I dash down one more alley in a desperate attempt to elude him, only to find it dead-ends. The alley is unusually narrow, with barely enough space for one car to traverse. My pursuer sees that I am trapped and a broad sinister sneer covers his grotesque countenance. His oversized hands are now on my throat, and I realize my end is near. Then, suddenly, out of nowhere, a white van appears slowly traveling down the alley. It barely avoids scraping the houses on both sides, I flatten myself as tight as I can against the front of one of the houses to avoid being run over, and the monster attempts the same, but his head is too big and as the van passes, his huge head gets caught and crushed. As I feel his hands loosen on my neck and his breath leaving him, I once again awaken, shaken and breathing heavily.

2008

It is a movie-like street scene. Wendy and I usually did not make presentations together, but in the dream we had been invited to participate in a small conference of select participants, presenting on novel work. The group gathered in what appeared to be an elegant, intimate library—a single room with warm wood paneled walls with rich brown tones, bookcases, and a striking, magnificently crafted dark mahogany long conference table around which everyone gathered. Wendy and I were first, and we presented our work in a complementary manner, each elaborating on the other's as we discussed our ideas.

Some kind of break—perhaps for lunch—occurred. The next thing I knew I was at a visually impressive intersection taking me to a broad boulevard lined by chic stores and restaurants with a beautiful background of rolling hills behind them. I was driving a large 1960ish sedan, and felt like I was in a scene of the old 1960s TV drama, "77 Sunset Strip."[14] Then out of nowhere a man came up to the driver's window of my car. He looked like someone I knew, though I couldn't quite place him. He appeared good-looking, but almost entirely in gray—his hair, face, and clothes. He stood in marked contrast to the sunny, blue sky day, generating an unsettling feeling from his unstable presence. Without warning, he pulled out a revolver, placed it against my window, and said "I am going to have to kill you."

I felt cornered with but moments remaining for me, but realized my engine was still on, and that I was in gear with my foot on the brake. I looked the gray man in the eye to engage him, and simultaneously floored the gas pedal to both create a roar and a jump start that I hoped would sufficiently startle and distract him, and in the same motion ducked down beneath the window out of direct line with the barrel of the gun. I also turned the steering wheel from this position, such that the car leaped over the curb and

roared down the wide boulevard. Bullets immediately followed me, shatter-
ing and moving through my rear and front windows. I felt a few bullets whiz
by my shoulders and forehead. As I was moving out of his range, I woke up
in a sweat.

Gene's dreams hit on certain images: the pterodactyl, the seal, the man with the huge head. In each of these dreams, these threatening creatures or strangers were trying to get him. His dreams were telling us over and over that there were these various kinds of pursuers and narrow straits, narrow spaces, narrow escapes. "Like Houdini," he said. Metaphorically, that was the whole point—the narrow escape of health. That is creative detective work. Dreams could be called the creative architect, for they shape the material and build a story that carries a message, but we have to be the creative detective and figure out the associations that make sense to us. Our dreams, our drawings, our reflections, and our reveries: our psyche generates this creative material for us. We can and need to work with it in our conscious mode to translate it and draw value from it.

The Authority of the Unconscious

In my work, we facilitate this process of mind–body imagery through an "intermodal" expressive arts process, going from one creative mode to another. A drawing may lead to a poem, leading to a sculpture, a sand tray, an enactment, or a physical movement. The aim is that the movement through these creative channels gives us an experience we can actually sense though our bodies. Paolo Knill, my friend, colleague, and mentor in the field of expressive arts therapy, theorizes that this process is based on the concept of *crystallization*.[15]

In crystallization what is important therapeutically is not just an insight itself, but rather that things come together on many levels and crystallize into an element of knowing, a surprise—and often more than merely a surprising insight. He calls it "the arrival of the third," meaning the emergence of a new imaginal realm. The same language is used at times to describe the new, shared ground of being in the psyche between life partners, or between a therapist and client, a doctor and patient, or an individual and God or spirit. Image also creates this new, original shared space in the psyche, working on many levels, crystallizing them into one: the unconscious, the imagination, the emotional body, the intellect, and the physical body. Image moves and guides a person toward wholeness. To work with evoked imagery, we dialog with image—we make associations, we talk with it, we move with it, we listen to it—to take in its energy. Each modality affects and deepens image, allowing the crystallization at a sensory, experiential level.

This process of association and exchange goes into what the British psychoanalyst Christopher Bollas calls the "not knowing,"[16] or what the English pediatrician and psychoanalyst D. W. Winnicott refers to as the "transitional phenomenon" or "transitional space."[17] We are forced to grapple and to make meaning with this ongoing and uncomfortable experience of uncertainty in our lives, and we often need a particular emotional environment to do it in. This practice of being with uncertainty is aided by creative engagement. The good news is that the psyche releases its creative resources through images and sensations. The bad news is that most often we are clueless as to how to respond to or work with this communication because it can confuse us. It is so cryptic and symbolic that we have a hard time understanding it, much less accepting it and trusting its authority. This "competent unconscious" draws from our wholeness of mind. It is intrinsically holistic.

In my clinical practice, the creative detective work that my clients do is inspiring. It's not easy work to venture into open inquiry and introspection, prepared to follow clues wherever they may lead.[18] The outcome is inherently uncertain, after all. Particularly for many older persons who are accomplished and busy becoming even more accomplished, there can be a perceived risk to new information or insight. A fifty-nine year old client, whom I'll call Daniel, was struggling to free himself from a highly enticing, highly lucrative business career that had seized control of his life. He had neglected other parts of his life: relationship, love, commitment, health. He described the feeling as a vortex of driven ambition, one in which he felt out of control in a chaos that was "all about confusion, blur, and anxiety." In our sessions, he drew furious tornado-like images that depicted him swept up into them. Then one day he told me that he realized he had been clutching to old habits when trying to find a new path, and his old habits weren't helpful. They only led him helplessly back into the vortex. He began to gain control over the seemingly random inner turmoil through experimenting with new external images as trial scenarios for new options in his life, allowing himself to experience how these images felt as he explored them. He drew a spinning vortex, anchors thrown off of it to slow it down; tainted and encapsulated hearts; and beams of light. His drawings began to reflect a new sense of balance and receptivity to constructive change, and one day he spoke of a sense of "before" having given way to a new "after." He described the feeling being as if an immovable beam of light had focused his attention previously on a limited view of what life held for him. But with his growing awareness of capacity for change, he felt that this churning had positioned a prism in his mind, directly in the path of that immovable beam of light. The light was now splitting into an array of new beams with different colors, representing the new emotional tones entering his consciousness about what was starting to appear possible for him.

Daniel had a well-cultivated inner voice track about his value and his accomplishments, and it was a very addictive track. It said: "This is my addiction and my hunger, to constantly reinforce my external accomplishments. I will keep you on this track." That inner voice—the pre-crisis personality style that he had clung to so tightly for so long—was a lot like the immovable beam of light, focusing his attention and energy on a narrow path of purpose. The image of the prism that broke the single beam of light into the full spectrum of possibility became a conscious tool for Daniel, a new lens for creative detection. Now his path was illuminated with new potential for engagement and expression.

In Gene's reflections on the Holmes quote, "you see but you do not observe," he touched on this aspect of our own (or doctors') filters on perception that often get in the way of our recognizing what is truly present in what we see or hear or feel. This is what I call the mind–body confrontation. I thought with Gene that we knew what the problem was, knew what we were treating, knew what we were doing. But then this "something else," what I called *confrontation with the psyche* in my Phase Diagram, showed up. It wreaks havoc on the system at a time when a person, who may be struggling through illness or crisis, is most vulnerable. The shift also can be moving on a trajectory that is foreign to us, at least at first, as in Daniel's experience. It is the time when most people try hard to stay in their role or stick to their strategy because their locus of control is shifting so rapidly. Learning this new language, a right-brain, non-analytical, germinal language of imagery and sensation, can be frightening, overwhelming, or exciting. Confronted with an image that is supposed to hold some meaning for us, say a prism shape, most of us would naturally question: "What does this prism shape have to do with my crisis?" or a patient might say "I came in here to get well, but we are paying even more attention to my pain." And yet, the power of imagery is that it speaks its truth in its own language of sensation, sometimes clearer than linear logic allows.

Narrative-illness writers, doctors, and patients themselves all tell us that it is our suffering that wants to be accompanied with care and witnessed by the presence of another.[19] These tasks are not the work of fixing what is broken, for as whole selves, we are not broken, though we may have parts of us that feel that way sometimes. But like the teenage boy who felt he would never belong to the blue people, we can feel invisible, erased, ignored from the truths of our experience. In a way, too, we sometimes withhold evidence from the "creative detective" in ourselves and in others who care about us. We may be unsure of ourselves in terms of what to tell, what we feel can be heard and understood, or what detail matters. Our stories can feel un-story-worthy to us because we may find that others are put off by them, or confused or worried by them. We end up feeling unheard. Yet, it is in the telling and retelling that we find not only ourselves but also the connections and clarity that the stories hold for us. Clues, clues, and more clues. We learn from one another, from each others' stories. They remind us of our responsibility as patients to continue to tell our stories, because we are the ones who can shed light on whatever piece of the human condition we know.

Caregivers in our increasingly strapped healthcare settings are confronting these stories, often ill equipped to respond to that narrative and accompanying issues of spirituality and creativity in people facing medical illnesses and major life transitions. We need to re-examine the shared ground of creativity, therapy, and spirituality, which at their roots have always been connected to health and medicine, but which have been, in our healthcare system, somehow disembodied from our care.

I think of Alice, a patient in her late forties, and mother of three young boys. She is emblematic of middle-age women who struggle with all that they have to juggle, all those they tend, and the sense of losing touch with the self, an unavailability of the self that accompanies the process. At forty, both her grandmother and, three months later, her mother died. In midlife, a mere six years later, she is trying to understand her life: loving a husband who is so different from her, and tending children so different from one another, knowing these are all blessings in her life, yet constantly feeling frustrated, as if loving family were a job, when in fact what she needs is to be fulfilled in other personal and existential ways.

She sees her husband, who is from Spain, as a difficult match. He was a kind of rescuer in their younger days, but she no longer feels that she needs to be rescued; she needs to be met and understood. Her therapy is very much about how we *see* (not just a visual seeing but a collecting of insights) into a person when we are available and connected and how we love to "see into" because it is a learning and sharing process. She feels that she is not able to see this way in her relationship with her husband because he thinks all day long in what she refers to as "a different numbering system," her way of saying that they no longer share a common frame of reference for their relationship and, as a result, their relationship no longer feels right to her. He works creating mobile software systems, in practical terms a language they once shared in their work together in the telecommunication business. They had done very well as business-intellectual-money partners. But as their business became a big company, and their children were in elementary school and their needs were more demanding on her time, her midlife evaluation came as a desire for an affair with a "soul mate type" and a desire for her own creativity in writing and filmmaking.

Her drawings require determined detective work as she attempts to see them clearly and glean from them. In her drawings, she is trying to show her deep sense of invisibility; the feeling of just not being seen.

Alice notes about our sessions: "I can come in and have a lot of disparate stuff and it's like I toss you stuff and we build a flashlight." That is her description of what we do in our work of art therapy. We reconnect to her creative center from which she can make all the decisions she is struggling to make. The decisions have to be made from that centered place. In the dark, we only see some aspects of things and we make assumptions about what we are seeing versus what is really there. But it isn't always the full picture. So, we build a flashlight because we need to shine the light on all the places we can find—the corners, the crevasses, the atmospheres—and confront what we see.

The flashlight. The prism. The dreams. We need all of them, at times to focus our attention so we can see the up-close piece that is showing itself, to look closely, and at other times to allow ourselves to see a fuller spectrum of our selves, our circumstances, and our possibilities, to try to look at as much of the whole as we ever can.

Art is a holistic language. Illness is a holistic language as well. The body does not separate itself from the psyche to express itself. Body and psyche may express themselves in different colors, shapes, textures, images, rhythms, movements, pitches, timbres, energetic tensions, spatial compositions, or forms, but they are both present. The psychiatrist and futurist Charles Johnston describes scientific thought as the focus on the smallest atom, which is fundamental to this thought; he writes that what is fundamental in spiritual thought is essence; and in creative causality, what is fundamental he describes as a formative process: "the story of how things come into being, mature, and transform."[20] The language necessary for this formative process is the language of imagery.

The process of being a creative detective is about what we have to uncover to do that, what we have to look for, and how we have to not only look but really see. Gene's fascination with Sherlock Holmes and the relationship to Freud in the *Seven Percent Solution* is really a metaphor for the complexity of this kind of detective work.

Gene's capacity to climb into his computer when he was faced with challenge was a familiar sight—his inner creative detective showing itself. Be it on our porch, in a messy section of his large office, at the hospital, in the chemotherapy treatment room, or in his chair in front of the lake, there he would sit, his notebook or computer in front of him, sometimes with closed eyes, sometimes with a finger tapping, phrases forming in his mind like his teabag soaking in his cup—slowly deepening, absorbing, lying still in the process of strengthening flavor. Most of us looked at him, but did not necessarily see that this really was what Gene's creativity was: tapping into the potential of his resources at exactly the moments in time when he was up against adversity. It focused him. It also distracted him, engaged him, and invested him with insights, awarenesses, and connections that only he could make. I know no other person who could climb inward with the same fervor and wisdom that he had, as if he and his mental arrangements were a cave of respite. It was as if he learned a way to look and—as Sherlock Holmes described—not just see, but observe.

The Authority of the Unconscious Speaks Aloud

Through his creative engagement of science, literature, art, and his own inner world, Gene became his own creative detective, making associations and meaning. In January 2009, when Gene's urinary problems became diagnosed as the long-feared return of the metastatic prostate cancer, there were various rounds of procedures necessary. His bladder or urethra was blocked by tumors, and once this happens, there are serious and potentially fatal problems for the kidneys. Gene needed a surgical procedure called nephrostomy, in which a catheter tube is inserted through the skin and into the kidney. A fine guide wire follows the initial needle, and then the catheter, which is about the same diameter as IV (intravenous) tubing, follows the guide wire to its correct location. At first, the tube is then connected to a bag outside the body that collects the urine. Later, to remove the bag, the doctor does another procedure to open the tube.

Gene's series of procedures, done on both kidneys, took months because he also had to start the aggressive chemotherapy at the same time. By the time the medical team went to open the second nephrostomy tube, we acted as though we were pros in this process. The procedure usually takes less than an hour, but this time it seemed quite a while before the doctor came to me. When he did, the first thing he said was, "He is fine. But today is your day to go buy a lottery ticket." He proceeded to describe to me what had taken place. It turns out that it was very difficult on this second kidney to insert the nephrostomy tube and to slowly push it until it reached the kidney. This is all necessary so that the tube will be secured in place inside or outside the body, and a stent, which is like a balloon on the end, is placed in the kidney. When the balloon is filled, it helps to hold the tube in place. For some reason, the blockage was such that it was very difficult for the doctor to push the tube through. He tried and tried and finally said out loud, "We'll have to stop. I just can't get this one in." Out of whatever twilight state of anesthesia Gene was in, he spoke out loud and the doctor heard him. The doctor said that Gene had piped up, "Keep trying, doc. I can take it." And who can explain it, but the doctor listened, went ahead another time, and this time he made it through. The creative detective within Gene had located the one necessary piece of authority at exactly the right moment, spoken to exactly the right person. As the doctor later said to me, "This was a chance-in-a-million moment."

One month later, there we were in the hospital, in February 2009, and Gene had started the frontline chemotherapy for prostate cancer, Taxotere.[21] He had high fevers and low blood pressure, and the doctors frankly gave us very little information as to what to expect. Apparently, these are familiar reactions to the drug, but we didn't know that. To us it suddenly just seemed like he wouldn't make it, not from the cancer itself but from some tangential unknown. I was reminded of the euphemism of the nonspecific in "died from complications of . . ." I could see now how someone could actually die from the treatment before the disease did them in. I could see so easily how much danger chemotherapy creates as it works to kill cancer cells.

I was sitting in the corner of the hospital with one of Gene's doctors, who had called me to come in to see him at seven that night. I didn't know he had already been talking with Gene. I was sitting with him by myself in the corner of the hallway and he was telling me, "It is going to go fast Wendy. It doesn't look good."

"What do you mean fast?" I ask.

"Five weeks," he says.

"Five weeks? How can that be? Look at him. He has been doing so well."

"When the chemo doesn't work, it moves very fast."

It made no sense to me. When you haven't been there, haven't seen what the doctor has seen, it makes no sense. But I could see that Gene's internist was upset. He was anxious. He was sad. From this place, he began to tell me that he himself had done an internship at Sloan-Kettering, and he saw this situation so often that he had made his own decision to do family work instead of oncology.

He gave me advice about going to a different cancer center than the one we were using in the community. The picture of Gene going away and living in a hospital bed in a faraway place, not living at home with Eliana and me, was beyond anything I could contemplate. And, even if we did, what were they going to do— give him a different chemo? We already were going to one of the top oncologists in the field in prostate cancer research at the Johns Hopkins Kimmel Cancer Center in Baltimore Maryland. He was a member of the Brady Urological Institute and a co-leader of the Prostate Cancer Program and the Chemical Therapeutics Program within the Cancer Center. Gene had been meeting with him for years now discussing what they would do if his cancer escaped the hormone treatments and he needed to do chemo. He had set up his team of thinkers long ago, and they were working together on the protocol. So how could we do any better than that? Why would we go anywhere else now?

But I didn't say any of that. His internist knew all of that. Clearly he was upset, and I was speechless. He quickly got up to talk to Gene about something else, some new thought he had. When I went back into the room to sit with Gene, we just held hands on the bed. We could hardly talk. We were living our life. Certainly those past times when we had rushed to the emergency room with high fevers or low blood pressure from the side effects of chemotherapy had pulled us out of our lives, but, in general, most days, most weeks, we were living our life. What do you say in those moments? We are speechless. Holding hands, crying, ashen, no color to our faces or our thoughts, we are stunned into silence.

I come home—a walking sleeping zombie—because I have to. Eliana has to go to school in the morning. I leave the hospital at 9:30 P.M. I come home and drop into a sleep that is so unreal I can't even move from it. In the morning, after I come home from carpool, the phone rings and Gene wants to know if I have taken her already. "Yes," I begin.

"Can you come in here? Come now."

I come in and he is a different person. What has he done? He has ordered the test results. He wants to see the data himself. He doesn't want the interpretation of the tests, he wants the test results, and since he's a doctor himself, he seems to have been able to get them. He has looked at the numbers and he has assessed, OK, here was the cancer, two weeks later he started chemo, and now it is two weeks later than that, and the numbers are not moving in a positive direction. It is Gene who tells the urologist and the oncologist and the internist that they may not be reading the data correctly. There were two weeks before the chemo ever started and you can't make the assumption that the reason the numbers are bad is related to the chemo not working. In fact, maybe it hasn't had enough time, because maybe the numbers are bad from the first two weeks when the cancer had nothing to stop it.

Then he tells them this: "Believe me, I am not in denial. I am very used to the swing between fear and hope, and I have had years of practice with this cancer hanging over me, but I am a researcher and what I can't stand is inaccuracy."

He was the one living in his body. He knew the diagnosis wasn't right. He knew his own body. He didn't feel he was dying. He looked at the data and he instructed everybody else to look at it too: to see *and* observe.

He was right. He took Taxotere for many more rounds and months. He was right that they hadn't given the chemo enough time. February was nowhere near enough time. Taxotere worked all the way up until we had to change in July to a different protocol because it wasn't making enough headway on his lungs. And then they were right: when Taxotere stops working, the fall is very fast.

But what they thought would be five weeks, for him was five months, during which he prepared his testimony as the star expert witness on the aging mind for one of the biggest legal cases in the country.

8

Coals and Diamonds

The Brooke Astor Case

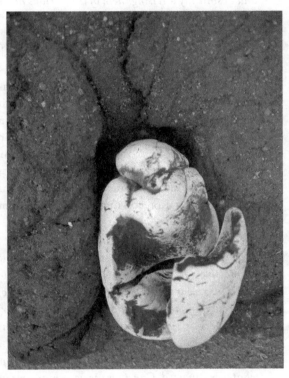

Figure 8.1 "Fitting into Our Niche" (2006), fired porcelain clay egg-puzzle with oxides set in mixed media sand/clay casting, 9 × 8 × 3 inches. Artwork by Wendy L. Miller, photo credit: Joshua Soros.

In late 2008, I was asked to provide professional testimony at the "Brooke Astor trial," a raucous tabloid-style courtroom drama that pitted the office of New York County District Attorney, Robert Morgenthau, then 89, against defendant Anthony Marshall, then 84 and heir to one of New York's oldest and most legendary fortunes, that of his billionaire mother, the celebrated socialite and philanthropist Brooke Astor.[1] Morgenthau's prosecutorial passion included cases of elder abuse, in particular those cases that would protect aging parents from adult children who sought to interfere with their wills when the parent no longer had the capacity to understand complex matters—including changing a will. Brooke Astor was over 100 years old and had developed Alzheimer's disease, when her son, himself in his 80s, fired the family lawyer and hired a new one. The outcome was new codicils to Mrs. Astor's will that ran contrary to her desire to leave much of her resources to charities. The DA's office conducted a search for their expert medical witness and selected me. This was just after the return of the cancer, and despite my advising them of this serious health change, they insisted on my continuing if I was up to it.

Gene was on a mission, for sure, fighting this battle, not just as a matter of principle but as a matter of legacy: his strategy was not so much about winning the court case as it was making the case for the science and for the dignity of family, as well as the self-affirmation that, with all that he was going through with his own sickness, he still had it in him to do his work and do it well. Throughout this period we were immersed and engaged with meaning, and that meaning allowed us to live through the impossible. Both of us were arranging and rearranging layers of information, trying to change meaning through high heat and high pressure, that same kind of heat and pressure that turns coal into diamonds: carbon pyramids of information copying and copying themselves into something new: a diamond.[2]

As time went on during this period, well into the summer of 2009, it was progressively harder for me to keep my energy up for more than two hours, and it was clear that I was probably going to be on the witness stand for an entire day. In fact, I was on the witness stand for three full days. But I had my helpers—Wendy and Alex took turns, each being with me for a day in court. Alex assured me, "Don't worry, dad, I will do everything to help preserve your energy—push your wheel chair, open doors, carry your bag, whatever you need. Consider me your manager in this prizefight you're in."

He knew the defense was going to try to disassemble me, and he was going to make sure I could keep taking the punches and come out for as many rounds as necessary. It made me feel even more fortunate in the midst of so many health problems that were challenging my good fortune that both of my children—Alex and Eliana—were loving and loyal. It was clearly rubbing off on Alex's children as well. His daughters, Ruby (5) and Lucy (3), were exceptionally loving to their 18-month-old identical twin brothers, Ethan and Bennett. Ruby and Lucy were very appreciative that the stork brought one baby for each of them, and the two babies were essentially the same. Alex had also sent me this picture of Lulu (Lucy) from a newspaper article. Lulu was in a one-mile race with a close friend, another 3-year old, and toward the end of the mile, Lulu's friend began to fatigue and stopped running. Lulu gently took her friend's hand and guided her across the finish line. The two 3-year-old buddies, hand-in-hand crossing the finish line, showed kindness and loyalty that gave me even more adrenalin for the ring in the courtroom.

I knew I'd be fine for a couple of hours, but if longer than that, I had no idea how I would do. As it turned out, I was on the witness stand for 8 hours each of the three days. The defense attorney who cross-examined me was like a pit bull. He tried to provoke me to respond with affect rather than maintaining a professional perspective. Having testified on Capitol Hill for 20 years while heading programs at the NIH, I was used to semi-hostile hearings, where members of whichever party was not represented in the White House would try to ask tough or embarrassing questions. It was part of the drill.

The pit bull (Brooke Astor's son's attorney) was not able to rattle me at all but I, in turn, did rattle him. He told me at one point, yelling, that one of the tests I cited as being important was criticized in a book that he waved in his hand. He then handed me the book and when I turned to copyright page, I found that it was 15 years old. I then calmly told him that any clinical book over three years old is ancient in modern medicine. The jury snickered. His body language revealed how embarrassed and furious he was.

I then referred to testimony by one of the lawyers the defendant had engaged for the signing of the codicils that contained the changes in Mrs. Astor's will. The attorney wanted to make the case as to how well Mrs. Astor was doing cognitively, even though she had already been diagnosed with Alzheimer's disease. He referred to a thank-you speech she gave at the Carnegie Institute upon receiving a major award for her philanthropy. He described her as giving the speech to the audience of 500 without notes. I, in turn, pointed out how important it was to look at a situation not just from a distance, but close up. I had a DVD of Mrs. Astor's speech, and had it shown in the courtroom. While it revealed that she did indeed give a speech to 500 people without using notes, it also showed on film a rambling and incoherent woman who had to be asked to stop talking. This was certainly a very different picture than what the attorney described.

There I was, making my own case, feeling at my best with the testimony, but feeling far less than whole with the effect of the cancer and its treatment.

I was testifying as the expert witness for the prosecution in one of the biggest public cases in America despite the ravages of cancer and the oppressiveness of its treatment. Alex was beaming and so was I through the tears in my eyes. We both fully understood that my time was very limited. We were both clearly making the very most of that time in the midst of the dark clouds and uncertainty that hovered around us, and we both saw and felt that the ominous darkness was eclipsed by the penetrating brightness of our closeness.

We knew it meant a great deal to Gene that Alex and I could see him this way, prevailing under these conditions, and be so proud of him. On my days with him, I sat in the back of the courtroom writing in my journal whatever I noticed. I wrote to keep my sanity, and just in case Gene needed something important that I might have seen or heard, I copied reactions and responses into my journal, not only reporting what I saw and heard but recording my own reflections. In the play-by-play of these days, the courtroom drama, the story of greed and exploitation of an elderly matriarch, became the parable for which Gene's science and theory gave new meaning.

Day 1: Alex accompanies Gene to New York City and gets to witness the first day in court when Gene gives his extensive presentation on Alzheimer's disease. Gene gave the court an entire medical history of Alzheimer's disease from four different perspectives: the workings of the brain in memory; a medical explanation of Alzheimer's in general; a medical explanation as regards Brooke Astor, shown from information he read from her friends, family, and other case witnesses; and a visual representation of his whole overlay of these three.

Day 2: Alex and I trade places; he goes home to his family and I arrive at the hotel to accompany Gene the next morning. Eliana stays with my niece in Jersey City. That day, I witnessed the cross-examination, which started after the prior sixty-six witnesses had taken the stand, the sixteen jurors and alternates had taken their places in the courtroom, and Gene's assimilation of the 12,500 pages of testimony he was given to read. I heard what the New York County District Attorney Office Squad's detective said in the car as he drove us to the courthouse in the morning: in all his years being in the courtroom, and that is many, he had never been so enthralled with an expert witness as he had been yesterday. "I could listen to you every day, Dr. Cohen," he said. "You explained it so well and made it so understandable to all of us in the room. That is a rare gift. Usually expert witnesses are talking to themselves. You were really talking to the jurors." This pleased Gene, of course, and was especially welcome in light of attempts by the defense to discredit the science and Gene himself.

At the start of the cross-examination, the defense attorney, Ken Warner, addressed Gene with a condescending tone, attempting to diminish Gene's credibility to the jury: "I am referring only to your opinion, *Doccccccctor* Cohen. Now, you were paid $400 an hour to read through the material, is that right, sir? That's quite a bit of money." The absurdity of this lawyer is unbelievable: spending this kind of time (the court's and ours) and money (his client's, of course) searching through Gene's bills, asking what he reads and how he reads, how much time he reads, how many hours he spends for this report and that report (saying nothing about the pit bull's own firm's legal fee of $150,000 per week!). They go over the itemized bills for over an hour of courtroom time. Relentlessly.

I say to myself, "Breathe, breathe deeply. Where is he going with this? If this is a lawyer's way of trashing a physician, what an absurd waste of time."

"I suspect you have never made this much money as an expert witness, have you, *Docccccctor* Cohen?" the defense attorney asks with the sneering tone that only further revealed his ignorance and his pointless, contentious small mind.

He knew nothing of the complexity of Gene's work life—the many expert testimonials Gene had done over the years. Nor did he understand the significance of this particular period in Gene's work life—the confluence of forces in science, medicine, law, and culture and social awareness that supported Gene's mission now. What I understood was that something larger than us had come in to support Gene—psychically, emotionally, intellectually, and financially. He had been given the laboratory of his dreams in the opportunity this case represented for presenting his science and doing so to huge media attention. I could see it, and I was proud and excited for him. At the same time, I feared that it was some kind of life "summing up" for him—too perfect that it came along right then in time, and too scary for me.

At the time, we were not living with a sense of him leaving (dying), and yet this whole project, as it got closer, became more and more Gene's singular focus. At every doctor's appointment, he would tell them about the case—that he had to be well enough for the case, that he had to organize his chemo around the timing of the court. The more and more he spoke of it, the more and more I feared it was all that mattered to him, and yet, of course it mattered. It was the thread that tied meaning and importance to his being. Yet it took up his time, his space, his thoughts, his sensibility—his energy. It focused him and it took him both into himself and away from himself. He wanted to give us, his family, the gift of being proud of him, and seeing him this way, we were.

He loved to talk about the case because it affirmed his abilities and diverted conversation away from the cancer. I hated to talk about the case because I feared it would eat him alive—as any obsession can when it saps your life force, and as it almost did when the defense attorney's stall tactics threatened to push the trial out even longer.

But Gene continued to use every question, every challenge, as a teachable moment. At one point the lawyer shifted from scrutinizing billing to diagnostic details, specifically Gene's view of the Clock Drawing Test, a fast screening tool used to assess dementia. Specifically, he discussed an analysis of its scoring used to assess Mrs. Astor's executive functioning, or capacity to reason or use rational thought. In this test, a person is given a blank circle and asked to draw the hands of a clock for a particular time. In people with dementia, this seemingly simple skill can be difficult, if not impossible. This has a sound basis in neuroscience, and the test has been validated and used reliably for many years both as a diagnostic tool and in research.

The defense attorney knew nothing about statistics, reliability, significance, or value. He tried to force Gene to take a subjective view rather than a scientific view of the test itself and of Mrs. Astor's drawing, which had telltale signs of confused ability. He spent forever on it, never making any headway from what I could see. It was hard not to wonder how, with such an ample budget for legal preparation, he could come so ill equipped to discuss even this most basic diagnostic tool. Shouldn't he have hired his own medical expert physician who knew the material he was using for his presentation? Sometimes the defense would highlight a certain part of the medical report, with no idea that directly underneath it was a more important piece of information that showed how faulty the defense's contentious thinking was. As a physician and a researcher, Gene had been reading these types of medical reports his whole professional life.

The defense attorney puffed himself up and clearly thought he had bested Gene when he handed him a book, entitled *Clock Drawing: A Neuropsychological Analysis*.[3]

"Have you read this book, *Doccccctor* Cohen?"

Perhaps he didn't think Gene had read it, and that that would undermine his credibility as an expert witness. I knew Gene hadn't read it, but I also knew why the point—and indeed the book itself—was irrelevant. Gene perused the book and pointed out its date of publication, 1994.

He responded, "This book was published fifteen years ago. In the medical profession, that is out of date." End of subject. The pit bull attorney's face turned red as a hot coal. Gene's face glowed; under pressure, the diamond.

Alex had nicknamed Gene "Rocky," for Rocky Balboa, the indefatigable boxer in the Rocky movies they had watched together over the years. And Gene was that. Here was this guy who did not look like the man I know; he was bald and shrunk, smaller and more fragile. We were moving him in a wheelchair around the courthouse in this Kafkaesque trap. At the same time, he was so much more of a big human being than these jerks running around being uncivil, rude, and, frankly, stupid.

My Gene was so sturdy up there, in terms of his psychological acuity, his capacity to not only withstand the demands of the situation but turn them into an opportunity. And yet, the contrast was undeniable: the extreme physical deterioration, the cumulative effect of the slow decline that the disease had brought about in more recent months. The medications had taken a toll on him, the light in this ancient courtroom was ghostly and the surreal sound of the lawyer's snide way of addressing Gene—*docccctor*—made me queasy. My heart pounded with the sudden awareness of his fragility. Listening, thinking, following this prosecutor's tone as he tried to trick Gene, trip him up by reading his own words back to him.

Gene stayed sharp in this cold room and he managed to swallow any of his emotional responses to this rude man. Lawyers are chronological, linear, focus on one point at a time, building an argument as if your information alone is the whole story or a concise piece to be considered in isolation. Gene's framework was to cut across frameworks—to synthesize and to discover. It had been his lifelong approach to science and life itself—his personality style. He had to talk over the pit pull's constant interruptions intended to stop Gene from explaining things clearly to the jury. Gene would begin a comment, only to be interrupted by the pit bull's intentional effort to distract—"You do agree, *doccccctor* . . ." or "Wouldn't you agree that. . . ." as he misrepresented again the facts Gene was sharing. But Gene persisted and made his points fully and clearly.

The bills, the clocks, the language, divided attention, lucid moments, individuality, wills, codicils, stages of Alzheimer's, capacity, performance, and consistency—all of it was odious beyond belief. It was enough to give one temporary dementia, a kind of courtroom Alzheimer's disease. From my notes, I wrote short phrases of facts:

> By 1953, Brooke Astor already had 38 wills and codicils, not counting the drafts she didn't go forward with.
>
> Her employees each were all supposed to receive $50,000 from her will.
>
> The codicil changes gave 49 percent that was originally deemed to go to her philanthropies, to her son, Anthony Marshall.

So many of these details made no sense, if only in terms of how families work. Mr. Marshall had been vice president of the Vincent Astor Foundation for twenty-six years before Mrs. Astor developed Alzheimer's disease. Brooke Astor had made her wishes quite clear in the years before she developed Alzheimer's: she had consciously and deliberately placed him in charge of some things, but not others. That he was trying now to overturn her wishes was, as the prosecution asserted, unseemly at best and at worst, criminal.

One of the attorneys repeated what had been established already: "Fifty-one percent would continue to go to her philanthropies, forty-nine percent would go to Anthony Marshall to provide to the philanthropies."

The defense attorney continued with this language, going over and over the difference between the Astor Foundation and the trust, pushing Gene and arrogantly reminding him of what he didn't know—though of course he didn't need to know it to know the science that he was there to present as an expert. But the lawyer kept pushing and pushing with more and more minute detail to try to show Gene up.

Gene is razor sharp in his ability to put facts together where they belong without getting lost in the details that would normally confuse a person. Gene said, "Since the second codicil gave the residual to Mr. Marshall and the 1997 will already provided the same decision, what was the need for these additional codicils unless there was something fishy going on in them?"

The jury opened their glazed-over eyes with the same smile that Gene characteristically brings out in people as he boils complexity down to common sense and reframes chaos into meaning. As Gene always said, "Let's not overlook the obvious." Right then, the lawyer held no trump card, and the discussion about the wills and codicils was over, just as it had been about the bills, the clocks, and Mrs. Astor's speeches. I was shocked over and over again, because I couldn't believe the lawyers would go to this much trouble with their information and have nothing of substance or even merely credible to support it.

Pride and strength sit a mere hairline from vulnerability and pain. Yet the brilliance and the strength of character—which is what Gene maintained through it all—beyond the lawyers and the defendant—that was the diamond in the room. Everything he knew and cared about—intellectually, clinically, ethically, emotionally—all came together to stand up for the value of human dignity in later life.

Meanwhile, there we were, in the courtroom where they grilled him for hours on end. And they didn't finish in the allotted time span they said they would. They wanted him to stay another day, and the pressure was strong to do that. But he had me, and I knew if it had been Alex with him, Alex would have responded in the same way. I turned to Liz Loewy, the attorney from the DA's special prosecution bureau, who came into the witness protection room to tell us what the defense attorneys wanted to do and how the judge was responding. I said, "Well, if someone is going to be held in contempt of court for not agreeing to stay over for an extra day, they can hold me. But my husband has an appointment in Washington, DC tomorrow morning for chemotherapy, and we are not missing it over a situation like this. That really would make this a criminal case! Mrs. Astor has been dead for five years, her son is struggling over an amount of money most of us can't even write on paper as a number, his lawyer has colluded in committing fraud, and we have much more important things to do tomorrow. We will not stay in New York for Gene to be on the stand tomorrow."

As it turned out, the court did request him to come back for another day, but it was not the next day, and we did go home for his treatment appointment. Alex came back with him two weeks later for his final day as expert medical witness.

They say coals are diamonds in the rough—perhaps diamonds are coals cut out of the rough. We are both coals and diamonds. We are raw and we are cut. We are dark and we are light. What it takes for brilliance to shine are the many cuts into the rough darkness.

I always thought that people who lose their spouses are seventy-seven years old or eight-seven years old. They are not fifty-nine. That is the internal belief or the developmental belief. Nothing in my life has come at its appropriate time or order: not the child, the husband, the work, the jobs, the fertility, the miscarriages, the adoption, the community. My growth is always a bit askew.

Because the process of Gene's chemotherapy was accompanied by his preparations for the Brooke Astor case, I knew that Brooke Astor had been widowed at in her late fifties and that she went on to live to be 105. But it is not how long I will live or not live that is on my mind. It is: How am I going to do this? How am I going to go on when nothing feels possible or in any way right anymore? I focus my imagination and engage in a huge creative project, working on a reunion with my extended family and on our family legacy project. Something in me is very engaged, transported even. And yet something else is lost and adrift as I sit in the courtroom: I am fifty-nine years old, and the synchronicity of my age being close to Brooke Astor's age when her husband died does not leave me.

I watch him. I look and I do see, but I am afraid to see. It is so clear that his life force has weakened. It's the reciprocity that keeps affecting me: the life force that is your social grace; the life force that has you answer someone's questions; the life force that has you participate and share and remember your part in things. All of it is not just weakened; it is turned inward. Everything takes effort and sheer will. I also remember the focus that comes with it though; the good news is that the internal focus is so strong that dreams, images, reverie are heightened, deepened beyond meditation. I see it happening to Gene. He is pulled inward. And in that process, it feels like he is leaving me when in fact, he doesn't have the life force anymore. He still wants to connect, but his light is flickering. This time, I'm on the outside looking in, and it's painful. It's painful to participate and to love while what is left of that life force is so self-absorbed—necessarily so for mere survival—that there is no more energy to be a social or interactive creature in the ways that we normally can take for granted.

Gene had set himself up in the little room off the porch all during the previous summer month of July 2009. It was the space that served as the filming room for our interviews for the family reunion material. It was sunny in there. He could see the lake, could see all of us, as he watched the daily events from a safe and quiet space. This was the first summer since 1994 that he was not in the lake swimming. We certainly couldn't risk anything going into his open nephrostomy tube, or further affecting his overall weakness from the chemotherapy. He sat in this room each day; starting out there early in the morning, he rested, he read, he memorized. He touched his balding "chemo head" with his fingertips, tapping on his baldness as if he could imprint his memorized information directly through his soft touch. He boiled down pages upon pages of notes from his reading and understanding of the testimonies, the depositions, and the reports. He color coded these boiled-down notes into further cryptic notes until, by the end of the month, just prior to the trial itself, he had it encoded into a two-page cheat sheet. He would then go on to do his entire testimony with no notes at all.

We could see him from the window as we sat around the dining room table, where we spent our time in endless family chatter, eating, talking, telling stories, and working on our own family reunion project. He was alone yet not alone. Usually when we are there at camp, we are together as a family. We go out in the boat or swim or drive to Camden, we run errands or visit with family. This summer, Gene was at one with his computer, with his Brooke Astor notes. He was very quiet. He answered in monosyllables. He was engrossed. He needed so much rest, so much food. He needed to be on his own time and space schedule and we were all aware of it. My cousin Andy cooked more and more clam chowder for him, filled with butter and milk, items Gene had spent the past thirteen years avoiding. Each of us brought food to him throughout the day, a kind of offering to help sustain him, body, mind, and spirit. Gene was on a mission, and it took all that he had, all that he was. It took so much strength to fight. It takes a lot of pressure to shine.

A Grand Legacy on the Docket: The Discovery Process

The flamboyant celebrity and high-society color of the proceedings were in sharp contrast to the dark medical tension under which Gene worked during this period. The backstory of the public spectacle was just the kind of society drama that the media loved, and that, too, served the mission in that it brought the science of aging, illness, and creativity center stage in the most literal sense. The cast of characters, the glitz and greed—there could hardly have been a more unlikely stage for a scholarly update on the emerging science of the aging brain and mental faculties.

The defendant, Anthony Marshall, at eighty-four, was heir to one of New York's oldest and most legendary fortunes, that of John Jacob Astor, the real estate and fur baron who was the great grandfather of Vincent Astor, Brooke Astor's third husband, and stepfather to her son Anthony Marshall. A background note: John Jacob Astor, the wealthiest person in the United States in the nineteenth century at the time of his death, had bequeathed $400,000 for the founding of a pubic library, the Astor Library in New York City, which was then consolidated with the privately endowed Lenox Library and the Tilden Foundation trust to establish the New York Public Library in 1895, one of the great libraries of the world and the largest city library in the United States. This was relevant as Gene saw it, because he felt it was inconceivable that Mrs. Astor would want to sever this unique historical and consistent cord of support on her part, as well as the part of the Vincent Astor Foundation and the Astor family going back to the nineteenth century.

The jury was made up of eight women and four men (and four alternate jurors), and they listened to nineteen weeks of testimony in the State Supreme Court in Manhattan. Gene was one of seventy-two witnesses, among them, key witnesses like Annette de la Renta (whom he had interviewed), Barbara Walters, and Henry Kissinger.

The eighteen-count indictment, including two first-degree grand larceny charges (numerous crimes over a six-year period), were brought against both Anthony Marshall and Francis X. Morrissey, Jr., a lawyer hired by Anthony Marshall in 2001 to do estate planning for Mrs. Astor after he fired her longtime lawyer, Henry Christensen III. Mr. Morrissey was charged in the indictment with forgery, criminal possession of a forged instrument, and scheme to defraud and conspiracy. Mr. Marshall was convicted of fourteen counts, charged with scheme to defraud, grand larceny, criminal possession of stolen property, falsifying business records, and other charges.

Big money was certainly at stake in this trial. Brooke Astor's fortune was estimated at $180 million when she died in 2007 at the age of 105. But something even more important was at stake as Gene saw it. Gene spent his entire career advocating a "whole-person identity" for aging people. His most important contributions to the field of aging were not only in the realm of science but in the realm of public perceptions, creating a paradigm shift from the sense of aging as a process of inevitable mental decline to aging as a process in which, despite certain declines, there is great potential for new leaps of creativity and productivity. Early in his career, he had led the charge to change Medicare to allow for reimbursement of mental health services beyond its original annual $250 limit; he had encouraged and supported research on the mental health of minorities, the impoverished and homeless; he encouraged the AARP to focus on mental health and aging; he was a key person to initiate and implement Margaret Heckler's (Secretary of Health and Human Services) focus on Alzheimer's disease during the Reagan administration. This case provided unusual visibility to continue his advocacy for the rights of the aging person, the dignity of family responsibility, and public accountability. The world was finally attentive.

Friends who loved Gene not only loved Gene for Gene, but they loved the way his mind worked. It's a funny concept. We can love the way someone looks, or we can love the way someone's heart is or the way someone makes us laugh, but when you love the way someone's mind works, that has its own different, special quality. It wasn't just that he was smart and kind, but that he had a way of framing things, and he worked very hard at framing things, to show their universality and relevance.

The Brooke Astor case pushed all of Gene's buttons. Because he had always been a cutting-edge thinker, and because he was an integrative thinker, he thought about things we were all growing toward in aging—as individuals, as an age demographic, and as a society. So in a way, that is what the Brooke Astor case was about for Gene: aging. Aging is something we experience like we experience jetlag; for most of us, it takes a while to realize we are, in fact, aging as we make a lot of assumptions about it. We don't really know much about aging until we get there or our parents are there or an illness forces us into it. We stay ignorant. For Gene, his access to Brooke Astor's material gave him access to a remarkable trove of data—the medical records, including doctors' and nurses' notes, hospital records, and clinical test results, then pages upon pages of depositions, conversations, presentations, the codicils, the housekeepers' comments, the perceptions of her dearest old friends. Here was an opportunity to delve into a special case study of everything he had spent forty years studying about the brain, about clinically working with Alzheimer's patients. All this at the same time that he was facing his own decline and his own illness responses to chemotherapy; his own aging independent of illness, and the impact of that illness on the aging process.

It wasn't just the subject of elder abuse or ignorance or rich entitlement; not just the narrow perspective of these lawyers; not just a misunderstanding of Alzheimer's. It was the multilayered impact and positive potential of it all. Gene became a teacher in the courtroom, teaching people how memory works, how science works, how neurology works, what our minds are made up of, and what happens when parts of that are taken away.

In a weird way, it almost seemed a metaphor, or perhaps simply an irony: Gene didn't have Alzheimer's and he had not aged in that way, thank God, but cancer is like that in that it robs you of something that was yours. You can be very bright and smart and have an amazing mind, but if you have an illness, even though you are bright and smart, your intellect doesn't get you out of it. It doesn't make you immune to the process of cancer and the effects of its treatments. And in the Brooke Astor case, even though she was bright and one of the wealthiest people in the country, those assets couldn't spare her from the illness and what it took from her. So to have that material, her material, be what sustained him, distracted him, affirmed him, the material that he was shaping at this time, at the same time that cancer was reshaping who he was, day by day, part by part—and the very work itself also depleting him—was a strange juxtaposition.

I observed Gene, read Gene like Gene read those files. Meticulously. And what I learned in my own discovery process was that he was the diamond in the rough, so far from rough on the outside, and yet inside, those of us who both cared for him and walked this journey with him, knew exactly how fragile he really was. We knew what capacity and spirit as a resource he pulled from—creativity in its highest form—the diamond of creative capacity. Everything he knew and cared about—intellectually, clinically, ethically, emotionally—all came together. This was an "encore" for him. I would have fallen apart as a broken piece of dark coal within five minutes of the pit bull lawyer parading his arrogance, disrespect, and unethical interpretations of data about which he clearly was uninformed. Gene patiently corrected so much of this man's presentation of information, simply so that the jury would have accurate information on which to base its deliberations and verdict.

Gene later wrote about one of the pivotal points on which the case rested: the nature of a "lucid moment." After the trial, in an editorial titled "What Is a Lucid Moment?" he tells the story from the trial: how the prosecutor highlighted a section of the medical transcripts to prove that Brooke Astor was "alert."[4] The lawyer didn't seem to understand that in medical terms, when a doctor writes in his or her notes "alert," it actually refers to a patient being awake, and as Gene wrote in his essay: "one can be very alert and very confused at the same time." The lawyer, in his questions and statements to Gene, set about to define the term in his own (incorrect) way—to suggest that "alert" meant something else, which is not a smart move when you have a physician on the stand. For instance, in one such episode, right below the lines that the lawyer had highlighted in those notes from 2004 were more medical notes, in which Brooke Astor's doctor, Dr. Pritchett, had indicated that Astor's thinking was "NG," which means *not good*. NG. In his essay, Gene elaborated on the point he made in testimony, which is that the mind holds contradictions—in this case alertness and confusion—and that it is essential for us to make fine discernments as we consider these in the context of aging and illness.

> One of the key issues that emerged from the defense was that during the signing of the two codicils that changed Mrs. Astor's will, she exhibited lucid moments. A lucid moment is a very poorly understood and very often misunderstood concept around which courts, lawyers, physicians, families, and individuals need to be better educated. A lucid moment is an elusive concept.
>
> In considering the nature of a lucid moment, there are two fundamental questions: What constitutes being lucid, and what is a moment?

Regarding what is lucid, there is much misunderstanding and consider-able variation in what experts and the public perceive about being lucid. For example, many family members seeing their loved one appearing alert, view this as being lucid. But in medicine, being alert simply means being awake; one can be very alert and very confused at the same time. For others, seeing a smile on a loved one's face following a given comment may also elicit a perception of lucidity, whereas, behind the smile may be a complete misinterpretation of the comment.

Also qualitative and quantitative distinctions so often fail to be made. A qualitative perception of lucidity may be the product of viewing only a fragment of lucidity, though experienced quantitatively by the viewer as constituting overall lucidity at that moment. Even healthcare profession-als and attorneys can fall into this perceptual trap. To really understand a will, its changes, and the ramifications of those changes—to possess what is technically referred to as testamentary capacity—one needs to be able to see more than fragments but the whole picture. If you want to take in an entire landscape, you don't want to look through a pinhole in a single sec-tion of window with several sections; you want to view what can seen within the entire window frame and all its sections.

In his decades working with patients with Alzheimer's disease (AD) and other dementias, Gene had developed a way to evaluate for the capacity for lucidity, based on the three major stages of AD—mild, moderate, and severe.

For healthy persons, their lucidity allows them to see the forest. For per-sons in the mild stage of AD, they can no longer see the forest, just some trees. For persons in the moderate stage of AD, they can no longer see the trees, just some branches. For persons in the severe stage of AD, they can no longer see branches, just a blur. At the time Brooke Astor's will was changed, an international expert on AD who had evaluated Mrs. Astor considered her to be moving toward the severe stage of Alzheimer's disease.

And what of the measure of a lucid moment?

A moment typically refers to something that is fleeting. In relation to time as well, too often qualitative and quantitative distinctions disappear when one is trying to determine if a lucid moment occurred. If a comment is made that seems in the moment to make some sense, somehow the experi-ence of that fleeting moment is transformed into an extended interval of lucid capacity for the duration of the encounter—even if that encounter is lengthy. To comprehend the complexities of a will and its changes requires an extended period of comprehension, not just a glimpse that can notice a branch without taking in the forest. More than a moment of lucidity is required.

One's sense of a lucid moment is often transformed or magnified through uninformed assumptions or a wishful moment on the part of the viewer, desperately searching for more than what actually meets their eye.

This question of "What is a lucid moment?" is hard to answer for anyone and can send any of us into deep reflection. Though Gene's editorial essay was about the court case, it certainly is a question we all ask ourselves when life throws us a curve ball and everything we know to be the recognizable identity of who we are amidst our home, family, love, and work lives shifts. We find ourselves asking: What is real? What is happening? How can I understand it? For each of us, it also boils down to the same question Gene posed: What really is a lucid moment? Gene always offered such compassionate windows into the workings of the mind and the heart. A kind of poetic response to the largest questions we ask as we confront realities that frighten and confuse us. As Gene writes, how we look is the real issue—through pinholes, or uninformed assumptions, while all the while we are desperately searching through our wishful moments for more than what meets our eye.

By the time his role in the Brooke Astor case was over, we were desperately searching for our old belief that Gene's own health could return to its pre-chemo state; that he would live to find out what happened in the case; that we would live to have our own lucid memories of how it had fueled his system with the rare atypical cells that his health needed; that his way of handling his situation would accrue like a stock investment. We didn't yet know that the chemo was coming to its end of options for us. We didn't yet know that there would only be another ten weeks of life. Do any of us ever know how long we have?

Was that looking through a pinhole? Actually, I think it was the opposite. I think that what happened when his cancer cells took over became the pinhole. His life was so much larger than the disease. Yet, our assumptions were, in fact, magnified by our experience—he had come out ahead so many times, so many years, so many ways, we hadn't yet imagined that it would be any different this time. Because, yes, we were desperately searching for more than what meets the eye.

It was the heart, the organ no one was even looking at, that eventually made the life-or-death decision. The hardening of the heart's encasement, the pericardium, the container, the protector of our breath of life, became the sudden limitation on his.[5] Strong, yes; even too strong, and in its strengthening, cutting off the space that the fragile heart needed in order to pulse. Eliana asked me, with the quiet hope of a child's science, if the doctor could just cut open the hardened shell so her daddy's heart could have some more room to breathe. I had to tell her he no longer had the capacity to survive that surgery.

What had saved Gene was now killing him. The truth of that dichotomy is the lucid moment of life and death's calling.

9

Mirror Mirror

*I now find myself looking into the mirror, as if the mirror can sum up
what has changed. In so doing, a lot of introspection and life review has
occurred. I'm looking at a series of twists and ironies that have unfolded
during my life.*
—Gene

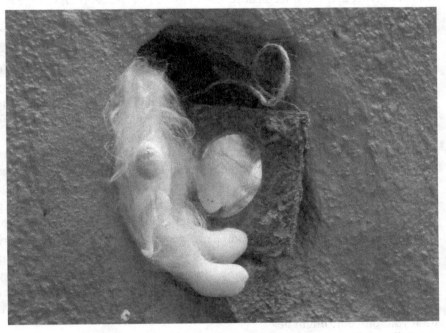

Figure 9.1 "Aging the Mirror of Mud Elegance" (2008), site-specific installation in
Costa Rica, painted adobe wall with cloth figure, and paper pulp mirror,
9 × 4 × 5 inches. Artwork and documentation by Wendy L. Miller,
photo credit: Joshua Soros.

As a child, I used to love this one mirror at my nana's house. Just calling it a mirror
doesn't really do it justice: it was a mirror-lined niche created by a built-in chest
of drawers. The niche was mirrored on all its surfaces: top, sides, and back wall.
I loved this mirrored niche because when I looked into the back wall and down

the two sides, I could see images of my face going endlessly down one side, and its reflection of the back of me going down the other side. Somehow, it was as if my face had its own hall of mirrors that went beyond pure reflections: the image of me was accompanied by a sense of being part of a history of faces, all mine of course, but those also of my older family relatives who had lived in this room and whose memories were ingrained in me. Sometimes I imagined that I could see them seeing me; or I imagined who they might see as me, or who I might see as I grew older, aged into myself. This niche revealed not only my physical self but also a maturing internal self, filled with myriads of perceptions, memories, and images already at work shaping the self I was becoming.

In the fairy tale "Snow White and the Seven Dwarfs," the queen repeats: "Mirror, mirror on the wall, who's the fairest of them all?"[1] The fairy tale sets up the allegorical mirror to ask: What does the mirror show us about ourselves? What do we see in our reflection and what do others see? How do our perceptions change and how does that change us?

We look up, any of us, from our busy day, or the sickbed, or the doctor's examination table, or a half-dozen decades of life we can hardly remember passing by, and we catch a glimpse of ourselves in the mirror and stop short. Who is that looking back? Which of our selves do we see there? How does the way others see us and define us shape how we see and feel about ourselves? All the different selves: the old me, the new me, the ill me, the healthy me, the doctor's me, the family's me, the worried me, the brave me; this is what shapes and what profoundly affects us. The notion of how we see ourselves—and how others see us—shifts our potential, for better or worse. Imagine that your doctor sees you as an outlier, a person who really has a chance, even against dark odds. Or sees you as a person who is uncooperative, not following the protocol, asking a few too many questions, showing up for appointments as difficult, stubborn, in denial, or in medicalese, "non-compliant." Just the thought of being seen by your doctor as troublesome, the worry that you'll be written off, adds to your burden; now instead of just managing illness or infirmity, you have to worry about how your doctor sees you. These differing views of you can change your own perception of yourself, how you might see and think about yourself and what your outcome might be.

There are so many ways in which our internal process can both distort and clarify our sense of our self and sense of possibility. As Gene suggested, at times our circumstances have us see through a pinhole rather than the larger window. This idea of our perceptions shaping our reality and our possibility applies to the way we engage life, aging, illness, and our innate creativity. We've seen how the metaphorical flashlight and prism are tools for exploring our thoughts and feelings in the context of circumstances such as illness or other changes that affect us profoundly. At times we can use the flashlight to illuminate and help us see what's in front of us more clearly: *What am I feeling?*

What am I doing to hide what is really inside of me? How do I handle the world under these conditions? Sometimes we need the prism to "split the refracting light into an array of new beams," as my client Daniel called it, and create possibilities that have been there yet were invisible to us all along. *What might I do differently now that I see how I am feeling? How might I ask for what I really need here?*

The mirror is the third tool in this metaphorical toolkit. Our mirror reflects not only what is objectively true (your eyes are brown, you have a scar by your ear, your head is bald from chemo) but our subjective self-reflections as well, the many hues and tones of our shifting perceptions and the meanings they hold or the meanings we give them as our awareness deepens. You might see in your eyes the joy or uncertainty or perhaps the fear of the moment; your scar may represent nothing more than a childhood spill on your bike, or it could be a reminder of some disturbing past or part of an illness experience unfolding right now.

Images provide depth as they expand meaning. Images and memories of past, present, and future, other people's perceptions of us, and our own perceptions of how they see us—all of these blend into the complex reflection we see in our mirror and take into our thoughts in the process of internal reflection.

There is always the moment we remember, the moment when we catch a glimpse of ourselves and we experience a sudden awareness. My sister, looking in the mirror when chemotherapy had taken all of her hair away, saw her face as our dad's face. Did this comfort her or absolutely terrify her? My mother had been given a prognosis of two to twelve years. Two years into that period, looking in the mirror when we walked into the ladies restroom at my great uncle's memorial service, she said very quietly to me, "Do you think that is the face of a dying woman?"[2] I wonder if what she saw was the natural beauty of her being, mixed with the evidence of her illness. She went on to tell me that others had always found her beautiful, but she didn't really know what they were seeing; to her it was just her face, the same face she had always seen. Perhaps when she caught that glimpse of herself, knowing she was ill, she actually wondered what the doctor saw when he looked at her. She looked at herself, but was so deeply connected to her own memories of herself, she couldn't "see" the face of a "dying woman" that intuitively she feared could be there.

At some point, we begin to see or perhaps sense in other ways an emerging awareness of the multiple selves that we are. The metaphorical mirror is the tool we use to integrate all the images of all these selves: past, present, and future, ours and others, the self as the disease's reflection, the healing self's reflection, and the reflections of aging and the living with age. The mirror is the container of the entire phenomenon of self-recognition.

Gene held the mirror up to the process of aging to think about his role and responsibilities as a physician in these processes. He used the idea of the mirror

*focus on youth, denial
physical attraction, power
prestige, famous*

reflection explicitly to talk about how society's view of aging had been distorted for so long, and his desire to call attention to that and, through his work, help bring about a shift in that perception.

> *I was a very young-looking 30-year-old when I was appointed the first chief of the newly created Center on Aging at the National Institute of Mental Health in 1975—the first federal center on mental health and aging established in any country. I was self-conscious about holding such an important position on aging with such a prominent appearance of youth. So a makeover went into gear—I grew a beard, donned a bowtie, and purchased a professorial-looking pair of glasses. Now, 34 years later, as the Beatles' song goes, "When I'm 64," my appearance because of the cancer has changed beyond that of normal aging.[3]*
>
> *In an article in Canada's major online publication, "Globe and Mail," following a talk I gave in Toronto, the writer referred to me as "a gleeful Father Time in professorial corduroy and bow tie." I also still had my beard and glasses. The article further described me as "due to health issues, he looks older than what the current culture expects for a man of only 64 years. He uses a cane and looks frail under a thinning nimbus of white hair." A far cry from my youthful appearance that I felt needed to be camouflaged in 1975.*
>
> *But the article also emphasized what my talk emphasized and what the writer felt that I myself displayed: "Ironically, the course of his own life has turned him into the best lesson in positive aging. . . . The aging brain isn't running out of gas. . . . It's shifting into four-wheel drive."[4]*

Gene reflected on the power of a medical prognosis to affect the way people see us and make assumptions about us in so many ways—just as the hotel clerk in Costa Rica had done in assuming that Gene was my father. This reflection of ourselves as others see us in the medical mirror presents a new challenge to the self, particularly if we are by nature an emotionally open and sharing person, as Gene was.

> *I think back to the several weeks following my initial diagnosis in 1996. Several health personnel involved in my treatment and close friends asked me what my plans were. In my mind, my reflex reaction to that repeating question was "I'm not dead yet, so I choose to live," meaning I certainly don't plan to withdraw or give up on what has been important to me. I learned that was a good choice when I was misdiagnosed with ALS. I figured to follow the same formula here.*
>
> *In contemplating my options, I recalled a remarkable essay by Stephen Jay Gould. Gould was diagnosed with an abdominal cancer—a*

mesothelioma—in July 1982. He later published an essay titled "The Median Isn't the Message," discussing his reading of the scientific literature reporting that mesothelioma patients had a median lifespan of eight months after diagnosis.[5] He described the research he uncovered behind this number, and his relief upon realizing that statistics are not destiny.

Following his diagnosis and receiving an experimental treatment, Gould lived for nearly twenty years before dying from a different problem. In my case, I felt I had to pay attention to my prognosis, at the same time recognizing that any statistic is accompanied by variation in the form of what statisticians and physicians refer to as outliers. Reality and hope are not incompatible.

I returned to work with nobody knowing my diagnosis. Only very close family, a few very close friends, and those involved in my treatment knew my health status. This was the same strategy I adopted when I thought I had ALS. For the time being, I wanted the opportunity to know my own thoughts and come up with a strategy without being overwhelmed by irritating comments, no matter how well intentioned they were.

I dreaded receiving unasked-for advice about what diet to follow, what vitamins to take, what alternative medicine interventions I should pursue, what so-and-so did that was effective, and so forth, even though I respected the value of many of these approaches in varied situations, especially that of complementary medicine. I also frankly feared knowledge of my diagnosis and prognosis would lead to adverse career consequences, even though my prognosis in effect pointed to my career along with my life becoming severely abbreviated. During my medical career and personal experiences I heard too many stories like what Max Lerner described in his book: "Very early, and throughout my illness, I tried to be honest about my cancer, with myself and others. I paid a price for my openness. As word spread, my lecture requests and magazine assignments faded away."[6]

Knowing that I would pay a heavy emotional price for being less open than I would have liked to, I also was wary of what Max Lerner described, especially since my research grant applications could reach a million dollars. Would the grantors really be as interested, I thought, if they knew I had metastatic prostate cancer along with its bad prognosis? At the same time I took steps to protect the grants and the funders by working with a very talented team that could certainly maintain the same quality of effort if I had to step back or drop out.

The mirror darkened as Gene began to experience the deep "dips" into terror-filled darkness. And yet, as he reflected on his experience he became aware of a dual nature of these episodes: both gripping him with fear and releasing in him a sense of relief and possibility—the pendulum swing of enantiodromia I described earlier. With his characteristic scientist's mind, both curious and analytical, he wrote:

> I returned to work very shortly after my diagnosis, and tried to resume activities, filling the day with them. It went well each day until I left the university to go home. When all the stimuli of the day that also served as distractions to my cancer thoughts waned, a darkness began to slowly descend on me. Sometimes it was so powerful, that I would have to pull over to the side of the road as the darkness completely engulfed me, feeling in total blackness sensing no life, light, or beauty around me. I would have sought psychiatric help then, but the descent into darkness though extremely intense was also brief—usually for about 15 minutes. It would then be followed by a steady emergence out of the darkness and a new feeling that there was something I might be able to do, accompanied by intense mental exploration of possibilities. And the mental exploration felt good, like a creative pursuit. This feeling was more engagingly powerful than any related prior positive feelings I had experienced, and I didn't want to do anything to lose it.
>
> I did wonder if I was becoming bipolar, but the deep dark dips, though dreadfully awful while in them, were transient and lifted into an elevating feeling that was focused. If the feeling had moved in a manic direction, disrupting my family life and work, I would have sought professional help. Instead, out of those elevated feelings came the realization that what I needed to do was something akin to my experience with developing a game to cope with the dark moods that followed my misdiagnosis of ALS.

Now Gene's passion for his work filled the mirror. He intended to create a new mirror on aging for society and for individuals to see themselves anew with inherent value and vast possibility.

> It was then that I realized my work had become all about creativity and aging, and no book had been written totally focused on that topic. Since I knew I always felt good writing, then researching and writing a book on creativity in my field of gerontology could reframe my days with a project that would extensively engage my thoughts, and provide a lovely process that would enhance the quality of my time.
>
> This strategy of creative immersion in my writing and work, combined with my strong circle of love at home, helped me to maintain a positive mood most days, despite the clouds that hovered around me and the circumscribed

free-fall mood dips late in the day. This period of my life following the diagnosis of cancer has proved to be my most creative in the research I have conducted and the books I have written—a powerful and poignant illustration of the influence of adversity on creativity, and in the second half of life.

Just as the queen in "Snow White" had to keep checking in the magic mirror about her beauty, so too with society checking about aging as we entered the 1970s, because when it comes to aging what appeared in the mirror over the next three decades took 3 very different forms. During the late 1960s and early 1970s, images of aging were at a low point in our culture. We heard phrases like "You can't trust anyone over 30" and "intergenerational conflict," and "age gap."

From my research I show that underneath the perceived age gap was operating a very real education gap that separated the generations. With the launching of Sputnik, the first vehicle in space, by the old Soviet Union in the late 1950s, the U.S. experienced an identity crisis around education and science, the race in each we felt we were losing to the Soviets. So a revolution ensued in the classroom that affected the young first. In 1970, at the height of negative feeling about older persons in American society, the level of education of the middle group in their mid-60s was less than a high school education—8.6 years. By 1990, that same middle group of persons 65 and older had greater than a high school education—12.1 years—and intergenerational relations had improved enormously.

Up until the last quarter of the 20th century, aging was largely equated with a series of decremental, unalterable changes with the passage of time. Significant decline with advancing years was seen as inevitable—our destiny. Dementing disorders were collectively viewed as "senility," a term than connoted the natural course of growing old. But by 1975 what the allegorical mirror revealed was the stirring of a fundamental conceptual change in how negative events with aging were being interpreted. The first of two major sea changes in thinking about aging in the last quarter of the 20th century was in process. There was an emergence of new hypotheses that attempted to explain decrements that accompanied aging not as representing normal aging, but instead reflecting age-associated problems—modifiable disorders.

For the scientist, the idea that a negative change is caused by a problem, and not normal aging, creates a new sense of opportunity to modify the problem. For the policy maker, this recognition results in a new sense of responsibility to do something about the problem. This sea change in thinking about modifiable age-associated problems launched the modern federal infrastructure of research programs on aging. In 1975, the National Institute on Aging appointed its first director, while the National Institute of Mental Health established a new research center on mental health and aging—*the first federal research program on aging established in any country (I received the great opportunity to become the new center's first Chief). That same year, 1975, the Veterans Administration launched their GRECC Program (Geriatric Research, Education, and Clinical Centers Program). Rigorous research on aging in effect did not go into high speed until the fourth quarter of the 20th century. The "problem focus" in turn led to the development of the field of geriatrics that soared in the 1980s and since.*

The transition from seeing progressive, unalterable negative changes with aging as being one's destiny with growing old to a new view of modifiable age-associated problems was a huge leap in itself. The culmination of the problem view of aging came with the concept of "successful aging," defined in 1988 as aging that reflected the minimum number of problems— the minimum degree of decline—as opposed to "usual aging" that reflected more problems, more decline. While this was happening it was too big a leap to go to the next step—to see that aging could be accompanied by potential and growth beyond problems and decline. But by the end of the 20th century, the view that aging could be accompanied by potential beyond problems was emerging. The "potential" focus of aging reflected the emergence of the second major conceptual sea change about aging and is documented in my book The Creative Age, the first book totally focused on creativity and aging, published at the start of the 21st century. The ultimate manifestation of potential with aging is creativity. By the start of the 21st century, the allegorical mirror was reflecting aging as one of the fairer of the fields in medicine.

Four major factors in particular stand out as affecting the changing image of aging in the allegorical mirror:

1. *The discovery of positive changes in the aging brain and mind that occur because of aging, not despite aging;*
2. *The increasing awareness that aging adds as it takes away;*
3. *A new view of aging as perhaps the best example of the whole being greater than the sum of its parts;*
4. *Growing recognition and understanding about what we ourselves can do to promote brain development.*

For so long science and society focused only on what was taken away with aging—that's all they saw in the allegorical mirror. But as our understanding of aging progressed, what was observed in the "mirror" changed. It is a poignant experience to read and write about a phenomenon, and then to personally live it—Carlos Williams' poetry about aging that adds as it takes away. But the phenomenon has actually been known far longer. It has been described as part of the human condition back at least to the days of ancient Greek mythology, which captured so many of the universal themes of humanity. These great myths contain that of Tiresias, a mere mortal wandering in the woods one day, thinking deep thoughts, with his eyes aimlessly wandering and inadvertently falling upon the goddess Athena bathing in the nude. Catching the eyes of a mere mortal viewing her naked threw Athena into a rage, and in her fury she blinded Tiresias. The other gods and goddesses questioned her, defending Tiresias as unwittingly being in the wrong place at the wrong time—certainly not a voyeur. They urged Athena to reconsider. She did, but she did not restore Tiresias' outer vision, instead granting him great inner vision. He became a great prophet and in his later years predicted the plight of Oedipus—exemplifying an old age that adds as it takes away.[7]

To make a difference

All of Gene's reflections in the metaphorical mirror culminated in greater clarity about his life purpose and passion. The images emerging in the "mirror, mirror on the wall" had continually changed in response to how others perceived him, and that had challenged his own perceptions of himself. It was clear that he was joyful to rediscover the man he knew looking back at him.

> *Finally, I came to appreciate what so much of my life and professional career have been all about—teaching, sharing information, and helping to improve the quality of life of others. This is what I do as a researcher and as a doctor. It is what excites me, fulfills me, and affords me the chance to make a difference for others.*

My parallel journey began as a deep education in illness that had begun some twenty years earlier, before I ever met Gene. I was thirty-four years old, struggling with a debilitating (though not life-threatening in the conventional sense) immune system illness that had the medical world baffled at the time. Chronic fatigue syndrome had yet to be recognized as a "legitimate" disease by medical science, and anyone who got it suffered not only the disease but also the ignorance and arrogance of those who looked at us in the mirror and saw us as medical malingerers.

In the early 1980s, it appeared that the disease was mainly infecting women in their mid-thirties to mid-forties. The illness was portrayed in the medical community and in the media as dubious. Since the disease struck women more often than men, the cutting stereotype was that chronic fatigue syndrome sufferers were anxious, self-absorbed, hypochondriacal women. Many were labeled depressed and hysterical; many were sent to psychiatrists. I knew that wasn't me, but it's hard to look at yourself in the mirror—literally or metaphorically—and see yourself truly, without the coloration of others' disparaging doubt and judgment.

There was growing evidence that multiple factors resulted in these similar illnesses. Since causes and cures were uncertain, patients became involved in diagnosis and healing. So many of the modern theorists on illness I read at that time—Elisabeth Kübler-Ross, Bernie Siegel, Carl Simonton, Larry LeShan, Larry Dossey, Stephen Locke, Norman Cousins, Marc Barasch, Jeanne Achterberg, Joan Borysenko, Rachel Naomi Remen, Ken Wilber, Kat Duff, Arthur Frank, Arthur Kleinman, Joyce McDougall, James Gordon among others—sought to redefine the meanings of health and illness, the doctor–patient relationship, self-image, and mind–body interaction.[8] Their new concepts helped me to cope with being ill through my thirties. They gave me the language and validation from other illness narratives while I was experiencing a pain that no one understood, and an isolation that no one could share.

The experience of being a patient, and the ability to articulate the experience, became important to me on my own road to health. Pain is blinding. It distorts our sense of our physical self, and it distorts our imagined self as well, in part because we believe it will merely be a temporary interruption. We may not imagine that it will give new meaning to our identity and we might have to permanently adjust to it. When we are well, we take our health or routine recovery for granted, but this new meaning emerging from pain begins to be reflected in small unfamiliar pixels of self. Like a digital image with a tick in transmission, the pixels of change in our identity flicker across our awareness, then seem to disappear, reintegrated into the image. For instance, I used to operate out of enthusiasm: that's who I was. But in the grip of my illness, when I tried to muster that cheerful and enthusiastic persona, I would get sick. I would look in the mirror and see the same face, but knew I was different now: a watcher and a listener. My strategy for handling this new circumstance was this: if I could hold onto my reality, feel a sense of control through recording details of my experience of this illness time, and through exploring psychologically my life patterns and habits before the illness, then I could give myself hope for help and change. Why? Because by holding onto the reflection of myself prior to the illness, I could believe that person was still there inside me. Like a bridge, the reassuring connection with my "prior self" gave me a way to move forward to engage my new and challenging reality, and in it discover my newly adapted and stronger self.

I was one of the lucky ones. I healed from chronic fatigue syndrome slowly and steadily over four years, and I was later able to build from my own experience and use it as a tool of investigation in my doctoral research in the early 90s.[9]

As Gene and I moved forward together in this current illness experience of cancer, my reflections, like the infinite images in my nana's mirrored niche, took me back to this and other illness experiences long past. The past teaches you what to expect of the present, what to expect when you look in the mirror. Gene and I, the scientist and the artist, both therapists who knew—as our respective phase models had illustrated—that positive growth and change are possible regardless of circumstances.

For me, the mirror of my illnesses, my reflections on my self in times of health and illness, held some important insights over time. Gene discovered these aspects of self- recognition in his own way, and my clients have described them as well. From that pooled experience come some fundamental insights about our relationship with our body and with our creative capacity as a wellspring.

We learn to feel betrayed by our own body. In my case, it was as if my body were victimizing me into learning what "weakness" means in a purely physical way, not an emotional way: drugged sleep, like a blanket of fog; swollen spleen, stunning me with its violent, sharp dagger-like pain; disorienting sensations of water rising inside my head, sloshing between my ears, magnetically drawing me inward; headaches, sore throats, body aches, loss of will or motivation to do the things that had previously been the inspirations of my life. Body weakness, body biochemistry, mind–body fatigue that is not tiredness but the result of a biochemical imbalance, and psychophysical stress—all of this felt like part of an invasion of something "not right" trying to right itself.

For Gene, the sense of betrayal was profound: he could not believe that a metastasis had been growing in his body without some kind of personal or medical awareness. He too felt betrayed by his body, his genetic constitution, and his original urologist, who appeared to have missed an opportunity to have discovered cell abnormalities in treating an earlier infection.

We also learn, or can learn, to trust the body and the symptoms that emerge for us as communication from deep sources within us—each of them a mirror into the illness. I learned to trust my body and experience my symptoms not only as pain but also as messengers to help me learn how to take care of myself. I learned to recognize them and to listen for them. What could trigger the symptoms? I began to watch, carefully, like a creative detective with the fine-tuned mirror of self-observation. Gene began to trust his personal experience and committed to sharing with others, knowing that they would benefit from knowing how he had handled it all and what had happened in his life.

I wrote in my journals, as Gene did in his, though our process was different. I kept two journals: one was a physical record; the other, a psychological inquiry. My writing voice separated itself from the voice of illness. I reported about "her" symptoms and how "I" would deal with this. When illness takes over, you can easily feel that all you are is the disease. This little bit of separation allowed me to have an observer inside of me who could see the me who was experiencing the illness. I learned how to integrate her voice:

> Mirror, mirror on the wall, who's the fairest of them all? Which self is the *observing-me* looking at the *ill-me*? Who am "I" now? My symptoms are part of me now. They are always there in the background. Symptoms

come now like messengers telling me when I am going against myself, when I am overstressed, when I need to rest, and when I am having "physical flashbacks"—a phrase Gene gave me to name the old memory channels of communication in my body.

We learn that the rhythms of illness time become a valuable source that informs our perception. In my case, I had already shaped something inside me, giving me an intuitive knowledge of this experience. Whether we like what we see or not, it is facing us all. The mirror of perception shifts and shifts, and progressively this chiseled perception reveals something new. In the context of our lives, our hearts, our psyche, our spirits, and our minds move into a changed rhythm of health. For Gene, this new rhythm showed up in his creative choices to write in tandem with me. This required a totally new approach to rhythm and style for him—one that offered the possibility of integrating story with image, personal lifestyle with professional lifestyle, and the surprising magic of shared experience.

Finally, we learn to understand the authority—the innate competence—of the unconscious image world. For Gene, as we saw earlier, his dreams took on a life of their own, reminding him of the imaginative power and energy of one's own aliveness. I experienced images in a different way than I had in the arts alone. My images connected me with a wisdom of the body, not outside of me but other than me, as though I was in the hands of something larger. I felt as though these images were physically there—as if they really existed inside of me. I found something visual, which was very important to me as an artist. Because chronic fatigue syndrome is virtually invisible and leaves you feeling invisible, it was strangely reassuring to find something "visible" within, something with such presence that I could hold onto it. The quality of the images was potent, as in my travels in North Africa, where I could float into the stark colors and shapes of the circular architecture in the Sahara desert, feeling surrounded and held. Or sometimes the imagery came with the opposite but equally powerful presence, like that of a metal bar across my chest, encrusted with old rust, pushing against my swollen spleen, scaring me into pain that was all too real. Little did I know then that over the next many years, illness would be the raw material I would use creatively. Little did I know that our mirrors expand and change in this way. Psychologically, I understood this as an integration process. But it could also represent a neurobiological process as well, a mechanism and capacity within us all.

When people ask about our healing, the focus is typically on the facts of the disease and treatment—what do we "have" and what is being done about it. But I believe the most important factor in healing is the intimacy and vulnerability one develops with oneself and practices with one's doctors. This is how we develop a sense of our own needs, and begin to see them clearly. We are deeply affected by the way we feel that we are seen by our physicians and others in our medical insider's circle. Their view of us affects how and what we reveal to them from our own mirrors. The clarity of this exchange is absolutely necessary for healing.

Do we have the time and flexibility of mind to discern the whole multifaceted experience, to locate the mind–body story and uncover what it reveals? The mirror is a depth reflector; it helps us see beyond the surface. This is the historical background that I brought to being with Gene through his "flight of the Phoenix," the term he used to describe rising up from the ashes of life-threatening disease. As if my own heart-body had been preparing me for my real love, which was with him, and for the challenges we would have to face.

Reflection Offers a Coherent, Affirming Sense of Self

A client with cancer, a woman who immersed herself in cancer self-help literature, was often helped and inspired by what she read. But she was thrown when she read and assumed to be true some bestseller-type book that basically held that we are responsible for our illnesses; that if we think positively and envision health, then healthy we will be. I take issue with that whole spectrum of literature and perspective—where we look in the mirror and see parts of our self to blame for a disease. We are not in some cosmic way responsible for our illnesses, and seeing ourselves as blameworthy is not helpful, not healing. We are, however, rightly called and challenged to become responsible *to* our illnesses. This kind of self-scrutiny to identify how we have participated in our illness—the confrontation with personality described in my Phase Diagram—is necessary for healing. Our task is to use reflection to learn our healing rhythm, or what is healing to us individually; to become more and more of our true self by removing what is not us.

In this process we may appear self-absorbed, but really it is an orientation, or a turning toward the self. It is shining the flashlight inward to find the "me" that best supports us through a challenging time. Such is the message of Sherlock Holmes and Freud: to be able to see and actually observe—to clean our psychic mirror so that we are able to see the full picture.

If we see our self as a patient only, that narrowed vision can close off our possibilities. It is by seeing our many selves that our possibilities are opened up, often in ways we would never foresee. For the larger story is that as I became responsible to integrating all that I had learned from my illness, I understood that there was a pattern in me that was trying to change, as if chronic fatigue syndrome were asking, *What is the relationship between wholeness and physical health? Find it.* Drawing from both Gene's and my experiences, opening up parts of ourselves to deepened creative potential, writing as a team about our shared insights and lessons, the mirror integrated for both of us the many "me's."

At a certain point in a life, through trauma of some kind (as illness often is) or through the natural movement of growth, the self needs more room to release its own energies. As these energies become available and move into awareness, like a sprout emerging from the ground, the structure of the personality is shaken. The movement of self is too strong for the space it has taken up in its more invisible stage. Different parts of the personality, which used to operate unaware of each another, now, through the release of the creative energies of the self, learn to recognize, accept, and harmonize with one another.

Mirror, mirror on the wall, who's the fairest of them all? Am I my symptoms or am I my health? Our symptoms, our experience, our memories and expectations: our reflections are part of us as we move forward. They are always there in the background. In the mirror, symptoms become messengers. They tell us when we are going against our self, when we are overstressed, when we need to rest, and when we are having physical flashbacks of memory.

In "Snow White," the wicked Queen could only accept one answer, one reflection in the mirror. As we engage the present moment, whether that is in health or illness, aging, or tending to loved ones, the mirror and all its infinite images become our friend. We need not fear it, but use it, to understand not only who we are in our bodies at this point in time, but who we have the potential to become, in sickness and in health.

Part Four

EMBRACING UNCERTAINTY

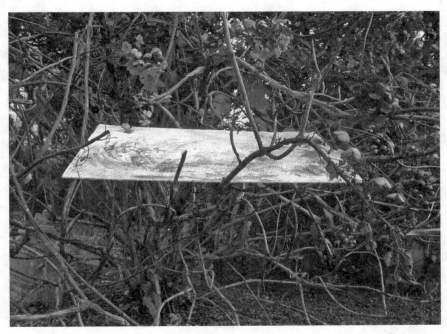

Figure IV.i "Floating in Nature" (2006), site-specific installation in Miller's healing garden, plaster sand painting on canvas board in branches, 18 × 24 inches. Artwork and documentation by Wendy L. Miller.

10

Illness as Partner

Intimacy, Vulnerability, Love, and Anger

The notes I handle no better than many pianists. But the pauses
between the notes—ah, that is where the art resides.
—Artur Schnabel[1]

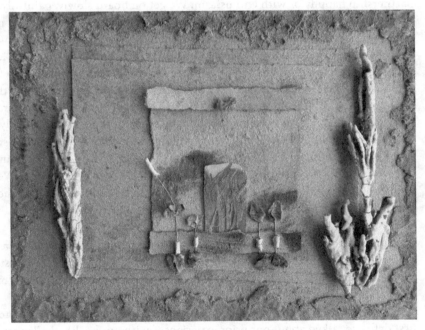

Figure 10.1 "Sandscape I: Family Pillars" (2008), paper, cooked sand, fired porcelain,
wire, and wood, 21 × 17.5 inches. Artwork by Wendy L. Miller, photo credit: Claire Blatt

It's hard enough finding the right partner to share our lives with, more challenging
yet to share our lives with our partner as we both intended, even vowed. Loving
partnerships teach us to accommodate and compromise, to accept the qualities
in another person that are unfamiliar to us no less than we celebrate the qualities

that are easy for us to cherish. We set out to embrace life as a team, navigate it together, wherever life leads. Partnership is both fulfilling and complicated. But what happens in the course of a lifelong commitment when we begin to realize that illness is also an additional partner?

Illness becomes our partner because we live together, in the body, in the family body, in time, in space, in intimacy, in the mirrors of our lives. This shared intimacy is the atmosphere of both the illness and the aging landscapes. An intimacy filled with the vulnerability of our joys, mixed with our sadnesses, our hopes mixed with our fears. Some of these vulnerabilities are internal, in our dreams and in our prayers; some are interrelational, in our friendships, in our sex lives, in our communications, and in our caregiving actions. We move through time, rhythm, and shared raw material as our psyches partner with their own truths.

How do we live with illness as partner? Most likely we do not accept this partnership happily or with enthusiasm. We get on board slowly, painfully, first even denying its long-term presence in relationship with us. As with so many significant parts of our lives, a relationship develops almost in spite of us. We enter filled with vulnerability. We are fragile. We probably feel exposed. Many people feel helpless, maybe even filled with various forms of resistance to these responses. For instance, we may act stoic, as if we are able to handle everything, or we may find that we quietly ignore certain aspects of our experience rather than admit we don't really know how to handle the situation at all. Clearly, our defenses are down. Old habits of personality persist, sometimes helpful, sometimes not. In these new circumstances, we feel opened in a way that can feel not safe, one that exposes more of us than we may be prepared to show. We feel vulnerable. Illness—whether ours or our loved one's—can weaken us, whether physically or psychologically, and often both. We are adrift in relationship to our own vulnerability.

Vulnerability is the crux of our challenge—the tender, painful spot in a now bruised life. Our question more specifically becomes: How can my understanding of vulnerability—my relationship with my own vulnerability—inform my relationship with illness as partner?

Gene and I were to live into this question from the very beginning. From our first date, we talked about our prior experiences with our health challenges, and our transitions moving forward from our first marriages. Our relationships with our own vulnerabilities, some spoken, some unspoken or unacknowledged, traveled with us into our relationship from the very get-go. Looking back on that early time together when we were living together, not yet married but engaged and, with Eliana as a baby, a family, we shared in Chapter 3 how Gene wanted me to consult with my family about marrying him, a man with a diagnosis of a life-threatening disease.

It wasn't just the death sentence draining hope, but the merciless prog-
nosticating that made it hard to focus on anything else—making it hard
to focus on life in facing a death sentence. . . . As the gravity of my situa-
tion further sunk in, I began to feel enormously guilty about what it would
mean for Wendy to marry a dying person. . . . Following her consultation
with her family, Wendy and I shortly thereafter did get married. On our
wedding day, we were able to maintain the wonderfully tight circle of love
and support by family and friends by having the ceremony and party at
our house. It included such highlights as Wendy coming down our winding
elegant staircase amidst soft lighting and music in her striking wedding
gown to the attendees waiting with anticipation, and not-quite 2-year-
old Eliana's impeccable job as ring bearer, to the music of the Elmo (from
Sesame Street) theme song, with her receiving an Elmo replica virtually
her size. The event was filled with intergenerational richness, such as my
6-foot-tall son Alex lovingly dancing with his 5-foot-high grandmother,
my mother, in her ninth decade. The warmth and joy of the ceremony,
dancing, and party, eclipsed the threatening crisis around my diagnosis
and prognosis, at least for the moment. Years later, when Eliana was 6, one
of her friends saw her in the wedding picture, and with a puzzled excla-
mation asked, "How could you be at your parents' wedding?!" Without
missing a beat, Eliana innocently replied, "You mean you weren't invited
to your parents' wedding?"

As Gene's notes in his journal reflect, illness was already our partner, alongside his joy on our wedding day and our decision to make a life commitment.
He so deeply felt and cherished this "wonderfully tight circle of love and support
by family and friends," and the fact that it all allowed us this joyful respite as it
"eclipsed the threatening crisis around my diagnosis and prognosis, at least for
the moment." We spent our wedding night not so far from home, in the dazzling
honeymoon suite at The Watergate Hotel, with a spectacular view overlooking
the Potomac River. Of his awareness that illness was our silent partner already,
he would later write:

While lying in bed there with Wendy, I looked up with the sensation that
the thread holding the sword of Damocles was strengthening; as Wendy
put her arms around me, I experienced our relationship as strengthening
as well. In retrospect, the most valuable recommendation I received during
the course of my cancer treatment was from Wendy right after our mar-
riage. Her attitude and spirit so complemented mine with a powerful ori-
entation toward living life, not succumbing to the dark clouds above us.
She saw only one choice for our family unit—to function as a family, living

life to the fullness, the best we could, not ourselves making us a victim of our circumstances.

I remember that conversation. I remember saying those words and meaning them. And I continued to mean them, holding them as a truth for every day of our life together. What I was to discover, however, was that living with illness as partner, living so intimately with my own and with Gene's vulnerability, would take us into a shared experience that deepened both our intimacy and our vulnerability in ways that were by turns comfortingly familiar and frightening.

Illness as partner forced itself into all of our decisions, not only about how we would choose to live but where we would live; knowing that this illness partner required health insurance was upmost in our priorities. In some ways, it was helpful to have certain decisions be clarified, but in other ways, it wasn't. I would often look at my friends and think about all the possibilities they were imagining for their retirement years, and it would create an internal panic in me.

Gene wrote, in 2009, reflecting back on the thirteen-and-a-half year course of his hormone treatments and how they struck him personally. He understood it all in epic terms as an assault on manhood that had been expressed in literature from ancient Greek times to Hemingway.

I was thinking about Hemingway's reflection that "A man can be destroyed but not defeated."[2] It made me flash back to my favorite book in high school—Hemingway's Pulitzer Prize–winning story "The Old Man and the Sea," especially now that people view me as an old man. I view the story now as an older man's will to survive—his perseverance to achieve an almost impossible goal while drawing upon fewer physical resources than he had before as a younger man. This story became part of my reservoir of images that contributed to a new theory about aging that I have introduced, suggesting that aging may be one of the best examples of the whole being greater than the sum of its parts.

I thought about my invited talks, and wondered how long I could continue to deliver them as effectively as has been the case. Here too I discovered a whole greater-than-the-sum-of-its parts quality. After a slower approach than usual to the podium because of my heightened weakness, I would feel that surge of adrenaline, and for the duration of the talk I would never know there was anything wrong with me; and fortunately the audience evaluations seemed to concur.

I thought about other losses, like my curly hair, which after what I refer to as a chemo cut became a bald head. With the image of my curly hair, I visualized Wendy's curly hair and drifted into the dark-side challenges to our romantic life. The romantic life of someone with prostate cancer who has been treated with hormones, like me, is not at all easy to talk about, not the least factor being the grotesque Dark Ages types of images that are generated. Prostate cancer loves male hormones—androgen, testosterone. Prior to modern medicine, one of the treatments was castration, to lower these hormone levels. Modern medicine put on white gloves and created what are euphemistically referred to as "androgen ablation" treatments through hormone-suppressing medications that, without the white gloves on, are referred to as "chemical castration," a major biological assault on your body. Sexual passion becomes severely challenged.

Back to Hemingway's reminder that you can destroy a man but not defeat him: I have become very sensitive about not giving up or allowing myself to drift into scenarios of self-pity or inaction where my cancer can further victimize me. But as my dream cycles have changed, my vivid nightmares have transformed into vivid daydreams that are typically positive and have slowed down time for me. They bring poignant rather long pauses to the notes of my life. In the passion scenario of my pause, I find alternative imagery arising as part of a new whole greater than sum of my parts. I think about it from the start when Wendy and I made love, the intensity with which our eyes engaged, and how good we felt in each other's arms. I think about my fingers moving through her curly hair and our embracing, and miraculously experience the gradual emergence, through a synergy of emotion and imagery, of feelings that have been suppressed by "state-of-the-art" chemistry. My daydream pauses move me closer to Wendy.

The art lies in how we handle such pauses, the pauses that live in between the notes of our lives, between our personal reveries and our personal angst. Loss and pain are unsympathetic partners. What happens in intimacy when the illness condition hangs over you in the bedroom, like a sword of Damocles? There are ways in which our compartmentalized thinking protects us from the emotional avalanche of loss and pain, and protection is what we need. Denial implies that it is an intellectual choice. The truth is there are internal screens, split screens of awareness, which protect us from the avalanche of raw sensation. Our perceptions shift to meet various illness realities and developing realities. But, in intimacy, in bedroom intimacy, the language is all about sensation, and there is no telling what happens. *The loss of spontaneity, the remembrance of love.*

Over time, we harden, or perhaps open, to be able to leave at least some part of us available as our partner is trying to dig out of the deep sea of love and lossness.[3] Lossness is different from loss or from sadness. It is an overlay of sensation that tugs at the body, leaving it outside of its own presence, leaving us outside of where we thought we were, reminding us that in no means is this experience fully in our own hands. Lossness is the movement of the pendulum swing going on and on over years of various changes and various states of sensation, change, and understanding. This pain is invisible to others. It does not appear to accompany our daily lives, but it sweeps over us like tidal waves in the most unexpected times and ways. During the intimacy of sex, where the closeness revolves, evolves, and moves through us, one or the other can suddenly be catapulted into a foreign private zone, a zone where communication can suddenly fall silent, where illness as partner silences the senses, or tricks them, sometimes cruelly, sometimes with pure and complete love. *The loss of fantasy, the entry of compassion.*

Intimacy is a very strong muscle, exercised with the fibers of friendship, care, and the ability to weather strong waves of distance, drowning, smothering, and recovering will. Intimacy is our life force. Lossness catapults us with the force of an orgasm, yet awakening the self into the fluids of change, adrift between darkness and light, with known and unknown parts of self floating away, surrounding us, pieces of one another struggling to keep the force field from magnifying us with its strength, like waves of grief, where we are thrown farther than ever into the hinterlands, never knowing we were signing on for these places in the journey called love. *The loss of libido, the stir of desire to make new.*

The sword of a diagnosis hangs over you at the strangest moments, accompanies you into the release of shared closeness and intimacy. I think of Joyce's Molly Brown and her *yes I said yes I will yes,* in her moment of ecstatic love and merging, open to it.[4] In our own moments the heart whispers, cries *yes, yes, I say yes,* and then, with no warning, the illness-body screams *no, she said no, she said no, no, no:* no opening, no merging, no allowance. The intimacy that hurts and harms and fears and screams. The intimacy that merges the hopes and fears, the longings and the losses, the pleasures and the pains. *I say no, I say no, I say no, no, no,* and an anger of surge, an anger of release, an inner place that even in its opening and loving and knowing, pulses against love, life, loss, as if it knows, while sensation itself does not know, cannot know, and will not know what is to come. And the love that surrounds the unknowing, sometimes, just like grand love, sometimes, surges on its own waves of intimacy; and in this illness partnership of soul love, it imagines, between us, an anger so huge that it bursts through Molly Brown's voice like an evil counterpart to the shared love and sweet intimacy. *No, I say, no, no, no.*

We Seek to Normalize Our Reality, Whatever It May Be

Awakening into the light of the day, we return to our individual boundaries of being. Do we even recognize that our vulnerability is accompanying us? We may experience ourselves as different; we may act with more hypervigilance; we may find that we insulate ourselves; compartmentalize; isolate; normalize; but do we even recognize that each of these strategies is really our vulnerability expressing itself? *The intimacy encoded between us in tender distance.*

Yet, our vulnerable, unprotected self ultimately reveals itself to us. It is new, this unprotected side of ourselves, and therefore new places open and close within us. At high speed, vulnerability can present as a blur. Fragile places; raw places; sudden tears; sudden strengths; sudden angers. And we have no choice. Illness as partner enters on its own terms, with a life of its own, a temperament of its own, and a community of characters and characteristics of its own. Whether we like them or not, love them or not, they live with us. Like most couples, Gene and I had different perspectives, different styles in the way we responded to things, and this included how we responded to this shadow partner of illness. He might turn to science and literary allegory, while I might turn to my art or existential contemplation. But the illness has its own say in so much of what happens, the timing, the environment, the circumstances, and the rhythm of the shared partnership—the now three-way partnership. *The loss of daring, the pause, the stop.*

Most of us, under the stress of learning to live with illness as partner, with all of its erratic "behavior," become hypervigilant. How could we not? We are designed by nature to be hypervigilant in the presence of a threat. In illness, uncertainty becomes the climate of our relationship with everyone and everything. We pay very close attention to everything so that no stone is unturned, no information is unseen, and nothing else can grab us from behind. To do this means we live with our finger on the fragile pulse of the hope. We protect ourselves; don't let anyone in who moves the story too far into a future. We don't let anyone share any kind of advice or information that takes care of his or her own anxiety rather than our needs. To fine-tune in this vulnerable way, we may need to isolate ourselves. We pace ourselves, monitor the flow of those we will let in, when we will let them in, and with what kind of information. We try to normalize what isn't normal in any way. We do this by creating a new normal, searching for the tiny moments when our vulnerability becomes our strength, our inner guide. We authorize our vulnerability to speak for us, represent us, to be present to us rather than hidden away as most of us do in ordinary times. This is such a shift that it can feel like a "twilight zone," as Gene described it.

> *My doctors were conveying to me that I had no future path, while the rest of the world with no knowledge of my condition was contacting me about program plans down the road. It made me feel like I was in the twilight zone[5] . . . gripped by a strange new sensation . . . paralyzing. . . . I was being barraged by menacing medians: "The median life expectancy with metastatic prostate cancer is low." "The median time to symptoms appearing is this." "The median time that treatment will help is only that." Again, all of the medians were minimal. As if median time meant normal time, when in their truth, all the medians were minimal, i.e., not normal. I had to learn what language to let in to find my own normal."*

Normalizing is often misunderstood as denial, when in fact it is the opposite. Normalizing is the attempt to accommodate the conditions of a new reality. The new reality is filled with the presence of life, death, aging, and loss, and our effort to accommodate that is a moment-by-moment managerial task. It is an enormously difficult task, and largely invisible to anyone else. The problem with the word *denial* is that it is so loaded with unconscious judgmental tone, and so subjective that any scientifically based meaning is elusive. As Gene pointed out, what is called "denial" can be maladaptive or adaptive.[6] At best, denying or tuning out fear frees us to take purposeful risks and face adversity. Most often, however, even those whose work is grounded in science use "denial" casually, often in what comes across as a condescending and demeaning way. In this casual lexicon, "denial" blames and judges us negatively for all the changes and demands we are trying to accommodate in order to keep going so that we can continue to live with our new condition, to live under new conditions. "Denial" implies that it is an intellectual choice, but so often it is not. Truthfully, how much information can we bear, yet continue to dare to do all that we have to do, to accommodate our new levels of need?

Our essential task is one of self-preservation—to preserve our deepest self and our loved one's self from being disappeared into the illness—and to do this, we deliberately focus our attention in a certain way, we selectively engage in certain information and ideas that allow us to stay in the conversation. To call that denial as if it's a refusal to accept reality is not giving us credit for the hard work we are doing to stay engaged in our reality. We deserve to be met where we are, not made to feel defensive.

During the same months that Gene was going through chemotherapy, we also needed to tend to the healing process of openings and wounds from various procedures on his kidneys. I learned to create different kinds of bandaging that stayed drier for him, making the incisions less sensitive, less infected, and more tolerable. He learned how to manage fevers with his own preventative medicines. He took his blood pressure before it would surprise him with high numbers. We learned ways to accommodate because we had to.

We were also managing the flow of more life and living into that life, for that is what enlivened him and that is what mattered: daily living. Preparing his materials for his webinars, writing the reports he wanted to finish for his grants, taking his autumn road trip with Alex, watching Eliana play basketball at her games, wanting enough energy to do and attend to these things—this was the life material that mattered to him. Ultimately, when all of the accommodations were not enough to counterbalance the onslaught of ill health, I could "see" how many organs were in the process of breaking down. By then, it was a natural sensing of this biological truth, communicated to us through his body. Looking back, in retrospect and knowing the end result, one might say we were in denial, but to do so is to misunderstand the reality of living life forward.

In Vulnerability Lies the Courage to Embrace Uncertainty

In Chapter 4, I wrote about time gained or time lost depending entirely from whose perspective we are looking, and I shared the story of Marty, who was elated to have a six-month reprieve from scans, while his family feared that that much time would be too long—that a closer watch was needed on his condition. The truth is that both Marty and his family were accommodating, managing, trying to normalize life, which, in fact, was moving between relaxation and trauma, again and again. Marty's family's natural response was to worry; they felt helpless to save his life and wanted his doctors to be more vigilant. Marty's natural response was to want to live well into his life without the cancer world probing and deciding for him if he should live or he should die. He wanted the right to live without becoming limited to or defined by his illness. This was vulnerability experienced from two different places in the family body—from Marty in his own way, and from his family in their way—quite differently for each.

One of my clients who has been struggling emotionally with his entry into his sixties has three friends who have passed away within the past six months. His own wife is a breast cancer survivor, so he clearly has up-close experience with the traumatic entry of illness as a partner in one's life. In his anxiety and pain over his lost friendships, he has turned the mirror inward on himself and his wife. Will they continue to be healthy through their sixties, seventies, eighties? In his musings about his friends, just the mention of a particular cancer brings forth so many assumptions—that a person living with cancer is dying all the time; that weakening and slowing down makes a person unavailable; that we may have completed all that there is left to say in our relationships. He and I have revisited these unexamined assumptions a number of times in different ways, opening the frightened places of vulnerability, existential awareness, and meaning. I say, yes, it matters to continue to communicate with our friends, whatever method is feasible, whatever amounts of fear it activates within us; that the assumption that our relationship with them is done, that we have said all we need to say, is worth questioning. I say, yes, living all the way up to and into the final breath includes the care and love of our relationships.

What is it that grips our vulnerable essence and tries to tell us that we are no longer wanted or needed by one who is ill or dying? What has us assume that their "going" means an end not just to the person but to our relationship to the person even now; that maybe we should "go" first from the relationship, slowly exit from our own reactions and responses? At times it is us, the eventual survivor, who declares through our own actions that the one who is ill or in grief has become an untouchable, invisible, or off-limits person.

We assume it is about their need, but really it is our own. We assume we have already said what needs to be said, but our discomfort speaks so loudly we can hardly hear what actually needs to be said. It is our own vulnerability and fear that tell us to step back, move over, defer to illness-the-partner or aging-the-partner and absent ourselves emotionally. To stay present is to keep company with the uncertainty of life, and it takes courage to do that. Sometimes we have no choice but to be on intimate terms with uncertainty. When we are healthy, we think we know how we will be or how we will feel or what we will choose to do if and when such and such might happen *to* us. But when we are inside of that "something" when it is living *with* us, everything is different. It rearranges us. It rearranges our priorities, our thoughts, our feelings, our needs and desires. It is from that place, that changed place, that we will come to make our decisions—not assumptions—but decisions and actions as to what we can and will do.

In the meantime, what do we do, confronted with the essential vulnerability of life? We dread it. We fear it. We think we understand it. We move it away as best we can. And sometimes we move people away just because they remind us how close it resides to us. We fear vulnerability as if it were contagious or will find its way into our life through osmosis, and that by distancing ourselves we might be able to escape the inevitable.

But when the crack opens, it opens us. We find ourselves praying, silently speaking to the uncertainty. Maybe this is what prayer is—a meditative voice that we both speak to and listen to at the same time: *May we each be dropped into this essence gently. If the innocence of our loved ones is to be broken, may it be broken gently. If we may live long enough to accompany these processes together, may it be lived gently. May we be able to let go when our time comes, as gently as gently moves.*

Caregiving as an Act of Certainty, "One True Thing at a Time"

There is nothing more intimate and vulnerable than the act of caregiving. It both pushes on us and pulls out of us everything we have. Caregiving is like being the captain of the ship, or the pilot of the plane. It is filled with so many responsibilities and actions. Yet there are deep gifts in caregiving, filled with all of the mystery of serving, returning, and accompanying our loved one.

A snapshot of my own caregiving day is much like those of others I know, if not in specific details then in the sheer ordinariness of it all: the emails, the appointments, meetings with Eliana's teachers and shepherding the schoolwork, the making of lunch, the morning drives, bringing downstairs now whatever Gene needs, getting his clothes for him, gathering what I need for my clients, making the tea, stopping for a moment in my studio and seeing if the clay piece has dried, covering or uncovering it, warming up my office, sitting with a client through their life, coming back into my own, returning to the house, making lunch for Gene, going to a doctor's appointment, sitting in the chemo room, picking him up, checking on how it went, having a conversation with the doctor, sitting at Starbucks with Gene after the conversations, dropping him off, going to pick up Eliana from school, having a conversation about what happened in her health class or what she wants to wear to the party on Friday, coming home, everyone going off to their own worlds, at the same time keeping a structure that brings us all back together for dinner (make the food, present the food, eat the food, clean up the food), all done by about 6:30 or 7:00 so we can begin to organize for Eliana to shift into homework mode.

This ordinariness, however, always proves deceptive in illness time because everything can change in an instant. One evening I stand at the sink, cleaning up the meal or whatever we have done, and I look across the family room to see that Gene is taking his temperature or his blood pressure, and I know he is weak at this moment. In my mind's eye, in that moment I see through a split screen that I have written about earlier, the feeling that all of our actions are a kind of preparation for the fire drill, for the fear of the pending emergency.

The split screen works this way: one option is that I am going to clean these dishes and put them in the dishwasher and move my way into homework mode with Eliana. The other option is that Gene's temperature is going to spike and redirect the evening and we are going to have to rush off to Sibley Hospital, and will I bring Eliana—or whom will I ask to come over? My mind flashes to the way pilots or captains have to see *everything at once:* all possibilities as critical decisions and potential consequences come before their eyes in one moment. And then if Gene's temperature is fine, the entire lineup of options shifts, I don't need the crisis plan right now, and I return to the everyday, relieved that it was just a fire drill, not a fire.

I watch Gene lay his tired body onto the couch to take a catnap, waking up and reading through a chapter in ninth-grade biology or geometry so he can help Eliana with her homework. The day ends in some kind of family tension because I have to get Eliana off the phone or computer, until finally, later into the night, I drop down into my own bed to fall into a book that I can't even read, or open an email that I can't deal with, or on a Thursday night, to watch a television show with enough medical tension that I can lose myself in those characters pushed up against the existential edge of mortality.

What is my relationship to my role of caregiver? Along with the deep sense of responsibility, love, and desire, an uncomfortable feeling begins to arise. It's not really resentment that happens in the caregiving role, but it is an awareness of an inequality, as if the world has narrowed down to the needs of one person. Your partner is still your partner in your heart, but caregiving becomes more and more of a presence—tending illness as partner.

The imbalance of it all begins to affect you. It begins to feel lonely. On one level, you are being asked to do everything, and you want to do everything; your love for this person is deep. On another level, you feel a huge responsibility, and that responsibility is yours alone. And then there is some other level, where everyone encourages you to take care of yourself, but your own needs and stresses and all that you are balancing are necessarily ignored.

Shift in Awareness from Illness as Foreign Invader to Illness as Partner

We used to look at cancer as coming from a foreign invader, something we had to get rid of. Now it is about normal cells that have somehow gone awry. How can we change an environment that for some strange reason has gone awry? I am not suggesting that we have causal power over the biochemical environment or that what we do causes cancer or doesn't cause it. I am suggesting that we have to be *responsible to* the situation once it is here. And that means ask, think, pay attention to whatever we can.

Gene is eating no fat. Cancer cells love fat. He is not going to give them any. Maybe this is not a war of killing but of managing behavior. If anyone can come up with a creative solution to behavior, it is Gene. Regulating and watching bizarre behavior is his forte. Beware, cells, you have come into the body of a psychiatrist, and a clever one at that.

Gene sleeps in the same way that I imagine cancer moving—like a drowsy sleepwalker in the darkness of the night. He closes his eyes on the couch as he watches some action show on the television. If you ask him what is going on in the show, he can't really tell you. TV is like an action lullaby that quiets his active mind. Then eventually he decides he is going to climb the stairs to go to sleep. He collapses on our bed or gently lowers his fragile body into the sea of comforters. We arrange and rearrange the pillows so that he can breathe, so that he can be comfortable, so that he can relax. Then a few hours later, I may check on him, and he is gone from that bed and into a different one. It used to be because he was restless and didn't want to keep me awake. Then it was that he needed his space to take care of himself and all of the bodily issues that he was adjusting to. Then he also needed me to feel rested so that I could keep the family schedule going early in the morning, the prep for school, the carpool, the lunch, the routine that begins our family day.

Now though, it seems I have to look in many rooms, in many beds to find which one he has inhabited and for which hours. He roams. He rests. He changes positions, lights, shapes, styles of bedrooms and mattresses. Too restless, too uncomfortable, too not right. Goldilocks and the Three Bears. Everything about cancer is not right, down to cellular discomfort.

And this discomfort is not just in his body, but in the family body. A friend of mine who lost her husband eleven years ago told me that losing a parent was so traumatic for her sons that everything trivial fell away. I know exactly what she means. Another friend, who taught me how to paint, has been faced with her own life-threatening entry of cancer. She says, "Everything in the world looks different to me now, in my micro-universe and in the macro-universe. I never saw how much suffering there was around me. I am in my sixties, as is my husband, and I thought I had lots more time for everything. Our children are both in college and I have to keep working. I have to keep it all going, but the process of managing everything through this foggy and 'shocked into silence' brain inside this landscape of total uncertainty changes every single thing I do and every single thing I look at."

Using art expression as a way into our experience lets creativity guide our inner work. Let me give an example of the way imagery can process the complexity of emotional, physical, and, frankly, spiritual elements. I have seen this same image from a number of people, with a different slant depending on the individual person's circumstances or storyline. On a piece of white paper a fragile thin line runs from the top of the page to about midway down, bound to a figure either holding onto the line by a thin connection, or having the line wrapped haphazardly around the figure's middle, or just barely touching as the line and figure come together.

The first time I saw it was from a woman in her late thirties, recovering from chronic fatigue syndrome, an ex-overachieving lawyer dropped for years into the limbo of being unable to work, a state of rest and recuperation, which triggered many early feelings of abandonment when her father remarried and created a second family.

Next was a woman in her late forties who drew the image after divorcing and fending for herself in a high-powered lobbying firm in Washington, DC. She had tried to maintain the same personality style of aggression as she had when she was married, forgetting that she was able to soften from this persona with her partner at the end of each day. Alone, she had a hard time transitioning, and the style seemed to have control of her, driving fast over her own feelings and responses.

A third woman, in her late sixties, was struggling with the judgments and assumptions projected on her from the members of her Christian Scientist Church as she turned to Western medicine—surgery, radiation, and chemotherapy—to save her from breast cancer. They shunned her for not entrusting her faith in her body's ability to heal on its own without medical intervention. On top of cancer, she had lost her spiritual community as well as her health.

All three, with different circumstances, different reasons, drew the same image. Like the feeling conveyed in Gene's image of the sword of Damocles, the thin thread holds, drops, or hangs a person into this uncharted territory of "nowhere." Sometimes it seems that the figure is so tired that it is limp; sometimes the figure is reaching and just missing or almost missing the line; other times the figure is out of body. Always the figure has a slight energetic feel, almost there or close to empty. The differences among depression, grief, and replenishment are so slight, yet so significant.

The process of looking at this picture together is almost always the same: first, honoring the intensity of feeling that accompanies the image. There is deep suffering and angst, a quality of "I am at my rope's end." Sometimes we cry together; sometimes we wonder how all this could have happened; sometimes we unconsciously slump in a way that matches the weary energy of the image. Eventually, it seems that the image captures our deepest feelings, bypassing the intellectualizing we might do and cutting straight to the core of feeling, which may, early in the struggle, be feelings of how hopeless and depressing the situation is.

That is the clue, the moment of transition, the psychospiritual confrontation with the psyche: *I give up.* And that is an opening. "Where is up? What is at the other end of this particular rope? From where do we hang?" Isn't our health always a thin thread? We may cry into the image on the page, but really, where does the image come from? The first time I asked the question, I did it with paper. I placed a second sheet of white paper above the picture as it lay on my drawing table between my client and me.

"What is that for?" she asked.

"I am wondering, what is at the other end of this line? What does it connect to?" The air between us changed, palpable as these moments can be.

"The other end? I never thought about that," she pondered.

"Why don't we think about that together, on the page?"

What is at the other end of the line, the thread, the rope, when we give up? Is it downward or upward that we give to? When we look up from where we are myopically focusing, what is up there? What are we connected to? To what, whom, where do we call out? What is the line of connection for us?

In each circumstance, the image that follows arrives unconsciously, like a third element between us. It arrives with such unconscious competence as if it knows its own wisdom. With the first client, the ex-lawyer, it was a simple green circle, slowly drawn round and round an orange center. A memory of something past, we both looked at each other with tears in our eyes, tears of recognition. It was reminiscent of something she had drawn a long time ago as an image of inner strength related to the kind of love and support her grandmother had provided for her. Here it was, the same image, smaller, more faintly drawn, but so clear, we both recognized it instantly. It was like a faint memory of strength, remembrance, a calling. "I am here," it seemed to say. "I have always been here. I have never left you." With the other two clients, they began to search for resilience and stability, inner strengths drawn from their associations to shape, color, and pattern.

Image can be a spiritual creative resource: a reminder in the darkness that the psychic gold is sometimes sitting right there in the center of the wound, not depressed, perhaps forgotten, untended, shriveled even, but alive and slowly still breathing, ready to be re-recognized. These small seeds of inner listening are our call to give up-wards, to reach for what remains, regardless of the circumstances. Give up, giving up-wards, reminds us that as long we are here, we are connected somewhere, to something, someone, somehow. *Give up* is our collective call and response we have with our knowing self, the voice of our intuition as prayer.

Deep Sustenance: Friendship, Partnership, and a Prayer

It is not just the intimacy between us that I am referring to, but the intimacy in friendships. I am embarrassed to say that I feel envy about my own friends' lives. Not envy as jealousy, but the definition of envy in every culture as the description of protecting our loved ones from the evil eye, or what is unintentionally transmitted through coveting something that someone else has. In Hebrew, it is called *ayin ha'ra*; in French it is called *le mauvais œil*; in Spanish it is called *mal ojo*. It is the kind of envy I feel toward the people who do not have the sword of Damocles hanging over their lives. Yes, I used to ask, Why me? Over and over, Why me? How could we have so much cancer and loss hanging around our family? Now I realize that is not exactly what the envy wanted protection from. The envy is the longing for the innocence, the freshness, the everydayness, the lightness, and the joy of just moving along into a future without the doom of future hanging over you. The thread not only hangs above you, but you are hanging on by a thin thread as well—internally, in friendships, in caregiving, and in loving.

We entered into a week in late October, just after Gene returned from his annual fall outing with Alex, where it was once again time to start another round of chemotherapy, and yet his system was so deeply weakened, we couldn't imagine how he could do that. It had been what we were doing for so long that we just continued to think he would do it. But the doctor stopped us in our tracks, suggesting it was time to stop.

Our community of friends step in and step up. They are on email talking with each other about what they can do and how they can help us. I said to Gene, we have to dream. We need a dream to know what to do. He's too tired to dream—he needs Ambien to sleep and I am too awake to dream because I have to keep waking up to come downstairs and make sure he is all right. And so my friend Cara, always with one foot in the transcendent realm and one in the physical world, dreams for us. She lives far away and this becomes her way to be near us. She dreams of angels, realms upon realms of angels surrounding us and protecting us, with a sound that is a deep kind of vibrational benevolence. At first she thought it was music, but then she said she couldn't even call it music, it was a benevolent vibration. It feels to me that she "sees" other levels of life, or I say she has the capacity to talk to God. Whatever it is, that is what she does. I don't do that. I don't have that channel open, but I can feel the comfort of it because I trust that in her. I feel the benevolent presence of it.

Perhaps Cara's dreams are the kind of communication some people would call prayer. Her voice of intuition sees or listens or trusts some thing that both calls her and responds to her. If this is prayer, here is mine: that this hammock of loved ones, this group of men and women who adore Gene and adore me and are totally rooting for him, rooting for the miracle, rooting for the atypical, the hero, rooting for their daddy, rooting for their pappy, rooting for their husband, their colleague and mentor, their doctor, their friend, that we do what we learned to do from Peter Pan when Tinker Bell's light was going out: Peter turns to the camera and says to the audience—all of us in our homes glued to the TV screen that night—that we should clap, clap our distant prayer, and we did.[7] We clapped and we clapped and we clapped because we didn't want Tinker Bell's light to fade. I just hope that every one of those realms of angels and every one of these loved ones in all of their places will clap and clap and bring this life force back into Gene. Give him the energy and strength that his body deserves: let us try another blood transfusion and more oxygen. Bring him back to his own light so he can make the decision that he needs to make, whatever that is so he knows: is he fighting, is he dying?

At a lecture I attended years ago, the psychologist Lawrence Leshan told me that he works as a radical activist.[8] He helps people fight for their life by mobilizing everything that matters to them all the way until the moment that together, we know we are not fighting anymore. And he told me that I would know that moment.

We don't know if this is that moment. But we do know we need that light. That's my call to prayer.

11

Grand Rounds

Listening and Hearing as Healing Resources of Creativity

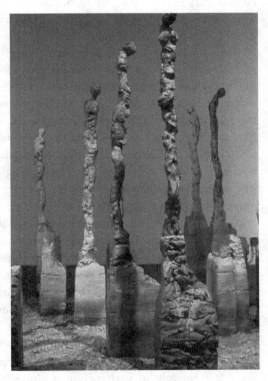

Figure 11.1 "Woman Building: Strategies for Standing" (1982), large room size installation at Southern Exposure Gallery in San Francisco, CA. Six out of twelve fired clay figures with oxide slips, each close to 5 feet tall. Artwork and documentation by Wendy L. Miller, photo credit: Joshua Soros.

Gene loved to teach. He especially loved to bridge the gap between traditional medicine and the humanities—finding inspiration for understanding the human condition not only through science but through art, literature, music, history, philosophy—even comedy. This was more than just his teaching style; it was the scientific lens through which he viewed creativity, aging, and illness. That is, we are so much more than our frailties or diseases, more than the sum of our deficits, and our wholeness itself has healing properties that are routinely missed by medical science, to the detriment of both patients and providers.

As a physician, a psychiatrist who worked closely with aging patients and their families, Gene felt strongly that in the practice of medicine, physicians and others did a disservice to patients by reducing them to a diagnosis (including, at times, a misdiagnosis or a missed diagnosis, as he knew from personal experience). By focusing so narrowly on particular types of clinical detail, as of course they must, they often overlooked the context for symptoms or suffering and tuned out the fuller human story unfolding before them. This, too, has clinical significance, for narrative is not simply a colorful accessory, it is clinical detail in story form, a patient's native language.

Gene's view of aging had long been that it is a developmental process "adding to" rather than "taking away" from creativity as a resource for health and healing. In his research he found that how we view ourselves and our potential, and how we tap into our creative faculty, can alter how we experience illness and aging—it can recalibrate us so that we can better cope with our changing circumstances. New coping creates new wisdom derived specifically from our experience, as well as cultivating vulnerability with strength, intellect with intuition. Neither creativity nor the expanding experience of aging removes life-threatening challenges, but they both do enhance our skills in facing them. These are the messages he sought to share everywhere he went.

As clinicians and professional partners we shared that view. As clinicians, we both knew that when illness takes hold and medicine has no cure, the illness experience, and even the death experience, continues to offer the potential for spiritual or emotional healing that can relieve suffering. Because that potential still exists, the common awkward or dissatisfying communication around the reality that is our life is a punishing psychological segregation at the most human level. This is true whether the communication gap involves family and friends, or the medical professionals who enter the picture, as we'll see in the next chapter. When you consider that care and healing are the whole point of medical intervention, the absence of thoughtful, caring conversation with those already suffering is unacceptable. The silence hurts those who are ill, but also hurts those on the caregiving side of the relationship. It denies everyone the opportunity to fully engage, to share an experience, to learn, and to be moved and changed by the people and the circumstances that bring them all together. In essence, the effects disable innate developmental potential and withhold the most natural healing resources from those most in need.

As professor of both healthcare sciences and of psychiatry and behavioral studies at the George Washington University School of Medicine and Health Sciences,

Gene was a frequent lecturer and drew not only from his research but also from his many years as a clinician and from his patients' and his own life experience. In his editorials as well as in teaching, he used analogies from nursery rhymes and fairy tales to illuminate potentials and biases against older people. For him, common folklore made profound points in ways that most people understood and appreciated.

To the body of instructive case stories that Gene used as a medical educator, stories that put a face on aging, illness, and creativity's healing power, he planned (with this book) to add his own. In fact, together our experience as clinicians and insiders in this particular case study made it a case about not only the individual body, but the family body as well, and we brought different yet complementary perspectives to the interpretation. Through the nearly fourteen years during which he and we lived with his illness, he also lived at the interface of his scientific research on creativity, aging, and illness. I lived at the interface of my clinical practice and research on the arts, medicine, and healing. Together, our worlds both diverged and converged, and the language between us cross-fertilized, creating a blended approach together.

In the medical Grand Rounds tradition, one presents a case to medical students or one's colleagues and other clinicians as a learning opportunity. In earlier times, the Grand Rounds presentation often included the patient for a hands-on examination by those in attendance and to answer questions they might have about the patient's illness experience. This is not so much practiced anymore, but regardless, the case study and discussion format offers clinicians a chance to step back and look closely at a case, interpret it, and apply the scientific and therapeutic theories and knowledge they consider relevant. From a purely medical perspective, so many aspects of Gene's illness truly did make it an instructive case history and cautionary tale.

Gene wanted his story told. He felt that he was always, by necessity, giving a partial narrative—this part to one doctor, that to another, this to one friend, that to another—and he wanted the whole story told, as he wanted this wholeness and coherence for every one of his patients and for every one of us. He saw in his clinical work and research how people's narratives were reduced by the culturally imposed limitations of stereotypes—of aging, of illness, of so many narrow interpretations by others. He wanted to empower others to feel ownership of their own wisdom, their life experience, and to feel their worth—that the whole is greater than the sum of its parts.

Gene intended to share his story and insights gained as both a physician and patient. He also understood from his work with so many patients, as did I from my own, that his case—our case—was emblematic of so many in which communication between the patient, family, and medical and other care professionals could contribute so much more to healing than it often does. With that intention and in keeping with the Grand Rounds tradition, what follows is the "case" as Gene saw it through the lens of his own experience and clinical understanding. In sharing his case openly this way, it was not Gene's intention, nor mine, to fault or complain about physicians; he wanted to share a perspective about how to look and perceive an older person aging into their wisdom, intelligence, and capacity. Just so with my own interpretation, which follows his.

Grand Rounds I: Presentation of the Case

AN ANOMALY IS SCIENCE, TOO

If consistent patterns and predictable outcomes are the bread and butter of science and medicine, anomalies are the essential ingredient of advances and break-throughs. The challenge is to stay alert for them.

In Gene's case, a seemingly innocuous prostate infection diverted even a capable specialist's attention from the more serious problem—prostate cancer—as it developed. So much so that by the time the cancer was detected, it had spread, metastasized to his pelvic bones, and was no longer the slow-growing, highly treatable disease that non-metastatic prostate cancer can be in the earlier stages. Then came the dire prognosis: given his high PSA readings, PSA of 360 and a Gleason score of 9 (10 is the worst), only one-third of men with metastatic prostate cancer survive five years. His doctors didn't express particular optimism about his chances of beating those grim odds. And yet, remarkably, he not only made it into the fortunate thirty-three percent who make it five years, he went on for more than thirteen years.

Despite this remarkable case of a guy who year after year proves the exception to the clinical assumptions in so many ways, rather than studying Gene's case to learn from it, some doctors' response was simply to label him a medical anomaly. Case closed. His hormone therapy had continued years beyond the statistical median because instead of dying, Gene continued to live and thus continued to be treated.

But how does a treatment for metastatic prostate cancer become the catalyst for a completely different disorder—a bone disorder—that eventually kills you? Gene would have to sort this out himself, which he did, and wrote about it.

Bisphosphonates are a class of drugs that prevent the loss of bone mass.[1]
Classically, osteopetrosis is a rare, typically congenital disorder, in which the bones become overly dense; this results from an imbalance between the normal ongoing formation of bone and the normal ongoing breakdown of the bone. Normal bone physiology keeps bones healthy by enabling ongoing

remodelling of bone that has a rejuvenating effect. Two bone cell types are at work here—osteoclasts and osteoblasts. Osteoclasts break down bone matrix. Osteoblasts generate new bone matrix. The work of both is necessary for normal bone health.

When prostate cancer cells metastasize to bone, they eat away at bone like aggressive osteoclasts. One of the medications I was on—an intravenous (IV) bisphosphonate—was used because it helped block the osteoclast-like effect of the cancer cells. Unfortunately, it also over time had an adverse effect on normal osteoclast activity, thereby interfering with normal remodelling of the bone. Because it was rare for someone to survive as long as I have with metastatic bone disease, it was rare for someone to have been receiving IV bisphosphonates as long as I did. Hence, I was the first patient my doctors saw with this long-term side effect—the abnormal transformation of my bones (in the end simply referred to as a metabolic bone disorder) by the extremely long use of the drug intravenously.

When the doctor concluded, echoing his colleagues' view, that "medically, you do not exist," he was saying that there were no other patients who had ever been on this treatment for so long; he and his colleagues had no data to study. Gene doubted this was actually true—that no other patients in his situation and on this treatment had ever outlived medical expectations. But he could believe that no effort had been made to document and study such outliers as himself. He knew from his experience as a scientist and clinician in the field of aging that assumptions can be limiting—almost always are—in that they can keep us from looking or seeing someone older with fresh eyes and open minds. He also knew this from his experience with the delayed diagnosis of his prostate cancer and how diagnostic assumptions based on incomplete data can lull even the brightest medical minds.

Then, with the sudden diagnosis and dire prognosis in hand, the medical conversation and assumptions about Gene changed just as abruptly and dramatically: it went from zero conversation about aging, disease, treatments, and the prospect of death, to a barrage of assumptions about what would happen to him, and happen in a very short time.

The internal conversation that accompanies these clinical transitions can take us to dark places and dilemmas that seem to offer only bleak options for action. How often do we feel comfortable enough with our doctors—or our loved ones—to share those feelings? Even later, in 2004, when Gene's leg broke, this was when he discovered that the medicine he was taking to protect his bones from further metastasis had in fact so hardened his bones that his femur, the largest bone in the body, had snapped. In the course of living though this injury, Gene noted, we are struck with a "double assault" on both body and psyche.

In my case I had to reconcile the double-assault on my body parts and psyche from cancer coupled with the side effects of cancer treatment, and ask what could I expect of my fragmented whole. The outcome was more than the surgical repair of my fractured femur and the medical treatment of my metabolic bone disease allowing me to once again face my cancer on my feet; it was the capacity to write a new book in the face of such adversity.

And what were my choices anyway? Do I continue the medication that was helping arrest the cancer, but in the process was making my entire skeletal system vulnerable to fractures? Or do I stop the medicine and potentially unleash the arrested cancer back on an aggressive attack? I felt as if I were in that Woody Allen scenario where he comes to a crossroads, contemplating which road to follow. He deliberates in his warped philosophical conundrum way, "Down one road is utter despair; down the other is complete desolation. I pray I make the right choice."[2]

This was the first time in my life that I looked back on my life, not in the context of experiencing a warm nostalgic memory, but in the sense of wanting to step back into my past to avoid the present and future. When I heard my favorite song, "Yesterday," on the radio, its words invoked a mood of mourning.[3] Fortunately, the sadness and self-pity did not stick. They served their cathartic purpose, allowing me to internally regroup, recognizing the fight was not over and that my responses to my prior flights as a Phoenix told me that here, too, there might be light at the end of the tunnel. It was at this point that I was most profoundly experiencing problems that can accompany aging, but William Carlos Williams' poetic refrain of the age that adds while taking away was never far from my consciousness. I just wondered what form "something added" would take now—in my life. At the time it was taking the form of the book I was writing (The Mature Mind). What was also taking form, but did not fully come together until after the book was published, were two new intersecting concepts that further focused the direction of my career: (1) the view of positive brain and behavior changes occurring because of aging, not despite it; and (2) the realization that aging may be the best example of the phenomenon of the whole being greater than the sum of its parts.

Despite the progress that has occurred in understanding aging, and despite the growing number of individuals aging well, many still view aging like a crapshoot with snake eyes increasingly coming up. Borrowing from Einstein, who asserted that God does not play with dice,[4] I would suggest that when it comes to aging, God or Mother Nature does not play with dice. Aging is not, as many suggest—"random." Science is uncovering an increasing order, rhyme, and reason to it, revealing that aging is about living with positive potential right to the end, and not rolling over to die. And this is where the two new concepts come in.

Grand Rounds II: Interpretation Through Gene's Developmental Lens

DEVELOPMENTAL INTELLIGENCE DEEPENS WITH AGE AND EXPERIENCE

Gene held that the great developmental theorist, Jean Piaget, had stopped short with his view that intellectual development is largely confined to the first quarter of the life cycle, culminating in what Piaget described as the fourth and final stage of intellectual development—formal thought—characterized by objective and analytic problem-solving, like mathematical thinking, with the capacity to come up with the solution.[5]

Fortunately, Piaget's students and followers did not stop there, especially with the recognition that despite the brilliance of many young adults in the formal thought stage of intellectual development, significant judgment gaps occurred, reflective of a still not yet fully mature frontal lobe in charge of executive function.

Postformal thought. What Piaget's followers found was a fifth stage of intellectual development that emerged in midlife, characterized not just by analytic reasoning, but synthetic thinking as well; not just by an objective focus, but also by a subjective orientation to problem-solving; not just with the goal of finding the single best answer, but with a recognition that sometimes there was not a single solution but competing, contradictory, or multiple solutions. It was a type of reasoning that provided not just a fine-tuned focus on the trees, but an ability to take into significance the forest as a whole. It was a form of reasoning that could balance attention to the well defined with the intuitive, a way of thinking that figuratively integrated through relativistic reasoning and dialectic discourse the heart and the mind. It was a more mature form of thinking that developed because of aging, not despite it.

The aging brain moving to all-wheel drive. In reviewing the extensive research on postformal thought, I was struck by what was being described as appearing to reflect a greater synchrony of right-brain and left-brain characteristics as described by Roger Sperry, who received a Nobel Prize for advancing our understanding of right brain/left brain differences.[6] I then learned about Roberta Cabeza's studies, reported in 2002, of how young adults and middle-aged adults use the two hemispheres—right and left brain—when carrying out the same tasks. Cabeza used functional MRI brain imaging techniques to see where the brain lit up when young adults and middle age adults were engaged in various tasks; MRI imaging was employed as tasks were carried out.

Cabeza found that the young adults did indeed use both sides—both hemispheres—of their brains, but depending on the task they used one side more than the other. For some tasks, the left was used more, for other tasks the right side was predominantly used. It was not as simple as some people being left-brained and others right-brained; they all used both sides, and the task determined which side was used more than the other. With middle-aged adults, something very different was observed: for all the tasks in general, the middle-aged individuals tended to use both hemispheres of the brain together, in a more synchronized manner. The asymmetric use of the hemispheres was reduced with aging. Cabeza then labeled this phenomenon the HAROLD Model, an acronym for Hemispheric Asymmetry Reduction in Old Adults.[7]

Initially this phenomenon was only viewed as a compensatory brain recruitment phenomenon with aging—recruiting brain tissue from another part of the brain to assist the brain with aging in the face of some lost capacity to continue to carry out the same task. It would be like using two hands to carry something instead of one. The same task would be carried out just as effectively and just as timely, now benefiting from bilateral involvement of the brain. For shorthand purposes, we can refer to this phenomenon as the brain, with aging, moving to all-wheel drive.

But I raised the question that perhaps there was more going on than brain reserve alone kicking in, though that in itself was an extraordinary development with aging. I asked if it were not unreasonable to assume that if you are recruiting additional tissue from another part of the brain for a task usually taken care of by tissue from a different area of the brain, that you also can get some of the added value—the added qualities of the new tissue being added. This would be analogous to an off-label effect for a medication, such as with aspirin where it was initially found to have the remarkable ability to lower fever and pain. But over time, numerous other uses for aspirin were discovered, such as its influence on lowering the risk for heart attacks and stroke.

I then went on to suggest that any activity that optimally uses both sides of the brain for a task at hand with aging is metaphorically savored by the brain—it's like chocolate to the brain. An example I gave was with autobiographical story telling. Older persons clearly like to tell their story and to share it as oral histories, reminiscence groups, memoirs, and autobiographies—which surge in number with the age of the author. I view telling your story as part of a new psychological growth phase with aging—"the Summing Up Phase." A new study by Eleanor Maguire and Christopher Frith showed aging affects the engagement of the hippocampus during autobiographical memory retrieval.[8] *When comparing young adults in their early 30s with older adults in their 70s,*

Maguire and Frith found that in the 30-year-olds, the autobiographical memory retrieval task primarily lit up the left hippocampus, while in the 70-year-olds the task lit up the hippocampus on both sides of the brain. The hippocampus is the part of the brain that is critical in initially processing new information and preparing the information for memory storage. The hippocampus has also been a major site of the brain where neurogenesis—new brain cell formation—has been discovered with aging.

Both the 30-year-olds and the 70-years-olds told their story equally well. Those compelled to point out deficits that accompany aging asserted, "It took using both sides of the brain for the older adults to tell their story equally well. In turn, I asked the question, "Are all things here really equal in performance? For example, do the older adults have the same amount of information to process in telling their story equally well?" Obviously, the older adults have considerably greater memory storage that they have to sort though, and given this to tell their story equally well suggests something [a capacity] more than equal. Moreover, I asked, "How many 30-year-olds do you know who passionately want to tell their life story?" The autobiographies on library and bookstore shelves are far more likely to be by older authors. Here, I suggest, is more than a brain recruitment phenomenon alone—it is an example of the added value of tissue, in this case from the right side of the brain—contributing to the desire to tell one's story. Among what we learned from Sperry's research on right/left brain differences is the role of the right brain in fantasy and intellectual curiosity apart from left brain analytic skills and facts that could enhance one's desire to tell their life story. Autobiography with aging optimally draws upon the qualities of both sides of the brain and again, I suggest, is like chocolate to the brain.[9]

Gene presented his reasoning and the "like chocolate to the brain" metaphor at an NIH staff scientific forum in 2005. He wanted to present it to the most potentially critical audience of peers to get their valuable feedback. Rather than the oppositional response he anticipated, the *NIH Record* the next day highlighted his presentation—to his delight, noting his metaphor of "like chocolate to the brain." Equally powerful was their response to his interpretation of this phenomenon of "all-wheel drive," which he believed kicked in during middle age, reflecting the neurobiological counterpart to the development of postformal thought with aging. In other words, he postulated that they were connected—that the increased synchronization of left and right brain functions with aging helped to enable this development of postformal thought. For him, both The HAROLD model and postformal thought represented positive changes that occur both in our brains and in our behaviors because of aging, not in spite of it. Gene continued to write about all-wheel drive and the whole being greater than the sum of its parts with aging in this way:

Related to the positive changes occurring because of aging, or more accurately, empowered by these positive changes, is the phenomenon of the whole being greater than the sum of its parts with aging. Aging may actually be one of the best if not the best example of this phenomenon. The key factor operating here is synergy that occurs with aging. Synergy is the interaction or cooperation of two or more components to produce a combined effect greater than the sum of their separate effects.

The movement toward all-wheel drive, especially as reflected in the rise of autobiographical story telling with aging makes the point. It illustrates the synergy that comes from this neurobiological phenomenon with aging—the enhanced synchronization of the working together of both sides of the brain, resulting in more than the two hemispheres contributing added brain power for the task at hand, but providing as well the added value of the unique qualities that each hemisphere houses and brings to bear to the collaboration between the left and right brain that comes with aging.

This is occurring in the second half of life when all of the major qualities of the mind are reaching their highest level of maturity—cognitive functioning with the development of postformal thought, social intelligence benefiting from accruing life experience, emotional intelligence, judgment, and consciousness including spiritual awareness. The individual maturing of all these qualities and their better integration with aging results in a new synergy of the elements of the mind, reflecting what I refer to as developmental intelligence (DI). Developmental intelligence shows itself as wisdom and reflects, with aging, the manifestations of the mind revealing a whole greater than the sum of its functional components. Figure 11.2 illustrates DI with the focus on an eye.

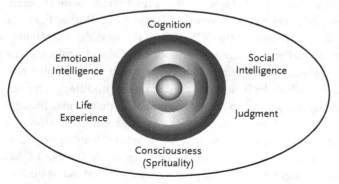

Figure 11.2 Developmental intelligence: the eye. Diagram by Gene D. Cohen.

Developmental intelligence (DI): *The maturing of our individual capacities for cognition, judgment, emotional intelligence, social intelligence, life experience, and consciousness (includes spirituality)—further enhanced by their improved integration and synergy with one another as we age. DI shows itself as wisdom.*

Let's look at our body as a work of art. Do we do justice to our understanding and appreciation of it if we focus on what is happening with individual parts and add up what we find as our picture of the whole? Do we do justice to our understanding of aging if we add up changes, especially ones we do not consider positive, and have these accumulated changes represent ourselves as a whole? That would be like breaking a painting down into parts, then analyzing those individual components, and judging the whole image by the sum of these individual elements. While this could apply regardless of age, with aging, society continues to hold the added expectation that negative changes are operating and that the whole would reflect such loss as well.

Gene liked to use as an example Leonardo da Vinci's *Mona Lisa*,[10] pointing out that you could analyze parts of the portrait in isolation—her eyes (and absent eyebrows), the curve of her lips, or her general expression—but what would the parts, or the sum of the parts tell you?

Is there an intelligence to her gaze? Is it an intense gaze? What about the missing eyebrows? Is there a touch of sadness? Is there a sense of disdain? Is there any sexual suggestion? How much information does this part give you? What do these parts tell you? Is her smile aloof? Is it alluring? Are we looking at a grin, happiness, disgust, or veiled disdain? Again, how much of the big or total picture do you get from a part or component? Do any of the parts truly give you a sense of the whole, even if you add up all the parts alone? Of those polled, 83% felt that Mona Lisa's predominant mood was that of happiness; 9% disgust; 6% fear; 2% anger. How would you describe her—ambiguous, enigmatic, engaging? Clearly the sum of the parts alone doesn't give the answer. The answer instead is in their synergy, and the synergy may be such that the answer is in a realm beyond the whole.

This was the point about creativity, aging, and illness that too often was ignored by all of us—our medical teams, our family and friends, and ourselves when discouraged. Creativity in connection with loss, specifically, could be considered the catalyst that *makes* the whole greater than the sum of the parts under any circumstances.

There is nothing romantic about loss—nothing at all. But it is part of the human condition that when loss occurs, and we can only go so far in restoring function that was lost, this is often not good enough for us. We become moti-vated by that inner push to attempt to transcend the loss—climb a new mountain—and in the process tap into capacity that we did not realize we have. This is the power of the human spirit. Loss occurs throughout the life cycle, but it clearly occurs more often in the second half of life, creating more opportunity for creativity to emerge in connection with loss and influence a whole greater than the sum its parts, where sum of the parts may not be working as well.

"SKY ABOVE CLOUDS": THE RIGHT METAPHOR FOR DEVELOPMENTAL INTELLIGENCE WITH AGING

In one of Gene's public talks in the Midwest, Gene mentioned that old metaphors for aging that depicted withering possibility were tired and patronizing: "it's the 'autumn of your life'; the leaves are falling off your tree; it's the 'winter of your years,' when the ground is covered with snow." He suggested that artist Georgia O'Keefe's "Sky Above Clouds" images were more apropos.[11]

> *It's what Georgia O'Keefe reflected in her "Sky Above Clouds" series of painting in her 70s. It is as if she is saying there is no denying the clouds that can occur with aging, but there is sky—blue sky—above the clouds. This is what I reminded myself throughout my flights as a Phoenix—that there can be blue sky above those very dark clouds. There is no denying that clouds can occur with aging, but what has been denied is the sky—blue sky—found above the clouds.*

As it happened, in the audience was a film producer on her way to New York and the Museum of Modern Art (MOMA). At MOMA, she visited the museum store and saw an item that made her think of Gene's talk—it was the "Sky Above Clouds" umbrella. She sent it to him as a gift, which he treasured and used routinely in his talks through the years to come. The producer, Melissa Godoy, along with her mother Eileen Littig, eventually produced the American Public Television film *Do Not Go Gently*, focused on creativity beyond the age of eighty.[12] Walter Cronkite narrated the film. Gene was the scientific commentator, and O'Keefe's inspiring image as a metaphor for positive change with age, and through illness reached an ever-wider audience. Gene carried the umbrella with him rain or shine, and never hesitated to open it to reveal the blue sky above clouds, he said "as a poignant reminder of the potential, and the reality of what is possible."

This idea that age and even illness can open possibility is present in so many of the stories of great contributors through the ages, and no less common in the lives of the rest of us. Among the most inspiring examples, one that helped sustain Gene through the most challenging moments of his own illness, was the sculptor

Beatrice Pearse.[13] In 1999, at a conference on creativity and aging in Santa Fe, Gene attended a juried exhibition by older artists. A colleague told him not to miss the sculptures of Beatrice Pearse, so he sought her out.

> *Beatrice was standing by her sculptures of owls, looking like a work of art herself, wearing a colorful smock over a long black dress. She greeted me with a welcoming smile and sparkling eyes. In discussing her work, she apologetically explained, "I haven't been an artist for long; I was a legal assistant all my life, and I didn't start sculpting until I was 94. I don't know what I did with those first 94 years!"*
>
> *Remarkably, Beatrice's vision was so impaired, she was designated legally blind. She grew up on a farm and was fascinated by the sight and sound of barn owls. Those images were burned indelibly in her brain. When she decided, on a whim, to try her hand at sculpture at the age of 94, she discovered a love for the feel and texture of clay. She remembered the owls and found she could see them clearly in her mind's eye, transferring that clarity to the sculptures. She started exhibiting her work and received positive feedback and recognition.*
>
> *About four years after meeting her, I received a letter from Beatrice's family. They told me she had died, but that she continued sculpting until a week before her death. Beatrice's story reminds me of Beethoven, who composed some of his most monumental pieces after he had become deaf. Beatrice lost her eyesight, but she continued to have a great inner vision of barn owls and other farm animals. Beatrice's story is a reminder that the inevitable losses that accompany aging need not provoke crisis or withdrawal from life. Hers is also a powerful story of the whole being greater than the sum of its parts.*
>
> ***The whole is greater than the one.*** *During the fourth of the four psychological growth phases seen with aging—the encore phase—we increasingly witness where an older person at advanced age serves to bring family and community together through reunions and celebrations. One of the classic cultural examples of this was with the old* Today Show, *when weatherman Willard Scott would feature each day a new centenarian who captured the enthusiasm of the country in the context of a celebration of long life. In these cases the phenomenon of the whole being greater than the sum of its parts presented itself as the whole being greater than the one—or the one affecting the many when the one was at an advanced age. This phenomenon was also seen with the Delany Sisters—Sadie 105 and Bessie 103, who described their relationship as the longest human relation ever. Their story,* Having Our Say: The Delany Sisters' First 100 Years, *became a* New York Times *bestseller, a Broadway hit, and a movie, where the two as individuals beyond the 100-year mark mobilized a great many with a sense of awe, fascination, and respect for a very long life.[14]*

While Gene continued to remain circumspect about divulging information about his own health complications, in large part concerned about the impact of predictable negative assumptions about his own work and life, he knew from his conversations with patients, colleagues, and audiences that peoples' personal stories held potent meaning for others. His own mother's story—just three days of it at the very end of her life—was a beautiful example of the very point he was establishing with his research and theory of creativity and developmental intelligence deepening with age. He titled it "When My Mother's Inner Light Began to Flicker."

My mother, Lillian Cohen, did great until she was turning 90, at which point she suffered a series of small strokes that sapped her memory. She then slowly began to fail, losing weight and becoming increasingly frail, despite excellent care in the nursing home where she wanted to be. But throughout her decline her indomitable spirit remained apparent. Her memory was minimal and her word bank even less, but whenever someone would approach her, her residual capacity was a tiny but reliable repertoire of engaging social graces—a reflex smile whenever someone approached, accompanied by "Hello, good to see you," and when they had to move on to another task, another smile and "Thank you, come again." The staff adored her.

On my visit to her 3 days before she died, she was asleep, immobile in her wheelchair, pale, her complexion sallow. She looked as if she were in a coma. The nursing assistant came over to transfer to her bed. She ever so gently lifted my mother, now so much lighter than her former self, and moved her very carefully and tenderly toward the bed. My mother remained completely motionless, with no clear sign of life, appearing but half her size when I was a young boy. A deep sadness and sense of loss swept over me seeing my mother this way. But then, just at the point of touchdown on the bed my mother's eyes reflexively opened, she spotted me, and an impish smile spread across her face as she uttered, "Good service, huh?!" The nursing assistant and I both broke into smiles, both of us unexpectedly uplifted and quite moved by her spirit that filled the room—a presence greater than the sum of her parts. Three days later my mother died peacefully while taking another nap.[15]

Grand Rounds III: Interpretation Through an Integrative Lens

INTEGRATIVE INTELLIGENCE BRINGS WISDOM TO HEALING

Gene's concept of developmental intelligence encapsulates the many ways in which we reflect on, take apart, and learn from our varied kinds of experiences—all aspects of creativity as we age, and in our illness experiences as well. We learn to see everything that counts and has accumulated in our lives. He provides us with the building blocks from his background in brain science: the two hemispheres of our brains and what happens as we age and move into all-wheel drive; the research in neuroscience; the various kinds of creativity in connection with loss; and the art of the synergistic relationships of developmental intelligence that lead us to a matured wisdom. He provides us with these individual components of developmental intelligence and shows us how as they mature, they become better integrated with aging. He discusses the synergistic effects and what individuals themselves can do to benefit from these phenomena.

Just as intelligence develops within us, observing all of the parts that Gene named, intelligence also integrates, meaning those faculties such as cognition, life experience, judgments, and spirituality synthesize with one another, and the whole becomes greater than the sum of its parts. That synthetic process is what I have referred to as *integrative intelligence*.

In the spirit of our shared Grand Rounds, I would add that art expression affords an opportunity to draw upon and integrate even more the different capacities associated with right- and left-brain manifestations. Our understanding of intelligence has been greatly increased by Howard Gardner in his elaboration of *multiple intelligences*—including "linguistic intelligence," "spatial intelligence," and "body-kinesthetic intelligence."[16] This concept has had a profound influence on how we understand and nurture different learning styles, not only for school children but for all of us as we grow older. A practical application of Gardner's research findings in the context of aging and illness would be, for instance, possibly the creative types of community-centered classes at senior centers or healing/wellness centers.

Art expression allows us to draw upon intuition and fantasy along with conceptualization and synthesis; it connects kinesthetic awareness with verbal expression. Our creativity, as this innate faculty or capacity, enables an integration of these diverse elements, thereby fostering integrative intelligence. When we merge Gene's concept of developmental intelligence, Gardner's *multiple intelligences*, and my own clinical work helping clients tap their power of creativity, the developmental enrichment is clear: art expression brings one's own language of sensation to the powerful voice of recognition and discovery.

In my studio, I am interested in the language of imagery as narratives of meaning, whose stories include both the body and the psyche. My sculpture studio and practice are set up like my artwork: a physical overlay, upstairs/downstairs from one another in a renovated carriage house behind my home. My clay figures live outdoors among the trees: a garden of souls forming. With my clients, I am a creative detective, walking with them through their inner landscapes, discovering and uncovering clues. This is my work in both art and in therapy, and in both arenas, it is our creativity that shines the light of self onto the parts or pieces that help us discover what most enlivens us. This is our individual way of being creative, and it often needs to be challenged so we can discover what conditions within us mobilize it. Whether it is, as we saw in previous chapters, Alice's symbolic flashlight or Daniel's prism, we all use "refracted or reflected light" to see from as many angles as we can, and from these vantage points, we find both the integrative process of creativity and the creative process of integration.

This becomes especially relevant when we are living with illness, aging, or adversity as a life partner because these circumstances force us to seriously tend our inner guardians, our immune systems. In so doing, we ask how healing is related to our creative expression. Under these harshest of circumstances, we need to mobilize our enthusiasm for what is going right in our lives, because this is what strengthens our systems. And so finding our individual ways and risking what it takes to live from these places becomes our task. It is a difficult task in that our systems have been "cracked open," through diagnosis or prognosis, and in this new place, we see everything differently, and we search valiantly to discover our own unique way of being creative. Why? Because we now are up against the awareness that everything and every moment matters. Each detail matters. Each part of our story matters. We must know and be present with what has meaning for us.

How are integrative intelligence and developmental intelligence related? Gene defined developmental intelligence earlier in this chapter as a wisdom which includes "the maturing of our individual capacities for cognition, judgment, emotional intelligence, social intelligence, life experience, and consciousness, including spiritual awareness—further enhanced by their improved integration and synergy with one another as we age." In essence, his was a biologically based theory of wisdom.

Integrative intelligence, as I see it, is what happens as a result of all the other forms of intelligence coming together, as the "star" model shows in Figure 11.3.[17] These intelligences take place in phases, developmentally integrating along the way. Integrative intelligence is the synthetic result of developmental intelligence—the awareness of going through a process of coming more and more into one's creative potential by using our resources, and by integrating the work it takes to move through the necessary developmental phases of inner and outer growth. This is what our illness journey represented, as it does for so many others. Both Gene and I looked toward the new scientific discoveries and links that both neuroscience and psychoneuroimmunology were bringing to the understanding of relationship within our bodies and minds. At last, this was science not separating us into parts, but seeing the patterns and relationships of various systems.

The task of holding polarities, differences, and diversity requires a creative focus. This type of focus is the encounter of directed focus in a particular arena within us. In Figure 11.3 this is shown by the straight arrows in the small outside triangles, which can be named as roles we play or arenas in our lives, such as

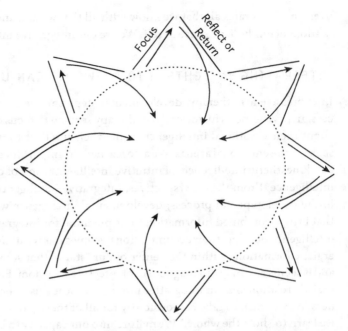

Figure 11.3 Integrative intelligence: the star. Diagram by Wendy L. Miller.

"family life" or "job" or a passion for something, such as swimming or writing. These represent the many parts of ourselves. This type of focus narrows toward the open point of the triangle, which reflects how we focus to learn more specifically about any part of ourselves. Then we need to expand our focus when we return to the center where we observe and orchestrate our insights, reflecting on what we have discovered. This expanded focus is shown in the star by the curved arrows, which save the information from becoming lost or trapped out in its own linear narrow focus by returning to the center with what we have learned. This action is a formative process, and it works to integrate our intelligence within the movement of the star model.[18]

The star represents a reflected focus that has us continually stretch out into new areas of interests, the triangles of ourselves, to deliberately avoid getting caught in the small limited space at the open focal point of the triangle. Our task is to remember to reflect and to return to the central circle of the star, carrying with us the new information, allowing the core authentic self to create its own combinations and synergies within the central space. This is our integrative intelligence. We can imagine ourselves standing at the center of any and all of the intersections that have contributed to our identity. We can place our identities within the star triangles, like a three-dimensional list of who we are. What tensions do we experience at these intersections? What new energies do we experience at these intersections? What has been lost, rediscovered, or newly found? This movement over time integrates all that we know with all that we are, and we evolve into the wisdom of our holistic sense of self. We are our integrative intelligence.

INTEGRATING INSIGHTS INTO "NEWS WE CAN USE"

In expressive arts therapy, developmental steps emerge in the therapeutic process. In psychology's historical past, therapy seemed to focus on educating people about their emotional intelligence, using their intellect to understand or make sense of the emotional arenas. We also learned the importance of body knowledge and kinesthetic intelligence, of intuitive intelligence, and of creative/metaphoric intelligence. From these perspectives, integrative intelligence would arrive later in the developmental process; developmental intelligence would be the vehicle that brings combined information to its potential for integration. So, as kinds of intelligence develop, their accumulation becomes our wisdom. But it is in the synergistic formations within the center of our "stars," that something new arrives, and it seems to catalyze a magnetism of integrated wisdom. For me, the art of synergistic relationships in integrative intelligence leads us to healing and to wholeness. As we learn to take responsibility for all of these parts of our development, we learn to "hold the whole." We mature into our capacity to hold the tension that exists when we hold just parts of a truth, half-truths I call them. Like cancer survivors who celebrate every birthday growing old instead of complaining about each birthday as a grim reminder of age, the shift in perception—how we think about ourselves—is a creative process that we can approach with intention.

We learn to take responsibility for aspects of ourselves that may previously have been unknown to us; in other words, we tend them, and in so doing, we move more and more toward the health of our whole self. This intelligence often goes unheard and unrecognized because to be able to hold the tension between various internal parts, we constantly tell ourselves stories that are partial or half-truths. For example, when we get lost and it triggers extreme anxiety and fear in us, we temporarily forget that each time this has happened, we are still safe; in fact we do find our way home.

My women clients in Chapter 10, whose stories of vulnerability shared the image of being at their ropes' end, really were images of finding their way home—finding themselves—in a complex process. We are often pushed up against an edge where we can no longer see beyond its myopic surface. The goal of healing, which Commonweal's medical director and author, Rachel Naomi Remen, defines as the *movement toward wholeness*,[19] requires that we recognize which ingredients are necessary for our half-truths to move toward whole truths. Integrative intelligence is the result of this movement.

Integrative intelligence is ultimately the goal of our creative faculties, and, as I have written earlier, perhaps when integrated, creativity and healing are one and the same. In art therapy, this process looks very individualized, as each person's images are unique; yet there are also universal images, shapes, colors, and symbols that we come to associate with healing and wholeness. Might these images be a collective call to bring forth a social awareness to respond to what we creatively know internally as we each face the crucial issues of our health, our times, and our culture? In Chapter 3 we met the librarian with melanoma who developed his own narrative about traveling down a hill on top of a treasure trunk, integrating and crystallizing the image of his physical markings on his chest with his inner child's image of a treasure trunk called a chest, learning when to open and when to close it. He was both practicing and developing a way to accommodate the rudderless feeling of facing random growths. It is not denial to have our metaphors carry us. If anything, these metaphors inform the necessary step-by-step actions that we take daily to normalize the extremes of living into our age and our health. To accommodate the changes in each organ, each node, each blood change, each biopsy needing wound care, each test, so that we can locate ourselves in our own attempts to live normally.

Learning to reflect in our own lives is really a creative and healing process. Helping each other exchange information provides us all with a deeper understanding of what we need for our own health. Alice, in Chapter 5, developed the image of the flashlight so she could discern and aim her angst and her insights. She also developed an image of what she named her "temperament model" of how people let pressure out according to their temperaments. She drew an image of cells following their DNA programming, creating pathways through pressure release. In paying such close attention to what she was seeing or feeling inside, she began to listen to her own complexity of pressured reactions to her children and husband. She began to creatively "play" with her temperament image as if it were a musical and biochemical instrument, with various tones for each of her sons, helping her adjust her own reactions to their temperaments: lowering the tone of her anxiety with one son; allowing another to paddle his canoe before facing his homework; harmonizing internally with her anger instead of having it escalate in direct conversation with her husband.

This can seem simple on one level, yet it is a complex challenge because we are changing our behaviors, and that requires a conscious and diligent effort. This is so important because we all wish to love and communicate as best we can in this relational exchange. There are two parts to that. One is how we relate to ourselves—listening to our images, recognizing their role as messengers of meaning, and using those messages to create a mind–body loop of exchange. The other is how we take what we learned and use it in our interaction with others. This process of creating relational exchange—an authentic exchange of feelings—might truly be a biochemical musical instrument, played between us.

Healing equals the movement toward wholeness in its own unique and individual ways. Imagery and art making are preverbal and direct experiences. Story, action, arrangement, and image transform energy. The language could take place as an interactive body among parts of the psyche (for example, a dialogue between body and mind; between feelings and body; between the outer world and the inner world). The language could also take place as an interaction between therapist and client (image/story creator and listener witness). Imagery and art making provide a context for the unconscious to be expressed and to provide its own metaphors of expression for release, guidance, sublimation, problem-solving, and healing.

CASE STORIES OF INTEGRATIVE INTELLIGENCE AND IMAGERY AS HEALING

My clients are continually coming in with parts of stories—sensations, feelings, responses, reactions, opinions, moods, frustrations, and judgments. In the course of the work, we aim toward a larger perspective, a way to observe the parts of the story so that they can all coexist. In my arts practice, images always appear. We don't always make them, but they always appear in our conversations. From where, we ask? Are they from the personal unconscious, a collective unconscious, a wisdom, a knowing, an unknowing? "Unknowing" as defined by the British psychoanalyst Christopher Bollas in the dialectic of creativity in living is "the loosening or unbinding of set ways of knowing and doing in order to discover new meaning." It is a creative attempt to loosen the bonds of any part of us believing that it knows the whole part.

The stories of hanging by a thin thread, looking only from one side of the paper; the green circle floating inside its surroundings of orange, recalling the unconditional care of a grandmother's love; learning to practice our own temperament models like a musical instrument—these images of health repeat themselves in a new context and thereby are seen differently. Some people ask: *Are our images supposed to be random? Am I supposed to be pleased with my images, because most often I'm not at all!* These are the types of inner places that people constantly explore in the quest to know from where images appear. These places are half-truths—one part of us observing another part. Yet, it is in the data collection of our images, the art of respecting and listening to these images, that we begin to have something from which to imagine: voices, gestures, movements, shapes, patterns, sounds, which guide us as we move with our imagination, or as imagination moves with us. This is an active process of whole making because as the images collect, cohere, disappear and reappear, parts of our stories get rewritten, retold, and reimagined in new ways. These new ways hold the potential for the larger story to speak and be heard. They become the ingredients we alchemically cook with so that our images mix together, get reshaped and reformed until a new image of understanding seems to come through.

For years, I have held peoples' images in my office, like an art orphanage—wonderful children we sometimes nurture and feed, other times we file away, seemingly abandoned, yet never really so. For months and months may go by in which an image remains on the shelf, and then a new drawing, a new painting, a new poem, a new movement brings forth a new meaning, and a new aspect to the whole story comes in. Suddenly, the earlier image vibrates with relevance. For me, images act as guides into a creative space, where we become receptive to the perceptual field where mind–body connections are experienced, and this integrated essential light of the self comes through, even if it expresses itself in a dark uninviting image.

Recently, for instance, I was facilitating a workshop for a retirement community. It was based on the existential conversation that the writings from this book explore. One of the participants was quite ambivalent about taking the time to be with us for the afternoon. Her husband was in the hospital and she was very concerned about him and about the possibility that this time, his health could be on a serious decline. It was difficult for her to hold back the thoughts and feelings of him nearing the end of his life. What would this mean for him? What would this mean for her? Who would she be? She couldn't imagine. What she did imagine as she held the soft claylike material in her hands was just how tightly she was holding on in all ways. Her hypervigilance and her fear were tightly wound inside and outside. She began to tell herself that she should be more open; she should try to learn to let go. As she molded her clay, the large image of a hand took its shape, with its fingers spreading out in openness. She tried to control the clay, to make it remain open, but in so doing, she began to feel bad, not just about her image but also about herself. She continued to tell herself she should become more open; she should try harder.

I had shared with her that I knew of no greater preparation and practice for being present with uncertainty than art making. Because the creative process is an immersion in improvisation, play, and the holding of unknowing, surprise, and mystery, we need to be very careful about our honesty because images never lie. As a matter of fact, I said, they know exactly what they want and they can rebel when they are misunderstood. She proceeded to kinesthetically experience exactly that. Her image wanted to be a tight closed fist—tighter and tighter as a matter of fact. As she slowly allowed the material and the image to guide her, or perhaps better said, to be respected and acknowledged for the image's own truth, she developed an intimacy with the material and with the hand. It sculpted into a fist, with white fingernails digging into its knuckles. Gently as she sculpted the tight closed fist, she felt a compassion spread over her, and as this compassion for the hand grew, and its state of tension, so its image and its meaning softened her, and she felt the power of compassion toward herself as she opened to the truth of her experience. Tight and holding on tightly was exactly where she was and where she needed to be; but in its closed state, it also held compassionate care and intimacy. She felt whole when she shared her experience with us. She felt that the wisdom within had honored her as she had honored it. And in so doing, they had become one. This is integrative intelligence—a wisdom that honored the truth and vulnerability of her experience.

Images do not always have to appear wise to be integrated and intelligent. Another man in this workshop was extremely unsatisfied with his imagery as he was making it. He went so far as to describe the quarry tile color of the material and the shape he was forming as "it's looking a lot like fecal matter." He expressed the same confusion so many image-makers describe as they are unsure where they are going or what image it is they are making. And yet, later he told us, when his image transformed into an enzyme, it had just "popped into my head. I am a scientist, and enzymes are what define our whole being." He was proud, and clear, and far from confused or judgmental. If anything, he was humbled into the honesty of his own question to me: "Where does this come from when truth just pops out like that?" His question softened everyone in the group, just as our materials had done, and we sat in a quiet knowing. Creative faculty? Human spirit? Healing? Life force? Whatever we may call it, it is not a mechanism per se, but something we can actually see as being defined in the identity of the self. It is something that gets released in us when we are present with it, and in that exchange something in us finds not only its own meaning, but its own healing.

"Being with" is what we have to do—easier said than done because, in fact, it is very hard to "be with" so many parts of ourselves when they are bumping into one another. Ultimately it comes down to a simple sublime catalyst of a moment. To be with our creativity, aging, and illness time is a powerful vulnerable, gentle, still, honest compassion. Alyce and Elmer Green, originators of clinical biofeedback, and physiological researchers at The Menninger Institute, combined the disciplines of autogenic training and biofeedback.[20] They have said that healing takes place in a particular brain wave (theta) state of reverie; that this state of reverie is the state of healing; and that it is in this brain wave state that we experience the holistic aspect of the arts where self-generated healing takes place.

This kind of thinking pushes me to imagine the chromosome of hope, wondering what happens when we tap into the cellular wisdom of our deepest integrative self. Might this be the fullest integrative intelligence of our experience? Might this intelligence be the true meaning of "the whole is greater than the sum of its parts," when our wisdom sees beyond the dark tunnel that tries to shrink us, moves us into all-wheel drive, where our creative faculties are like chocolate to the brain?

12

Elements of Style for Doctor/Patient Communication

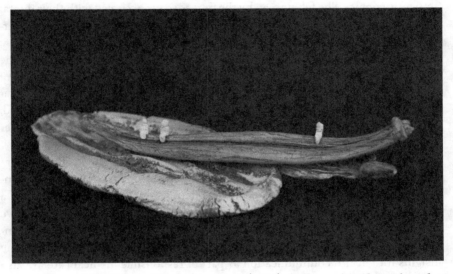

Figure 12.1 "On the Edge of Listening" (1982), fired porcelain clay with oxides, 6 × 14 × 2 inches. Artwork by Wendy L. Miller, photo credit: Joshua Soros.

Aging and illness can be uncomfortable subjects for any of us to talk about, but we must. In a sense it is just that simple: we must. At any age, and whatever our walk in life, our fullest development as human beings depends on engaging the realities of life—the people, the moments, the big feelings, and small stuff—because avoidance stunts our growth. As we have just seen in the previous chapter, integrative intelligence—the way we grow through experience—flourishes through connection, reflection, integration, and action. Communication is vital to health, wholeness, and healing; without it, we wither.

As professional partners, Gene and I shared the view that doctors, of all people, should be able to communicate with patients and families with respect, perceptive awareness, clarity, and compassion; that it's not asking too much for a well-educated clinician to view patient communication as a basic skill. Medical education, which historically gave short shrift to the healing potential of the doctor/patient relationship itself, has begun to embrace this more holistic engagement. But in our journey through Gene's illness, as life partners, we experienced this disconnect between the medical conversation and the holistic reality of our lives nearly every day. From feeling reduced or invisible as individuals in a doctor's eyes, to the medical errors based on incomplete assumptions or carelessness, these things hurt in deeply personal ways. The larger picture of this communication style that "disappeared" the wholeness of a person also spoke to us as conscientious clinicians.

Antoinette, in Chapter 5, well aware that she was dying, yearned simply for authentic contact. She felt unseen by the nurses so preoccupied with their digital screens that they overlooked connecting with her as a person—a still living person. What she needed most was recognition. She needed her dignity to be seen, beyond the clinical data to be analyzed or measured or compartmentalized. She deserved having her wholeness, fragile as it may have been, witnessed instead of being rendered invisible to those not so attuned. We all want and need to feel that we matter. We need to feel that we are "of the world," that we are seen, accepted, and appreciated in the eyes of others, however age or health changes may alter us: this is basic to our human makeup.

We have been talking about potential throughout this book. The doctor/patient relationship, like any other, is about remembering that potential and conveying it. But because the doctor/patient relationship affects every aspect of a patient's resources for healing, from cell to soul, it carries special power. When we commit to "do no harm," that includes harm by omission in the healing relationship, however unintentional. We'll look at that in this chapter, knowing that any insights into health communication as part of responsible medical care are also useful to all of us.

"Elements of Style"

Gene long thought the classic composition and grammar guide, *The Elements of Style*, by William Strunk and E.B. White, would be an ideal approach for outlining communication skills for physicians.[1] *Here's how to say it. Here's how not to say it.* Or, to borrow from the title of a classic parenting book, a physician's guide: *How to Talk So Your Patients Will Listen, and How to Listen so Your Patients Will Talk.*[2] He liked the idea that a simple guide could have a comparable impact on doctor/patient relationships, especially when the patients are adults and partner in meaningful conversation if given the opportunity and encouragement to do so.

Gene knew what he was talking about, tapping into his personal experience as a patient, and our experience as a family interacting with an extensive cast: doctors, nurses, physical therapists, surgeons, anesthesiologists, pathologists, radiologists, cardiologists, receptionists, patient navigators, hospital administrators, nutritionists, dieticians, home healthcare aides, hospice personnel, insurance handlers, and other system administrators.

Art of medicine is to Convey Caring for the person

My own experience as a patient could easily fill a volume on what not to say or how to say it poorly. It's the difference between the art of medicine and being artless—the gap between good bedside manner and the lack thereof. It is also the dilemma of physicians facing the communications double jeopardy of dealing with patients facing death and aging. I would be remiss as a physician in not sharing my personal experiences as a patient with the goal of better educating and sensitizing my colleagues to dealing with life-determining illnesses and aging in doctor/patient communication.

I want to point out that on the whole those providing my treatment have been very thoughtful and caring. But just as encountering the use of split infinitives is like the sound of fingernails scraping a blackboard for those attuned to grammatical precision, many comparable medical communication errors make a patient sick to their stomach, and faint of heart, too. Some of the errors were slight, one by one, but the steady drip could be exasperating. At the same time, there was the occasional egregious offender, like the "Bludgeoner" I mentioned earlier, from one of the country's leading cancer research centers, who emphasized my death sentence. The Bludgeoner determined that I needed to hear from him just how limited my days really were, despite my advising him right from the start that I was a physician who thoroughly understood my diagnosis and prognosis. But Doctor/Patient Communication 101 had left him on hyper alert for patient denial and for the need to intervene and set me straight.

The Doctor/Patient Relationship: An Opportunity for Growth

Relationships hold the capacity for our deepest caring. Why do we believe it is so rare for our doctors to truly listen to us? We come to our healthcare providers in need, usually with a pain or a fear or even a diagnosis. We feel we are facing something alone. The doctor/patient relationship is first and foremost an opportunity—to come out of isolation and into shared communication. There is an element of relief built right into the relationship from its very start; that together, some kind of relief will occur. There is an expectation that through being heard, we will be understood, and through being understood, we will know what to do or how to go about doing something. That's quite an expectation, especially

That fear, helpless, rage are all normal human responses, to help accept our own experience, to feel validated

at a time when medical doctors are often pressured to keep appointments brief and discussion prioritized around symptoms and symptom relief. We may want that genuine sense of relationship with our doctor, but we are also accustomed to the fact that we often don't get it.

We certainly approach our psychological clinicians—psychiatrists, psychologists, therapists, or counselors—very differently, with an expectation that they will in fact be there to support and bear witness to us. I love the intimacy of my clinical practice. I often hear other people talk about working without having an immediate sense of the direct impact their work creates. It is the opposite for me. I am held accountable in every hour I spend with my clients because they have entrusted me with their confidence that something will take place between us in that hour that is meaningful to their life. I can't know what that is or what that will be, but I can commit to awaiting that, to being present in any and every way that I can, so when I have an opportunity to get a glimpse of what that might be, I am actually paying attention and I can *do* it. Usually it is giving praise to what my client has in fact just said or noticed or felt. As I have described earlier, I am both a creative detective and a psychic historian. I remember and I commit to remembering when we are together. That is an element of my style of being and listening in relationship. My clients have asked me to engage in a meaningful psychological conversation.

Kasey's Story: The Art of a Life Examined

I met Kasey as a client—a patient—more than twenty-five years ago. Her pain was in her personal life, in her marriage, and in her personality style of passivity, resigning herself again and again to her disappointments and invisibility. She had divorced her first husband at a time when doing so left her without custody of her two young children. She grieved this break with her children deeply. She had remarried, and moved out of state with her new husband and his family, but she did not always trust that the ways in which their love expressed itself took into consideration her needs for security—financially, emotionally, or supportively.

In art therapy, she drew with pastels, and sometimes it was so painful to watch her draw, I could hardly bear it. She would clean each pastel, slowly and carefully, so all of its edges of smudged color from any prior use were removed before she made a mark with it on paper. The process was slow and tedious, at least to the observer.

She had been a weaver, then switched to a career in healthcare, and on her own time she pursued diverse interests, from art classes to professional development trainings; yet these experiences, though interesting to her, never quite filled an empty feeling within. She did find something satisfying in our therapy work together and remained committed to that. Over time, she joined everything my practice offered: the experiential supervision group we ran, our "art as meditation" group, and my women's studio art group, which she attended for eight years. Through these group settings I came to know her in a totally different way, as she grew and our work together catalyzed a change for each of us in different yet evolving ways. Our communication changed when we collaborated—in this context she was innovative, not passive at all. She studied the ways in which material was designed for use and she learned the process for using it, from liquefying pastels, to building a beautiful sand tray collection, to transforming her weaving skills into "soul collages." Her grief over the early attachment losses to her children transformed—and informed her about grief—as she spent more and more time with them as young adults and new parents themselves. Her personal challenges informed her, as did all the stories of challenge and life that she exchanged with her mentors, doctors, clinicians, and others, including patients she worked with in her professional capacity in cancer support retreats, teenage grief groups, and hospice.

I came to know her as the seeker she was. That quality had been masked by her early personality traits, and I had not fully recognized her "seeker self" in its early path toward integration. It was through the mirror of our relationship that I came to recognize this about her. This is the potential of any relationship, including the doctor/patient relationship: if we allow ourselves to see the wholeness in one another, our understanding grows, and so do we.

In our women's studio art group, our collaborative work evolved into narratives we called "artlinks"—merging elements of written story and image from all of us to explore life's big themes and then make the story accessible to all, wherever they might be in their life journey. Artlinks was a catalyst, "chocolate to the brain," as Gene would call it, for creative adaptation to changing life circumstances. Our seasoned exchange of ideas, psychological conversation, and image making was our form of doctor/patient communication, in a group setting no less. It provided us with the freedom to creatively interpret and reinterpret each other's words, images, and ideas and develop them in our own ways. In this creative exchange, not only did the images grow, but we each grew, not only in wisdom, mastery and community, but in our shared love and care as well.

Kasey's growth was extraordinary to watch: her exquisite attention to detail, her persistence, her quiet endurance, and her color-coordinated fashion style all added up to a kind of elegant grace. Our time together became the holding container not only for our work and communication but also for this holistic growth and vast possibility within us.

Kasey died last year. She was diagnosed in her early seventies with breast cancer. She had completed the entire protocol of radiation and chemotherapy treatment, supported by her wonderful community of friends and colleagues that she had built throughout the years of her self-inquiry and soulful exploration. She and I celebrated when her treatment protocol ended, her stylish wig worn graciously, her hair slowly re-growing. Then, as happens sometimes, the unexpected slippery slope came—unexpected by all of us, doctors included. Her lungs filled with fluid. We thought it was a side effect of the chemo, but she was in serious pain and was hospitalized. Tests showed the cancer had metastasized throughout her spine.

In the hospital, surrounded by her husband, friends, and colleagues, she asked me for exactly the help that she knew she needed. Our communication was certainly that of doctor/patient, but also much more. Our relationship had evolved: I grew to respect her persistence and care deeply not only for her wounds, but for her strength. Not all doctor/patient relationships come to this, but the ones that do are unique, for both doctor and patient. These relationships have not only been through the shared healing crucible of illness time, they have also entered a transformational process and catalyzed one another.

At one point, Kasey most vulnerably, strongly, and honestly asked me: *"Will you be my guardian in communication with my husband?"* She asked me not only because she trusted me, but also because she knew how I had midwifed Gene through his death; she knew I had been her partner in health communication for nearly three decades. And she knew and trusted that my care would survive all else—that I would not abandon her in her deepest places; that I would not allow her deepest needs to go unmet or unheard. I would take care of her in every way that I could because fundamentally, she had invested in my role in our relationship for years and with it came her right to deserve this care from me, and I knew that as well. This is doctor/patient communication at its best. Yes, time and continuity help; but it is the willingness to believe that we all grow, that we all develop, that we are all, in our essence, kind, caring, and deserving of the care we need, regardless of how we might have initially asked or conveyed it—that dignity and respect are what work at its best. *"Can you make sure I will not be in pain? Can you make sure that my husband understands how to do that? Can you make sure that even if he is concerned with other aspects, such as where I should go or whether hospice will charge us for my care or whether we can afford it, that I will not be lying quietly here in pain?"*

Not all of that was said in words, but it was all certainly said in spirit: clarity, need, decisiveness, courage, focus, affirmation, command. "Everything trivial falls to the wayside," said my friend in an earlier chapter about the time after her husband died, and losing a parent was so traumatic for her sons. For Kasey, the fact that she felt seen, heard, and held in compassion through this passage strengthened her resolve as she approached death. This is the real "will" in us—the will to live fully ourselves, true to ourselves, even as we die.

When the moment presented itself, a group of us advocated for her, right there in the hospital: we rallied to locate our referral for the best pain specialist, we rallied to communicate with the nurse, who at first thought our request was changing the doctor orders; we intervened on behalf of the voice she needed. We did not walk away from her as she was fading. We stepped in. It was a Friday afternoon at 4 PM in a city hospital. We knew we had to work fast because we were facing a weekend at the hospital. By evening, the pain specialist was administering what she needed. By Sunday, she was transferred to hospice so that she could be cared for and prepared for a weeklong regimen of pain relief. After the very first round of pain medication Monday morning, she closed her eyes, coming in and out of consciousness for days, allowing everything to happen around her, yet opening her eyes to tell us about her peacefulness. I knew on Thursday when I visited her that her time was short. When she passed that night, I also knew she had made the choice to "give up-wards"—to pull from those inner resources in the psyche, the transpersonal qualities of peace, acceptance, renewal, and serenity; in essence to listen to the heart's desire. What more growth or healing could any of us ask for in anyone—in ourselves and in our relationships, whether those are doctor/patient or other caregiving relationships? Only that our caring is strong, and strongly received, up to our final breath.

In her 2014 acceptance lecture for the Gene D. Cohen Research Award in Creativity and Aging, Rita Charon, the physician, literary scholar, and pioneering voice in the field of narrative medicine, shared that doctors know they should follow up with a family after their patient dies, but do they do that?[3] Hopefully, yes. But, she went on to say that what the family really needs is for us—the physicians, the therapists and counselors, and others—to check in on them two and three years later, when we in fact can find out how they really are doing. I spoke at Kasey's memorial service at the time she died. And I call Kasey's husband every six months to say hello.

A year after Kasey's passing I called the other woman who had been in our studio art group and invited her to come with me to commemorate Kasey's life with a ritual of parting with an unfinished clay piece Kasey made—a piece that had never been meant to be fired in the kiln and thus remained hardened clay but still porous. At the time Kasey made it she had allowed sediment—"physical sentiment," if you will, in the form of watery clay "slip"—to harden into a small anniversary cake image, with a beautiful ceramic cat and beaded necklace of hope resting on its top. For twenty years, she had used my art orphanage as a holding place for it. We carried her unfired clay piece to a stream and set it free in the moving water. We watched the dry clay slowly and gently absorb water and break down, returning to its essential nature: earth. This way, too, we said both hello and good-bye to our friend and colleague and honored the wholeness of her in life, in death, and in her self-expression through her relationships.

To Be Heard: We Must Ask Our Questions, Tell Our Stories

What kind of conversation do we ask our doctors to engage in with us? What are the elements of communication that we bring into our encounter? The doctor/patient relationship is really an inquiry into what matters. How we each listen, how we speak, what we share, what we talk about, how we react, how we absorb information, in essence, is an opportunity to find out what is needed, and that can only be done through each of us listening really well.

Sometimes the words or the symptoms are not the key topic. The topic is that a crisis of some kind is occurring, be it big or small. Its story may meander through many types of descriptions: a racing tone or a repeated phrase about one's aching knee or a continual movement of picking at skin on one's arm. Its presence is in the room with you and all the language in the world is not going to take it away. Best to dare to respond to it, to say, you don't need to wait outside the room, come right in here and sit with us. We each respond in our own unique ways to crisis, and yet there are patterns that, if you're a doctor or clinician who works with many people, you can see and understand some meaning they may hold. We count on our healthcare providers having enough experience to help us see those patterns, even if they are just patterns in our own way of responding.

When I first visited my doctor with symptoms of chronic fatigue syndrome, I didn't know what I had but knew something was seriously amiss in my body. He picked up on my anxiety right away; he closed his office door and asked me what I was afraid of. I was able to speak of my greatest fear—that what I had was a brain tumor—and because I shared my fear, he was able to clarify for me why a tumor was not the issue, and then we could go about the business of figuring out my next step. We would search together for more pieces of the medical puzzle of my condition, but he had communicated that he cared about more than that. He cared about me. He was able to recognize what mattered to me, calm my fear with a specific conversation about it, and move forward with me. This way of doctoring recognizes what has potential for meaning and exchange when the two of you are together.

Narrative medicine teaches us that the question our doctor needs to ask is something like: "Please tell me the story of your illness, beginning wherever you would like. I am here to listen to you."

In her book *Narrative Gerontology: Research and Practice* and from her wealth of knowledge and research in narrative gerontology, the noted gerontologist and professor Kate De Medeiros writes about "telling the right story."[4] There are so many ways in which misinterpretation or miscommunication can occur between the teller and the listener. There are also so many issues of power that arise with words: power, authority, belief, attitude, praise, acceptance, and judgment—the list goes on and on—all intertwined with meaning. And yet it is in the hearing and telling, the listening and responding, that our identities reveal themselves.

Rita Charon, physician-author of *Narrative Medicine: Honoring the Stories of Illness*, professor of clinical medicine, and director of the program in narrative medicine at Columbia University, describes how she opens the conversation with her patients. She knows there are many ways for the story to be told and has come to decide that the best way for her to gather the information is with this simple statement: "I will be your doctor, and so I have to learn a great deal about your body and your health and your life. Please tell me what you think I should know about your situation."[5] She then listens, without writing notes, but rather absorbs all the information coming to her from her patient. She listens for not only content but also for the way it is expressed—the emotional tone of it, any details that are repeated again and again. Many of her patients are deeply moved because this is a first experience for them—being heard and having their story held in this way. Together, they co-write the story that becomes her notes.

Physician, educator, and author of *Kitchen Table Wisdom: Stories That Heal* and *My Grandfather's Blessings: Stories of Strength, Refuge, and Belonging*, Rachel Naomi Remen, through her work at Commonweal and the Institute for the Study of Health and Illness, developed a course called "The Healer's Art," which she has brought to more than eighty medical schools across the country and around the world.[6] She teaches medical students to do what in my star model would be called reflected focus: to focus on and listen to the values that first encouraged them to become medical professionals and to return to themselves, strengthening that sense of calling to serve in truly compassionate care. The topics in this course include deep listening, presence, acceptance, loss, grief, healing, relationship, encounters with awe and mystery, and self-care practices. If you think that most of these refer to patients' concerns, think again; these are aspects of life—including doctors' lives—that affect how they relate to their patients, to their colleagues, and to themselves.

Remen reminds students that today's sophisticated medical centers, showcases of medical research, teaching, and practice, are based on the model of the great ancient temple described in the writings of Cicero, in which a statue of Venus, goddess of love, dominates the courtyard. Remen reminds medical students

> that for all of its technological power, medicine is not a technological enterprise. The practice of medicine is a special kind of love. I tell them that our lineage can become our strength. And our healing.[7] (*Kitchen Table Wisdom*, p. 164)

Marc Agronin, geriatric psychiatrist and author of *How We Age: A Doctor's Journey into the Heart of Growing Old*, writes about his doctor/patient communication with older adults in their 80s and 90s and past 100. He refers to lessons difficult for a doctor as "lessons from fire," describing the "guarded sadness" of psychological trauma that some of his patients carry. One such story from a Holocaust survivor taught him that, over time, the sadness becomes a stand-in for the actual losses of loved ones:

> Sometimes the perpetual sadness of many older survivors is not to be healed but shared. . . . Any attempt to ease this emotion may be a threat to the painful but beloved remnants of memory. What some survivors seek is not medicine or therapy but the attentive presence of a doctor and others to serve as the next generation of witnesses.[8] (*How We Age*, p. 254)

I am reminded of a client of mine whom I wrote about earlier in reference to her life seeming to hang by a thread. She had been abandoned by her community of Christian Scientists when she chose to go to a doctor. They felt that she had lost her faith. When she went to her doctors, it was extremely hard for her to tell her story or express what her concerns were. Her doctor attempted to fill the space, if you will, with his story of what she was to do. He didn't know how to interpret her hesitancy, her fear of authority, her inner ambivalence about needing the medical world. And yet she had so much to share if he had just been willing to offer his presence as witness to her full story of pain. When she passed away, neither the medical community nor her Christian Science community was there for her. It was her family and family friends alone.

How we create communication together matters. I would want a Gene Cohen, Marc Agronin, Rita Charon, Rachel Naomi Remen doctor—one who understood deeply that not all illnesses or sadness or grief can be healed, but they certainly can be expressed and listened to. This sharing brings witnessing to one's story, to one's identity, to one's life. We live in community, not in isolation. We have no idea where our own story, our own health, our own identities will take us if we tell our stories and ask, insist, on being heard.

Kasey's story took us to what amounts to a scary place for many if not most of us. And yet we went there, learned more about her struggle and her strengths and sat with the details of her story, including her death and the streamside ritual a year later in which we commemorated her life and her courage to live it fully. Our own stories may scare us at times and we may hesitate to share what we know and feel, not sure anyone else will be able or willing to go there with us. But these stories show us what can happen when we do.

The narrative that develops as it is shared and elaborated in the doctor/patient relationship is created between the two. First is the expertise of the patient as a listener to his or her own symptoms and concerns, and reporting it from inside the experience. The doctor then contributes clinical experience and knowledge, but also the skill (when it is developed) to absorb this information with the deepest respect for its holistic meaning. Together they create a new and fertile dimension of understanding between them that neither would reach alone. Because without cross-fertilization, nothing grows.

Gene's MD Elements of Style: The Power of Hope, Humor, and Wholeness

Gene saw this basic human desire for meaning and wholeness portrayed in time-less themes of great literature, philosophy, and expressive arts, and he sought ways to make the big ideas more pocketsize through metaphors and models that could help people see their own potential. When Gene was particularly stressed or exhausted from the medical marathon of his cancer or its treatment, he would return to his writing, where humor, beauty, and creative expression restored order to the uncertainty of his universe, and of his life.

As scientist, psychiatrist, public health activist, and a voracious explorer of creativity across disciplines and the lifespan, he had an extraordinary wealth of knowledge to share. In his thoughtful, creative approach to serious subjects, Gene's integrative intelligence allowed him to engage effectively with a wide range of people and audiences in whatever "language" or communication style resonated for them. As an expert witness and communicator, he moved easily from courtrooms to Congress. As a clinician, he was a passionate advocate for every patient's health and dignity. He drew on humor and the chemistry of his relationships to create substantive commentary on medical topics, and was especially devoted to medical education.

With a physician colleague at the George Washington University medical school, he co-taught a course on physician–patient relationships and skill development including doctor/patient communication, difficult communications, cross-cultural communication, taking spiritual histories, caring for the caregiver, and ethics. In this course, they created innovative projects and program ideas about medical education, teaching, and research. Friends as well as colleagues, they also played off one another "doing shtick" as if they were a vaudeville team.

Gene often said that his model for doctor/patient communication was George Burns. He liked to share Burns' comments about shifting from a stand-up comic to "lie-down comic" as a wonderful example of the agile, aging brain, and medically relevant, too. Burns' humor—drawing from the intellectual texture and wisdom that only life experience can bring—embodied Gene's view of aging as "adding to" our inner resources.

When he thought, however fancifully, about an "Elements of Style" for physicians, his was motivated by his and his family's hurtful experiences, and as a geriatric psychiatrist, by his patients' experiences. In contrast to my experience with my physician's thoughtful concern and question when I came in about the chronic fatigue symptoms, Gene found that some doctors focused almost exclusively on clinical data to the exclusion of his or our well-being. Others didn't recognize the emotional content or implications of a clinical issue and rather than exercising their empathy or their intuition with him, they simply made assumptions. As is often the case when no meaningful conversation is involved, their assumptions limited their understanding of his situation and his concerns, and of his own capable mind as a resource for healing.

In his journal entries and his conversations with me, particularly as the middle years of his survival continued and he sometimes felt that doctors were still expecting him to decline or not live fully as he was, Gene expressed his growing sense of frustration, and sometimes exasperation and anger. He felt that truly, in the minds of some clinicians, there was nothing more to be learned or understood: not about him, not about his disease, and—perhaps most sadly to him as a scientist and physician—not about what had enabled him to live so long and well. As he outlived his prognosis, he began to feel he had outlived interest by medical science in identifying what was working and the potential that might hold for a cure, if not in time for him then for others. These feelings and ideas found a home on the page and between us, if rarely in conversation with those whose comments or silence left him discouraged.

Gene felt that insensitive comments during his office and hospital visits were the exception rather than the norm, but when they did occur, his stomach churned. He felt that these comments often reflected the professional caregiver's goals rather than the caregiver's contemplation of *his* goals, and it left a lingering bad taste for him as he considered other patients in this position.

> *Caregivers beware of emotional buttons and know from whose perspective— yours or your patient's—you are bringing up sensitive issues without realizing it.*

By focusing only on parts, it is easy to miss the whole, or misunderstand it, in effect overlooking opportunities for meaningful exchange. In Gene's case, while much of the medical conversation focused on clinical aspects of the disease, the impact of a different struggle took its toll unrelieved.

> *A decade earlier when I received a very poor prognosis for metastatic prostate cancer, what especially ate away at me far more than the death sentence I received was the agonizing feeling that I would be abandoning a family in need of my help. My father, Benjamin (Ben) Cohen, had been diagnosed with Alzheimer's disease, my mother was overwhelmed with his care and with the needs of my disabled older brother, Franklin, who lived with them, and Wendy and I had recently adopted our daughter Eliana, who at the time of my diagnosis was only not yet 2. The situations at my parents' home*

required and benefited from my daily calls there. I felt then that my parents and brother would all outlive me, and that I would therefore no longer be available to help, my absence adding enormously to their huge burdens and challenges. I was sick inside, far more than from what my disease caused. The thought of not being available to my 2-year-old daughter and wife compounded my despair. A decade later, when according to all the medical texts I did not exist, I did indeed exist and I was there for my family, through the deaths of both parents and my brother Franklin, as well as looking out for my brother Joel. I was also seeing Eliana growing into a very fine person and beautiful young woman. During the time of my parents' and brother's death, my son Alex and his wife Kate brought four new babies into the world—my four grandchildren—Ruby, Lucy, Ethan, and Bennett; the fourth is a new Ben Cohen.

Assumptions limit any of us from understanding what a person is going though. Medicine's continued hyper-focus on the image of "cancer as a battle," for instance, seldom sees this internal picture. The patient's visualization of this relationship with the disease may not be that of a violent warrior at all, but rather one of working in a more compassionate, collaborative way with the body's healthy cells to restore balance and harmony throughout by cleaning out the aberrant destructive cancer cells. Gene's guided imagery was that he cleansed those cancer cells by imagining the love he felt for his kids and later his grandchildren. That love was nourishing and sustaining: healing. Without respecting or even fully knowing the patient's perspective, insensitive comments are made; worse still, tacit decisions are made that determine when and how an individual should "fight" or "surrender" to fit the assumptions of others. These profound missed-understandings only add to the burden of one whose inner resources are already taxed.

During one particular visit to a medical research center some distance away, where Gene went periodically to check in with a particular specialist in prostate cancer, the nurse updating his health history made a casual comment questioning why, with the expertise there, he didn't just transfer his care over completely to the center. The inference was that it would certainly be more convenient to have all his records in one place, although she didn't think to ask how convenient or inconvenient this would be to her patient. Gene let it go—didn't feel like explaining or defending himself and his choices and the fact that he had chosen his medical team for a variety of reasons that were important to him. Then when she had finished bringing his history up to date, she mentioned this again, more pointedly this time, as Gene recounted the conversation later. "Over time, with the course of your condition," she said, "you may want to consider coming here for all your care."

Her message was in one way purely practical. But it carried an assumption with it—complications and death on the way—and that's what Gene heard. To him, the message was: "You know, you're only going to get worse now, and it would probably be best for you and the rest of us if you were to come here for all your care." Gene considered this "an unintended arrow," nothing intentional on her part, but hurtful. These kinds of comments—casual, clinical, unconsidered—only heightened his sensitivity to them. He once described them as a "reality assault," not because he felt assaulted by reality, but quite the opposite. These people and their comments ignored his actual reality and superimposed their own assumed version.

> Since diagnosed with metastatic prostate cancer in 1996, I have seen many physicians and visited many facilities for consultation and treatment. Upon passing the decade mark and being advised that according to all the medical textbooks I didn't exist, I shifted my focus of major concern to long-term side effects of my treatment, especially following my femur that fractured as a treatment consequence. During three of these consultations, while expressing my dismay about this situation, the physicians verbally or nonverbally conveyed impatience about what they apparently considered whining. (A cousin of mine once sent me this clever quip about the medical definition of whining: "What doctors describe as ongoing tough questions they cannot answer and are uncomfortable about being asked.") They couldn't understand my perceived fretting, since I had lived longer with metastatic prostate cancer than any patient they had known. Shouldn't I be grateful? Two of them—one more than the other—felt compelled to give me their view of a reality check with their version of, "Do you realize how long you have lived with metastatic prostate cancer, how lucky you have been?"
>
> Of course I feel grateful and lucky—like I have won the lottery! But does that mean I should be satisfied with the fact that nobody knew what to do, since according to the medical texts I didn't exist and there was no experience with how to proceed with my case? "Would you feel comfortable with that if you were in my situation? If the treatments were breaking your bones, would you feel lucky? Do you feel that, since I have lived longer than anyone you know with my condition, I should break open the champagne to celebrate my doctor's historic treatment success and accept the fact that I have lived longer than anyone expected—as if that's good enough?"
>
> As you can gather, I was worked up with this misapplication of the lecture from Doctor/Patient Communication 101. But I wasn't finished. This feeling had been building in me for some time, and they pushed the wrong button. I went on, "Moreover, since I have turned 60 are you looking at me differently because of my age? If you were talking to a 26-year-old who had a lived for 10 years with a seemingly untreatable cancer, would you react to him the same way, not understanding his concern and complaints when he saw others of his age with so much life to live?

You're talking to a gerontologist here. Do you know that in contempo-
rary society life expectancy is the same at age 60 as it was at birth during
the height of the glorious Roman Empire, and that is just a statistical state-
ment, with hundred-year-olds representing the fastest growing age group?
How much time do you think I have left? Or, like all the medical texts
where I don't exist, do you feel that a cancer simply enters an indetermi-
nate remission? These are the questions and concerns behind my demeanor.
These are the legitimate medical questions and concerns. And frankly, this
spirit of inquiry does not seem to have impeded my progress to date. Do you
think I should quit now? As my doctor, what can you advise me about these
concerns?"

Gene was trying to have this conversation with his medical experts, but he felt that his spirit of inquiry was often met with silence. They just didn't know what to say to him. He later wrote:

It was always a baffling question for my doctors, and for me their difficulty—
given the unusual circumstances—of contemplating an unusual (e.g., posi-
tive) outcome, was exasperating.

At one level, his doctors were responding to him as a treatment success, but without recognizing that in his mind, survival was not the full conversation that he needed. As I mentioned in Chapter 9, Gene found affirmation and inspiration in an essay by Stephen Jay Gould, the influential evolutionary biologist and author who taught at Harvard. In "The Median Isn't the Message," Gould noted that, while respecting statistics, he also wanted to show their limits: that statistics are not destiny.[9] Gould himself was diagnosed with cancer—an abdominal meso-thelioma that the scientific literature at the time gave patients a median lifespan of eight months following diagnosis. Twenty years later, Gould was still alive, later dying from other causes. Gene felt that medical literature should be documenting cases like Gould's, and like his own.

Gould's piercing essay helped me deal with both my dread and my focus,
with Damocles' sword and the horse-hair. At the same time, what I offer as
an example of postformal thought, others might assert is denial. But denial
is ignoring the statistics, not denying their status as the truth, the whole
truth, and nothing but the truth. They weren't the truth with Stephen Jay
Gould, nor, as it turns out, with me.

Doctors are not immune from societal views of aging influencing their percep-tion of what is possible for older patients in terms of treatment goals and outcomes. For Gene, these limiting conversations were infrequent, but they definitely took their toll. Sometimes after such an encounter, he would have one of his notorious nightmares.

And finally, we return to where we began, with hope, another important element of style, which has shown up from many different perspectives throughout this book.

> Hope is not a manifestation of denial; it is not a signal that someone needs a reality check. It is a wonderful human quality that needs to be properly responded to, in a manner that reflects the art, not the artlessness, of medicine. . . . Life-threatening diseases that hover over us often make us wonder about how friendly or unfriendly our universe is, a blurring of the rational and the irrational, what's meaningful and what's meaningless, and the difficulty in distinguishing between reality and absurdity.

Creating Our Own Elements of Style

We have come through this chapter to true integrative intelligence. From Gene's original theory-based concepts of developmental intelligence and my own of integrative intelligence, we have moved through Gene's perspective of the doctor/patient relationship as a doctor himself, then purely as a patient, finally to my further observations, being able to reflect more clearly now after having seen so much through my own clinical and personal experience. We have considered the doctor/patient relationship as the developmental catalyst it can be when we each open up to a different experience of ourselves in the context of this relationship.

This is in fact what the "elements of style" are to me: first, reflection and the search for meaning that we are entitled to define for ourselves and redefine as we move through life. It is also a sense of care and service to one another—the desire to give back what we have learned through the crucible of our own experience.

In 2005, one of my favorite artists, Maira Kalman, created an illustrated version of Strunk and White's *Elements of Style*. Her wry visual images in relationship with some of the grammatical sentences make me laugh. She has brought a joy to the tedium of grammar and structure. In this same vein, I would like to imagine myself as having that same capacity—not to illustrate here in paint but to metaphorically illustrate the doctor/patient relationship as a mutual exchange of wisdom—the integrative intelligence of both doctor and patient—through creative expression.

The elements of style in doctor/patient communication in an art therapist's office look different than those in a physician's office, yet each of us—clinicians and clients or patients—can and deserve to find this quality of relatedness with one another.

I like to imagine that this exchange, when we are "met" well—seen, heard, validated—mirrors back recognition to our cells, our chromosomes, and our souls. Met with hope of recognition, we heal, thrive, and grow. If there really is a chromosome of hope within us, its purpose is to remind us who we really are. Recognizing who we are is not simple because it changes constantly with our experience and because a lot of outside noise—perceptions, doubts, judgments— gets in the way. This embedded chromosome, imprinted in our coding, actually already has the knowledge of who we are; it has everything we need to find our way home to ourselves.

In relationship, we activate this innate ability, for with it comes our capacity for imagination—opening to any and every possibility of our identity. Whether we are doctor, patient, family, or friend, we owe it to ourselves to trust that coding, even as it continually responds to us and others. Keeping track of what is authentic is what carries us into true communication, where our wisdom is both developing and integrating all the time.

Part Five

CONGRUENCE

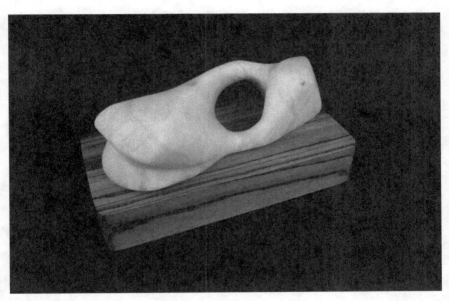

Figure V.i "Whole Hole Resting" (2003), alabaster stone carving on mahogany stand, 5 × 10 × 4 inches. Artwork by Wendy L. Miller, photo credit: Joshua Soros

13

Heartsong to the Inexplicable

A Calendar of Days

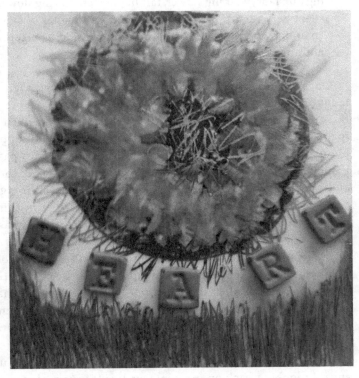

Figure 13.1 "Heartsong" (2011), encaustic wax collage painting, 5 × 5 inches. Artwork by Wendy L. Miller, photo credit: Joshua Soros.

Moments become prophetic only in retrospect. This one is from that morning in December 2008, nearly a year before Gene died, a mere few weeks before we left for Costa Rica for our winter break. I woke up in the middle of the night, compelled by these thoughts and feelings, which I wrote about in an earlier chapter as a kind of unconscious competence—a forewarning from some place of inner wisdom. Now, suddenly, one morning almost a year later, the thought that had haunted me now panics me:

> I have a feeling that my husband is not going to make it. I can't say why. It is just a feeling, a fragility, a quiet between us. A dark feeling. Twelve or thirteen years ago, when the cancer first appeared, I had a feeling that he was going to make it. No reason really. As a matter of fact, it was against reason, but it was a feeling, and it has proved to be true. So this feeling, this dark quiet feeling scares me. I feel myself seeing him fade, walking slower, talking slower, sharing slower, something silent between us. It is not a knowing; as a matter of fact, I think it is an unknowing, a loosening of something inside, a perception based on nothing yet everything.

Once again I know something is shifting. And yet, even now the intense focus on life crowds out the prospect of death. In the stark reality of daily life, the sensation is one of standing knee-deep in the tide when the tide is turning. The current of everyday life that once carried and supported us pushes by us now; we can feel the current pressing against us, past us, leaving us behind. Time slips like sand from beneath our feet faster than we can adjust and right ourselves. The language of disease washes through our conversations, a strange dialect in which talk of patently alarming things—metastatic cancer, nephrostomy tubes, new choices for chemotherapy, as if it is all something we desired—is as fluid and familiar as English muffins and jam. We feel as though we are swimming through the minutes of the hours of our days, doing our best to keep from being pulled under by change that is both miniscule and gigantic all at the same time. Just like the tides change everything about the movement of the water, our world is changing around us and we can neither stand firm nor find the flow that moves in a promising direction. On one level, these details take us more into the individuality of our story; on the other hand, the story could be anyone's, the changing tide a universal experience. In looking back on moments we live through, we see a larger context; the onslaught of details sometimes clarify and sometimes blind us. The universality is that as we live, we each also die, but what do we really know about that process? Gene liked to say, "The story is true; only the facts have been changed." The details of our moments may be different from those of your moments, and yet the story they tell is a story so many of us know or come to know in the last weeks of a loved one's life. The story is true, only each of our individual facts have been changed.

The Unbearable Lightness of Being

WHAT LIFE LOOKS LIKE

Gene comes home from his camping trip with Alex in mid-October. This is the father/son fall trip they have been creating for themselves for years. There was no way he was not going. I couldn't imagine how it was going to happen, and yet, it did. Alex arranged an amazing journey—rented an RV and decked it all out to be ever so comfortable for his dad, like a traveling living room. He drove Gene throughout Maine to the most beautiful harbors and coastlines. He equipped his traveling van with everything Gene needed: extra blankets and jackets, hats and gloves to keep him warm, extra tanks of oxygen, which he didn't even know yet how to use, but he knew he had to have them. Arriving at the airport in Portland, then making their way back to Alex's home in Lincolnville, Gene became so tired that when he entered their house, they all took one look at him and thought he was actually going to die right there on the couch as he slowly laid out his entire body system into its long overdue need for rest. The pre-journey had already taken its toll and given them a clear and immediate picture of exactly where Gene now was physically. Five days on the road, his son escorted him with equally as much love as gasoline, bringing beauty, love, and comfort to his dad's weakening adventurous spirit. *For him, with him, I can do anything*—internally said by each of them, I know for sure. I know that if you could bottle that much love, respect, willingness, and will, you would have a formula for something extraordinarily vital in family life. Sometimes when you can't see beforehand the toll that the psychological and physical assault is taking, you need to have a journey like that one. Even though that was the last one.

AS AWARENESS SEEPS IN, DECISIONS TAKE FORM

Thursday, October 22—I make a decision to take my artwork in to be framed. I have this realization that Gene may not ever be able to walk to my studio again to see the art pieces I have been doing all year so I decide that I will create an art show in our living room for him—first step, get the fragile pieces framed. Gene goes to Sibley to have his scans done. I pick him up. He is exhausted. We go to the oncologist's office for blood work. They keep him longer in the chemo/transfusion room because his heart rate registers an alarmingly high 125. The nurses call his doctor who says they should increase the oxygen level up to five rather than keeping it at two. He is resting. I am worrying. I leave the office, feeling annoyed at the nurse, even though I don't really understand why I feel that way toward her.

THE STRANGE COMFORT IN TRYING
TO KEEP NORMAL NORMAL

Friday, October 23—I go to work. I know something is changing, but I don't want it to change and I am hoping that I can will it to stay steady by staying on track in my own work life.

Saturday, October 24—I am scheduled to go to a conference in Maine and present the footage from the Legacy film project. I will only be gone 24 hours. My friend Carol is going to stay here with Gene. She is the only person both Gene and I can imagine staying here. I haven't left him in such a long time, except in Alex's hands for their trip, and yet I get on the plane and go with just Carol and Eliana at the house with him. He and Carol worry a number of times during the night about making a decision to go to the hospital as his breathing has become very bad very quickly.

THE ANGER THAT ACCOMPANIES AWARENESS

Sunday, October 25—I arrive back home early evening. Gene is sitting on the edge of the couch, Carol nearby. He doesn't look like himself at all. He is totally drawn inward. He tells me that his entire focus is on his breath. That is all he can do. I find out the next morning that when oxygen is increased to a higher number, as he had to do, that we need to activate the humidifier on the machine, adding distilled water, so that the nasal passages don't dry out, which is painful and makes breathing harder. Now, I come to know belatedly why I was annoyed at the nurse. Why didn't she give us the necessary information as to *how* to increase the oxygen? I am frustrated that neither the nurse nor the oxygen delivery person ever explained this to us. We have had to learn with Gene as the guinea pig, suffering through the process. What is the matter with these professionals?

REALITY AT THE INTERSECTION OF MEDICAL
AND FAMILY SHARED AWARENESS

Monday, October 26—We go to Gene's oncologist's office to see him first thing in the morning and discuss the next round of chemotherapy. He tells Gene that it is okay to stop chemotherapy; that he has fought a long hard battle; that it is time for comfort palliative care. I don't remember the rest of the day. It surprised and silenced both of us.

Reflecting back, I remember words and phrases about the various chemotherapies and about how information like learning the use of the oxygen had ever so slowly seeped into my consciousness of understanding, like the drips themselves of intravenous chemotherapy. In the summer and fall of 2009, when I see Gene walking slowly and breathing hard, I don't know if it is good for him to continue to walk up the stairs when he is weakened and exhausted or whether it will cause some kind of collapse somewhere else. But the doctors don't seem to follow my train of thought or worry. They have their own agenda or maybe there are so many sides to the prism of experience that we each see through our own faceted angle. Or perhaps we don't give them all the information that we see. I listen. I wait.

Finally the doctor clarifies it for me in something he says to kind of sum up as we are leaving his office: "Oxygen is a good thing to have so that we do not put added stress on the heart."

I finally get the rearrangement of facts that I need to make sense out of our situation. "Thank you," I hear inside. That is the heartsong, the state of reverie as the state of healing.

The doctor named and claimed what I couldn't tame because I didn't know what to call it. His naming helped me aim not only toward hope, but meaning; he made sense out of something that had been swimming around like lost cancer cells in the dark of the night, like my restless husband searching for the right bed. This is the heart of the matter: I am like a Geiger counter for complications caused by the treatments rather than a Geiger counter of understanding for the natural course of the illness. When the doctor finally explained that the oxygen was reliev-ing the stress on Gene's heart, I finally understood what we were doing—why he needed oxygen—and I could put that information together with what I was see-ing. Gene's need for a small backpack of oxygen to walk up the stairs at night had been his only use of oxygen previously, and the doctors' previous comments left the impression that it was "the lungs" that needed it. I hadn't understood the full process unfolding, what was happening or what clearly would happen in our very near future. The doctor's explanation suddenly crystallized the information for me. I could think clearly again, with a sense of direction. Now I could aim this clinical information in a practical way to help Gene. For instance, before, I was never sure if the exertion of going up the stairs was good for him or dangerous. Now I see that wherever he goes, whether walking or otherwise up and about in any way, we need to make sure he's not straining his heart. That one clarifying comment from the doctor has recalibrated my inner sense of what Gene needs and what to do.

Suddenly all concerns and conversation turn to another kind of chemother-apy, Mitoxantrone, one which specifically focuses on the lungs. "*The lungs.*" How quickly we separate the clinical conversation from the human conversation. I mean *Gene's* lungs. By separating his needs down to a body part, like his lungs, the clinical conversation is already scary. It separates us from the relational con-versation. The clinical conversation is precise in medical terms, but in human terms, it is detached and frightening. Are we supposed to shift from one perspec-tive to another? Do we try to live in both realities at the same time? How do we know what to listen for in order to make choices?

Tuesday, October 27—Gene and I are discussing his getting a blood transfusion today. The oncologist had told us that if Gene is ready to stop chemo, it's all right with him; as a matter of fact, he suggests two options. One is to go onto weekly chemo; another is to go for his comfort. We are so stopped in our tracks. He is too weak to make such a big decision. We are not ready to make this shift. We see that his body is struggling, but we have been in this fight for eight months now, added upon thirteen years of preparation, and it is the air in which we breathe. We sleep, we problem solve, we decide on the most immediate next step. We can't think when his brain doesn't have the nutrients it needs. We decide that a big decision like stopping chemotherapy deserves more blood, oxygen, and fluids, so that a decision like this can be made out of knowledge, not out of exhaustion, and fear. That is the step we will take. We call Sibley for a blood transfusion. They schedule it for Thursday; but he has to go in tomorrow for cross-matching of the blood.

Wednesday, October 28—I worriedly send him to Sibley with Al, a volunteer driver from Kensington, the first time I have ever sent him with a driver rather than with me, family, or a friend. He stays all day for the transfusion, and Al chooses to stay with him. What a lovely responsive man. I am working with my clients, and then I pick up Eliana. We come home; Gene has not bounced back. Usually when it is the chemo that has weakened him, after a transfusion, he is like a different person. I could bring him in to Sibley as a limp rag, but then he would come out himself. Not today—all that blood and fluid and he is still so weak. I begin to understand that it is the cancer not the chemo that is weakening him so drastically, but the formation of this understanding is still ghost-like in my mind. Too unreal to be real.

Thursday, October 29—I take him to the cardiologist appointment that the oncologist wants. I didn't want to use his time with more appointments; I felt he needed to stay at home and recuperate. (I am still using words like "recuperate.") But physicians diligently follow the referrals of other physicians. And so Gene, the physician, wants to follow through with the appointment. I take with us the tank that I think has enough oxygen but since we have never used oxygen before as "necessary," just as "in case," nor have we ever used it at such a high rate as he now needs, we run out of it right there in the doctor's office. I am so stressed, and have no idea what to do. I want to just turn around and take him home.

The cardiologist asks me what I want to do. I explain why I am so nervous and his staff looks all through his office for more oxygen; one tank after another is an empty. As they search, I watch Gene lying on the doctor's table. He can hardly breathe. It is frightening—for Gene, certainly, and for me, too. Finally they find a full one. The doctor suggests that I go home alone to get another oxygen tank so that Gene will be safe going home when the examination is finished. One won't be enough to see him through. As I drive and try to breathe through my own fears, I pull myself out of it, thinking, and frankly knowing, that somehow there is protection and love all around us, and there is no way he is going to die in the cardiologist's office while I am off driving to get him what he needs to live. There is no way that could happen, I think, and yet there is no reason to assume that.

A friend once told me how naïve she felt when her father, who had leukemia and had been growing steadily worse for a few years, died suddenly in the hospital from an infection he'd been battling but surviving for months. They were going to discharge him that afternoon; and then his heart simply stopped. It wasn't just that his death was sudden, she said. It was that he lived across the country from her and her husband and children, and he had planned to come visit in a couple of months; somehow his travel plans seemed to ensure that he'd be around to do it. And then he wasn't. All I knew for sure about Gene as I drove away was that he was struggling to breathe on his own and if that single tank from the office ran dry on the way home, he would not make it without more. So I drove away to get what he needed to live, needing to assume that he would.

Silly as it may sound, as I sped home, what came to mind was what I wrote about earlier, here in the real moment of living through the experience. I called out to Mary Martin as Peter Pan. She was my call to prayer in the fast car ride to retrieve more oxygen. I imagined everyone we knew clapping the light of protection into Gene's life force, so that he could breathe, so that something in him that he so needed would be lit up by this love.

When I returned to the cardiologist's office with a large full tank of oxygen, Gene was sitting in the waiting room, in a wheelchair, with the oxygen tank they had found. He hadn't even heard the results of what the doctor found, so unlike Gene, but such a sign of what it meant to be using all of his available energy just to breathe. I asked for an explanation from the doctor before we left. He said that Gene's pericardium—the outer layer of heart tissue—had hardened around his heart. They could try to operate on it but the doctor thought we should just let nature takes its course because, given Gene's condition, he believed that Gene would most likely die on the table.

It is not us, then, who make the decision what to do. It is his heart. As we drive home, Eliana calls from school to say that she is feeling really sick and she wants to come home. We go to the school to get her. We are all together, and all of us do not feel well. At home, Gene rests in his favorite living room chair with Eliana beside him. He tells her what has happened. That night I call the internist, because Gene's coughing is growing worse and his breathing is very difficult. I wonder if he should take something for his cough or what we should do. The doctor tells me that we need to call hospice tomorrow because any over-the-counter congestion medicine could have adverse effects. We have only just accepted that the decision has been made to have no more chemotherapy, and no surgery, and now they want us to call in hospice. Time decisions seem to be on a fast treadmill. Calling hospice means to me calling the people you call when you know that you're shifting from chemotherapy to palliative care—pain management. That is all I really know about hospice, and all I hear when it is suggested.

Friday, October 30—In the morning, I call Alex and tell him I think he should come now. He was already coming on Sunday, but the days and the changes are moving so fast, I feel he needs to come right away. I know he is the father of four children, and I can't be positive what is happening, but fortunately, he doesn't ask for or need such clarity. He just changes his flight and arrives later that night.

Reb David had been planning on coming to visit in the afternoon to hear about Gene's trip with Alex in Maine. Instead, as soon as he arrives, Gene tells him about the deeply discouraging week filled with medical shocks. It is clear to Gene that his body is failing, but more significantly, he says: "My spirit is broken." We both know this is unlike Gene. Reb David makes a plan with us to dispel the darkness and comfort the spirit by creating an evening of music and loved ones to fill our home. We agree on Monday night. We agree I do not have to feel obligated to invite our whole community. It is only for whoever Gene would like to be there.

It is Halloween night. I answer the door to young ones dressed for the holiday, their tiny joyful spirits. Gene is curled up on the couch in the living room. Hospice arrives that night, with the angel nurse Marco, who puts one drop of morphine under Gene's tongue and brings relief to Gene's body, spirit, and grateful eyes in one mere moment.

Saturday, October 31—We have the planned big luncheon with Gene's colleagues and friends from the National Center for Creative Aging and the National Endowment for the Arts: Paula, Susan, Gay, Phil, Alex, Eliana, and me. We were supposed to have it at Paula's but I asked that everyone come to our home instead. It is absolutely wonderful, and Gene quietly holds court at the head of the table. Our hearts are made buoyant by the amount of love, beauty, nourishment, and exchange at one dining table. The luncheon was like a celebration almost. He'd been through this horrendous week, hospice had come and given him just a slight bit of medicine, an amount we thought was just the beginning of a process with them that would take place over months. But at the end of the day, joyous as it had been, it was clear that the week had done him in. And now we had to learn how to titrate the pain medicines and we were yet to do a good job of it.

CAREGIVING AND LOVE REVISITED

Sunday, November 1—Gene rests but he is very weak. He has slept in the hospital bed in the sunroom. Jim and Laurie come over and help him eat some breakfast. He thanks Laurie for continuing his research with the family and his Alzheimer's game, "Making Memories Together" at the VA Hospital. Jim shares with him the notebook he created that chronicles his own work at George Washington University. Alex and Eliana go off to a day together—the zoo, of course—their favorite! Then in the afternoon Jaime and Laurie are here and we walk Gene out of the hallucinatory state from the morphine. He now spoke with me through cryptic images as his way of informing us that he was returning back to himself internally. "I'm at the Betty Ford Clinic" equaled "I feel drugged."[1] "Now I am at the Halfway House" meant that as he was coming through this, with more food, water, conversation, he was coming at least halfway around. "Now I am at Martha's Vineyard" referred to the famous journalist Art Buchwald, who had to send hospice home because he was not dying (this took place on Martha's Vineyard).[2] Our understanding of one another and one another's language is so apparent. I am deeply worried about the narcotics; they have eaten up our whole day just returning him to himself. I had no idea how few days we would have, but I didn't want him suffering or not present for any of them.

Then, from a different part of my life, Laura comes over bringing us a huge basket of food. She gently whispers in my ear, "I understand," and I know, she is one person who certainly does.

Monday, November 2—Alex and I are viewing the experience with the pain relief drugs in different ways. Both of us are realizing that Gene really is slipping from us. Alex is literally carrying his dad in the shower and onto the couch. He is viscerally seeing how helpless and weakened his dad is. I am so grateful that he is here, and yet so saddened that this is where we are. The nurse came yesterday with the social worker, but by today, I am feeling overwhelmed. Gene is in pain. Gretchen comes during the day, and lovingly rubs his neck, as she and Alex get a chance to connect. Reb David and a group of friends come that night to sing in our living room. It is very special. Gene can still talk, but his voice is weak; he smiles as his favorite songs surround him. We share the couch nest during the singing. Later, he sits up with Jim and Walter. The quiet talk of male friendship, as if everything is all right.

DYING TIME: YOU KNOW WHEN YOU KNOW

Tuesday, November 3—Gene comes into the kitchen in the morning rolling himself in his office chair. He tells Alex and me that he is very, very lethargic. Alex tells Gene that he loves him, that he will miss him greatly, but that it is all right for him to go. By "go" of course he means let go, let go of the struggle, let go of life. Just as I had to do with my own dad, I understand what Alex is doing, and how hard it is to be in that moment. They stare at one another, with gentle love and intensity. Gene then switches his gaze to me. He asks me if I think he is dying. I think so many things, I can hardly speak. I have to say yes though, because I know Alex is right. I know that is what I am supposed to say, but am I ready, do I feel that? No. Do I see it happening to him? Yes, and he looks up at me with his most intimate trusting eyes, and he asks me, "Do you think I am going?" And slowly, out of my mouth comes "yes."

Gene says he needs to go lie down on the couch. I think I need to lie down too, Gene. It was all so big. It was so big. The awareness that he needed oxygen to get air. I did not understand that all the oxygen would still not be enough, not just to breathe, but for that big beautiful brain to have enough oxygen for his system. So much had broken down and we had adapted and adapted and adapted. There are so many medical ways to shore up failing organs. We bargained, I guess, and we had made it work—imperfect, yes, but we made it work, whatever function there was left to work with. We'd accepted. And yet, "the lungs," his heart, bladder, kidneys, everything was breaking down, and still, still, his will to live was stronger than all of it. All the way up until—as we would learn soon enough—a mere seven days before he went.

That will people call the will to live, it's the strongest muscle in the body. I used to study that: how to activate that will, how to help the immune system, how to mobilize healing, and, yes, I totally believed as Gene did that creativity is the finest medicine in the world. Now I had seen it in action with him, so intimately, so dearly, so courageously Gene. We hold onto each other, in quiet, back at the couch nest from which he never rose again. Someone comes to the front door at this exact moment, but I can't leave Gene's side and I can't think what I would do or say to anyone—at that moment. Alex answers the door and after a brief conversation closes it; the someone has left. I learn that it was my dear friend Ellen, who had driven in from an hour away. Ordinarily her loving, spontaneous visit would have been just part of the (happier) comings and goings of the day. But she had no idea of the turn things had just taken, and Alex had no idea how far she had driven. Only much later did I explain to her why she hadn't been invited in. Days later people would just go around the back porch and come in that door and hang out in the kitchen together, still giving us our privacy or the quiet of only one person at a time with us in the living room, but that moment on Tuesday was the turning point: we were in uncharted territory. This time the final frontier.

Later, on the phone, I find myself revealing to the hospice social worker that I do not like the new nurse. I do not trust her. She has offended me over our discussion about the medicine. That first night when the wonderful nurse explained all of the medicines in the pain management package, Gene said we could throw away the Haldol. As a psychiatrist he was very familiar with the use and side effects of that drug and he knew he did not want to use it. I did as he requested, and threw it away, but now, five days later, when Alex and I are not sure how much morphine or Ativan to use, and what is the best combination, this new nurse suggests we try using the Haldol. When I explain to her what Gene had requested, she points out that that was what he said when he had his full faculties, but he is different now. This upset me to the core. It was our task to honor his knowledge, requests, needs—*his passage*—and ignoring his instructions now was not the way we were going to do it.

"Would you like to fire her and have a new nurse?" the social worker asks. "I have no intention of hurting anyone's career or making a decision like that," I tell her. "I just don't want that person in our sacred space." This conversation was disheartening, but a new nurse comes and I appreciate it. My nephew Ben begins his vigil here, staying at the house with us. Suzane brings us dinner. Andrea and Marsha stop by with fresh flowers and a tiny purple Buddha. Gene's friend Walter comes each evening with his floor fans so they can move the air, which helps Gene's breathing.

Wednesday, November 4—I am in angst. I call another woman from hospice that I had heard about. She is comforting. Rebecca is here during the day. Everything is very slow and intimate. There is no longer any desire or ability to eat; food, so long a sustaining ally and focus in our anti-cancer vigilance has vanished from consideration. Water is now just a sip and Gene takes it through the straw. Martha comes over, helps at the dining room table with the pile of bills. Friends are doing tasks in different part of the house. Laurie and Claire have come over one night and sorted through bags of mail. I cry a lot. Joshua shows up with his new girlfriend. They are like a breath of fresh youth to me. She has flowers and a pineapple. They go to take Eliana out of school for half the day and to bring her to her piano lesson. Shira comes over at night. She brings her friend Priscilla, who works with a different hospice agency. They stay long enough and talk with me enough for me to understand that my angst is that I need the medicines to balance Gene's lucidity with his comfort—that is the task and the tension, and it took me a while to understand it.

Thursday, November 5—We do a better job with everything medically. Visitors have come around the porch and go into the kitchen so they are in a separate world from us. We are in the quiet space in the living room. Alex and I explain to the new nurse Jodi that our perceptions of the medicines for Gene are different from one another; that we are not seeing the balance between lucidity and comfort in the same way. I am afraid that too much medicine will disorient him or make him uncomfortable. Alex is afraid that we are prolonging suffering for his dad if we don't give him enough medicine. The wife and the son: we are both doing our job as well as we can to protect the Gene we each love. Finally, we experiment carefully, and we are able together to move him into a gentler state. We all live by the couch nest. Alex sleeps on the floor by his dad. I can go upstairs for some hours to rest. Walter sits vigil with us each evening. Alex leaves the house for a few hours, finally taking the space to call his wife Kate. Ben is in and out, helping with whatever we need. Both my sisters are coming. My sister Julie comes over tonight. She had arrived days earlier from her home on the west coast, but went to a hotel in Silver Spring because I was so adamant about her not coming. I was trying to ward off any end approaching and yet it kept approaching. My keeping my family of origin away could not keep him alive, though I tried so hard to keep him alive. When I was ready to call her, she wanted to be a mere twenty minutes away, not a plane ride from California. She was right.

Eliana is finally home—school is out for the long weekend.

In the middle of the night, 4 A.M., I realize how slow his breathing is and I lay my cheek up against him as I do and I whisper into his ear. "Please do not go tonight. I know you are leaving, but please do not go gently on this night. Sandy is coming tomorrow. I am not ready. Eliana is not ready. She is just home today, able to not have to focus on school. She is just starting to move out of that mode. She is home, with us now. Give her a little time, sweetheart."

Gene wants music. How did he convey that to me? He kept pointing upward. "You want to go upstairs? You want me to move over?" Everything else I guess, he shakes his head. No. Music—the music of Pavarotti, up, he is pointing up, "Louder?"[3] I ask. Loud, that is what he wants. As I play it, he keeps moving his hand upward until it is loud enough. He turns, kisses me on my head as I lean into him. He holds my face in his hands. It is his last kiss to me.

Friday, November 6—He is not in an awake state all day. We keep the medicines very even. My sister Sara arrives. My friend Emily comes over to help. She does my laundry. Life is going on in the back part of my house without me, and yet for me. Eliana goes to the supermarket on her bike to buy cat food; some kids hassle her and knock her off her bike. She comes home crying. She had tried to call me, but I wasn't answering my phone. She calls her boyfriend, crying. He and his family call and come over. The police come to see what happened, as her wonderfully protective brother Alex had called them. It is a kind of drama that frightens my whole being. But she is all right, shaken up, but not hurt in any way. A mailman from the post office had stopped his truck near her, and the boys then ran away.

The evening air in the room begins to change. Friends arrive. Walter comes again with his wife Tova. Sandy and his wife Fern fly in from Chicago. His closest friends are all here. Sandy plays piano—the room is filled with music. Then Eliana plays piano, for a long time; it is her gift of music to herself and to her dad.

Gene is peaceful, very peaceful.

Saturday, November 7—We all went to sleep a little after the midnight music. I go upstairs to be with Eliana in her room. I want to make sure she is all right, but I end up falling asleep with her on her bed. Alex sleeps on the living room floor by his dad. Suddenly I awaken—it is 3:15. I have only been gone from Gene's side a few hours. I go quickly to him on the couch and I put my hand to his forehead. Gene is hot, and I begin to realize his breathing is so slow, so slow that I can believe I can feel it stop. It is not there. It becomes my breathing that I hear. I listen and I stay close to Gene's face. I breathe. I am confused, yet not. Finally, I wake Alex up, and say, "I don't think he is breathing anymore."

We wait. We listen. We are quiet. The loud sound of quiet. The stiffness of Gene's head, slanted against the pillow. We decide eventually to call hospice. I go to awaken Eliana, but she doesn't want to see her dad like this. She doesn't want that to be her final memory. She had no idea then that there would be no other time to ever see him again. I wanted to protect her, but instead, I allowed him to be taken from the house without her seeing him. I didn't know that was not the right thing to do until she told me much later that she was angry he had been taken away without her saying her own goodbye. I should have awakened her even if she only watched from the steps as they took him away. When hospice arrived, they declared death at 5:15 A.M. but I know it was 3:20 A.M.

Everyone who hears Gene had cancer for nearly fourteen years assumes that he fought for his life through all of those years of cancer living inside him. On one level, that is true, but on another, it is so far from the truth. Living with illness—the emphasis is on the word *with*. We live with, we wake up with, we accompany with. The word *cancer* is accompanied by an assumed imagistic language as well—the language of the fight/the battle/the race. The truth is we come up with material ways to accommodate what has changed in our life. We do this all the time, regardless of illness or age. It is the process of living.

In truth, we love our life everyday, every moment of every day. We all make assumptions and these assumptions play with our brain and our minds, as if they know how or for how long or in what manner we will live. We don't have a clue what anything looks like or will look like. We want to know, but we live our lives in constant uncertainty. When we are healthy, we think we know how we will be or how we will feel or what we will choose to do IF and when such and such might happen TO us. But when we are inside of something living with us, everything is different. It rearranges us. It rearranges our priorities, our thoughts, our feelings, our needs and desires. And it is from that place—that changed place—that we will come to make our decisions—not assumptions—but decisions and actions as to what we can and will do.

Assumptions never reveal the essential vulnerability of every single one of us. And what do we do with that vulnerability? We dread it. We fear it. We think we understand it. We move it away as best we can. And sometimes we move people away just because they are near it. We fear it could get into us through osmosis, as if we might be able to escape the inevitable.

But when the crack opens, it opens us. For the first time in memory, I reach for a prayerbook, and we find ourselves praying through the words of Abraham Joshua Heschel:

> In no other act does a person experience so often the disparity between the desire for expression and the means of expression as in prayer. The inadequacy of the means at our disposal appears so tangible, so tragic, that one feels it a grace to be able to give oneself to music, to a tone, to a song, to a chant. The wave of a song carries the soul to heights which utterable meaning can never reach. Such abandonment is no escape, for the world of utterable meanings is the nursery of the soul, the cradle of all our ideas. It is not an escape but a return to one's origins.[4]
>
> To become aware of the ineffable is to part company with words. The essence, the tangent to the curve of human experience lies beyond the limits of language. The world of things we perceive is but a veil, its

flutter is music, its ornament science, but what conceals is inscrutable. Its silence remains broken; no word can carry it away.

Sometimes we wish the world could cry and tell us about that which made it pregnant with fear-filling grandeur. Sometimes we wish our own heart would speak of that which made it heavy with wonder.[5]

What is it that really heals when enormous craters have plummeted into your heart? What art form can return to us all that has been taken? How does creativity strengthen the broken? Grieving certainly feels broken. This is the truth of our experience—when everything slips away, the search is constant for what remains.

Gene died surrounded by music. Songs by our friends filled our living room where his weary body rested on the couch we called his nest; his friend of over forty years, fellow father of geriatric psychiatry, arrived in time to serenade from our piano; his son, camped out for weeks in a sleeping bag beside him on the living room floor, just as he had done as a young boy. Well into the late hours of his last evening light, our then fifteen-year-old daughter's piano reverie calmed him asleep. There is no beauty here, just truth. Creativity? Healing? It is our only call, our heartsong to the inexplicable, where the silence reverberates somewhere in our hearts.

Final Entry: The Voice of Grief

11/9/2009, MEMORIAL

I can't remember feeling clear in any way, except when our whole family was in the limousine going to the memorial service. I spoke to the kids and the grandkids. I knew then what was needed, and I needed to make it clear to them so that they could be all right with what we had to do on this day.

Even twenty-one years apart, Alex and Eliana have this connection as Gene's children. When Reb David asked them which poets Gene liked, they couldn't name names, but they both knew to recite the same poem. It was the A. E. Housman poem he had taught both of them when they were children. Together they practiced it in the limo as we arrived graveside:

When I was one and twenty
I heard a wise man say
Give crowns and pounds and guineas
But not your heart away.
Give pearls away and rubies
But keep your fancy free
When I was one and twenty
No use to talk with me.

Generosity of Spirit

MAY 26, 2010, ANNIVERSARY OF OUR WEDDING

To Gene:

Seven months have gone by. You were diagnosed March 1996. You lived well with this cancer for over thirteen years, then you lived under the direction of its chemotherapy life for almost a full year more. That means it was longer than anyone expected—anyone in medical science at least. Those years look like a really short time now, like a shooting star, like everything flew by so fast and who can remember anything anymore.

This is our day. Eliana's boyfriend came by and gave her a dozen roses today, as it was a two-month anniversary since they met. He had another dozen for me for my anniversary.

AN AVALANCHE OF IMMEDIACY

Pressure. Pressure by people, by bills, by the phone, by emails, by appointments, by needs, by work, by school. Everything feels disorganized, as I am no longer able to sort anything. Everything is everywhere because if it moves from its place, it is gone. Out of sight, out of mind. What mind? If I move it, I can't find it. My mind has moved to a state my friend Michael calls "grief dementia," where the brain is not working as it used to and everything seems to slip from the mind. Rita called it the formation of new plasticity—that in the trauma of grief, every single one of our cells needs to go through reconfiguration. Both explanations have helped me, since everything was moving through me with no imprint or memory. It's as if the trauma of grieving leaves no remnant of ourselves from the experience, so it is very hard to find our recognizable markings.

That is the existential story as well as the physical, practical one. My mind is elsewhere. It cannot sort. It cannot listen. It cannot take in information that is not pertinent to the task or the moment. The physical system is not prepared for the grief state. The grief state is not prepared for the outer world. Nothing really is right anymore.

My days are spent frustrated over the paperwork and conversations about estate, probate, insurance, bills, credit cards, lawyers, Verizon, the Internet, AmVets coming to my porch to pick up the furniture and the enormous number of bags of trash, clothes, and other contributions that Kate and Alex helped organize from Gene's office, and not showing up for some stupid scheduling mishap. Incompetence throws me into high gear, and I can't communicate anything except my frustration over that. It is impossible to get through the death doorway, no matter how many times I fax the certificate, even when I call and use my husband's name as my own, all I can move are small centimeters through the blockages. The wall of paperwork is in itself built brick by brick with death death death. A moment of compassion, hundreds of moments of frustrations.

I am left with the tasks, the headaches, the misinformation and incompetence, trying to breathe under the avalanche of immediacy. Our own systems are outside of time, the papers define a me that is without me, without him, without a past or a future, without the password of entry or the correct answer to his security question, *"What was the name of your first pet?"* The indignity of it all brings out the worst in me.

Out of Disbelief Time

Fall 2010—Eliana is in Bethesda with her group of friends from her new high school. She was going to hang out between four o'clock and eight o'clock, so I chose to go to the movies with friends so I wouldn't have to drive back and forth. Around six o'clock, she considered leaving and going home. She said it out loud, but added that she knew her mom was busy so she couldn't come and pick her up. One of the new friends said, "Why don't you just call your dad?" She burst into tears.

The surprise of the grief waves—what place can we go, what dad can you call, what do we do with all the basic assumptions that people make, the life that people assume, that we had the luxury of assuming for such a long time, or really now I see was such a short time. Death marks so strongly. End of this chapter. End of assumption. End of innocent time. She doesn't remember it now, but I know that last year when she was still at her old school, she told me she wanted to change schools for many reasons, mostly because of the academics, but also because, she said, *"My friends are children. They don't understand me."*

And to me, her pain was that I was not patient like her dad. Losing one parent separates the combined front of parenthood into the individual styles of each one—and she was left with just mine. She no longer felt normal because, she said, *"I do not have my father and all I can do is yell at my mother."* She wanted to scream out her truth, which was that I couldn't understand her pain. And she is partially right: I have great fear that she will make terrible teen choices now with this huge loss. And yet, even in the words of her anger, she looks out to protect me and to take care of me. She and her friend Maya include me and check in on me when they are together shopping or having dinner. She wants to be strong and help out. She wants beyond everything to make her dad proud of her, and one way of doing that is through her support of me, even if she has to shout it out. Something in me prays I will be able to trust her to make good choices.

It is difficult to enter another's pain because we are always looking from our own perspective. We look but we do not see. This is what she saw: *"You lived with him forever, but because I am only fifteen, I only really have a few years of memory with dad. I don't remember anything from the years when I was a little girl and I haven't had any time to think about him, only to think about school."* She no longer felt normal. Nothing was normal. Sadness and loss send everyone astray.

The Un-generosity of Grief

I've learned a few things about grieving. Grief is stingy. There are no reserves, so giving is a difficult concept. A griever can give to a good listener, but cannot listen well herself. Reserves are too depleted to focus and care and follow another person's storyline.

A grieving person's heart is not available to open. It feels the vibration of care and community but it is wounded and therefore using all of its own blood flow to heal. Not broken, wounded; not needing to be fixed, wounded; not contagious, wounded. Grief is traumatic. We have no control over our autonomic nervous system—it responds and we respond to its response.

It's hard for a griever to initiate—it's impossible to know what one needs or what will work or who is best to be around or where to go or what to wear or if it will feel better or worse. It is all so unpredictable.

It took me all four years of my daughter being in high school to understand why I felt so disconnected, angry, and outside my own skin. Of course, I knew I was grieving, but only during her last semester did I understand that I was not generous in my heart or in my spirit and that I needed to find a way to open that even though everything in me had no interest in being open, had no desire to open, and frankly, couldn't bring myself to do anything more than what I was doing.

Finally, at the very end of her high school years, my generosity came forth in helping to create a night club prom for the class, and finishing the year off with a great party here at our house, bringing a tent to the yard, using our beautiful porch, and catering a wonderful meal. We celebrate the moms, the dads, the teachers, the friends, and the capacity we had mustered to bring forth our generosity of spirit for the best graduation party we all deserved.

The Existential Voice

There is a huge community of care around me. What a wonderful source of support, gratitude, and love it has been. The shared presence of listening is the real gift a friend gives to another.

The existential feelings mix with my heart and my mind. Are they a spiritual calling to know how to navigate through these waters? Who helps us understand? Who accompanies us? What do we need along the way? My sisters' words are close by, every day. I hear them. I know they care. I know they know. My words accompany me as they try to hold a mirror for me. My friends see, and they tell me what they see, sometimes, or they ask me what I see. Alex and Kate are in the magnetic field, pulsing with us as we all try to stay in our lives, yet need to move with the movement of our separated lives.

But there is an edge to the grieving process that is hard to articulate or speak of out loud. It seems to comfort friends to see or imagine that I will be okay. They like to envision another chapter that awaits me. This thought is perhaps really more comforting for them, but not fully for me, because thoughts and images of "new life, new passions, and new people" feel very unsafe to me. I don't want to be moved out of the now and into a then. Gene died way too soon, and imagining some other future pulls me away from the pieces of our life that we built together. These are the pieces that are sustaining me, holding me by that very thin thread.

Grief is not, emotionally, a safe zone. When we have walked the full distance of responsibility and caretaking, giving all that is necessary to our loved partner, all the way up to the moment of his death, to turn around and choose to walk it with another is not a step I would take right now.

People start quickly talking about the "hope" of a new companion, a new sexual partner, a new friend for you. A new companion, new attention, new possibilities of being loved and cared for by someone may truly comfort some people, but for me, it feels very unwelcome. I could define it by saying that Gene was rare, because he was, or that Gene was my true love, which he also was, or that Gene was my husband and the right husband for me. I could say I can't imagine loving again like I loved him, but I don't think any of these are really the reason for what I experience. It's much more of an existential dilemma than that.

When you go the whole length of the path with someone, not just the path you imagine or plan for, but the real one that happens to you, you intertwine your lives, and experience all the changes that come with that new formation. Why or how could you imagine trusting and believing in starting over and doing it all again? We know that we each are going to die, but that language makes it sound like I am merely afraid of newness, but that is not it at all.

To me, what is comforting is to honor the deep intimacy I have whether my husband is still here or not, and I don't want people asking me to replace that intimacy. I don't want to build a shrine to a past, nor do I want to be told there is a future. I want to stand in what is and has been and be allowed to have it still throb with its own breath, its own memories, its own legacy. I want to take in the beauty of the creative life we actually built.

Yes, he has passed over, passed into, passed away. What in me has passed? What in me has passed me by or passed over me? What in me wants to say, "I pass," to any images of what my healing should look like to someone outside of me? What in me dares to take a stand, right here, and say out loud that what we think is love and intimacy hasn't even come close yet to what we will be asked to hold when the soul and essence of love is placed in our hands and we are asked to breathe life, which is the ending of life, into our shared soul partner?

The Gift of Dried Flowers

Gene gave me very interesting bouquets of flower arrangements —they are made of a mixture of dried flowers and grasses, tightly bound together, and arranged in small containers of wire, wood, and a kind of moss (probably a synthetic moss) material. I seldom see them anymore in stores, but a small shop in our neighborhood, called Cottage Monet, used to carry them. They are unique looking, probably European made. I never thought too much about them, or about his aesthetic, as he also bought me bouquets of live roses. Recently, though, in thinking about creative faculty and unconscious authority and competence, I have found myself looking at these arrangements, as I have one in my living room, in my bedroom, another in my office, a fourth in my office waiting room. I pass them every day and always enjoy the weird sense that he gave me flowers that do not go away. Flowers that live in their already departed state. Flowers that transcend the tending of life. Flowers that make me feel he is still bringing beauty and love into my life.

Could he possibly have imagined this when he chose to buy me these? What was it in his aesthetic that made him choose these types of dried-flower arrangements? Could he have thought about the fact that they would live forever? And if he did, or didn't, how is it that such a strange dichotomy of life and death sits everywhere I look in my daily life?

What We Were Supposed to Do

There was never any doubt that Gene was somehow sent to me, and I to him. We were supposed to grow old together. He knew what we all would need. He had been thinking, studying, writing about aging ever since his youth. We were supposed to develop our potential together. We were supposed to show people their strength and power of creativity. We were supposed to harvest everything that he had seeded. We were supposed to rock on our porch swing together beneath the wisteria. We were supposed to have a cabin at Point Lookout and be the coolest old people ever, with grandchildren coming across the way to visit us from their seaside home. We were supposed to play cribbage into our old age. He was supposed to show us where the most creative retirement communities were cropping up all over the world so that we could make art and have our friends with us, navigate the best features of the home part of a nursing home, play more games, and finally have reverie time where he and cribbage would be my partners, and inside I would return to the adolescent beginnings of my boy-girl love, right up to the bitter end. We could count on one another, and so could everyone we loved. In the same ways that he had set up the right people for all of our friends and their parents, he would do it for us, and we would walk together.

14

Eating Fried Eggs

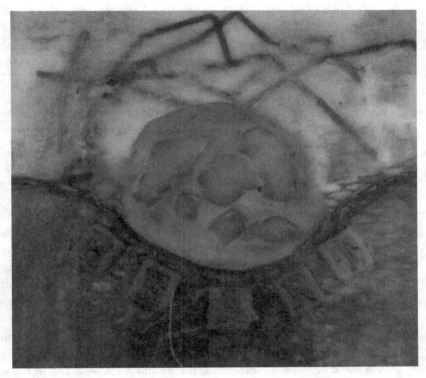

Figure 14.1 "Heart Fried Eggs" (2001), encaustic wax collage painting, 5 × 5 inches. Artwork by Wendy L. Miller, photo credit: Joshua Soros.

"Play cribbage," the dream said. To love, play cribbage. And so we did. We strategized, we counted on one another, we listened to what everyone told us, but we created our own tactics as we came to develop together, closer to each other.

How does a widow see her future? What does she see in the present? What language is she asked to adopt as she moves into this unwanted identity, using words like "late husband," and "widow"—words that basically say *dead dead*

dead over and over again. The obituaries, tributes, and news articles arrive on my desk: "Dr. Gene D. Cohen, considered a founding father of Geriatric Psychiatry . . . one of the founders of the field of Creativity and Aging . . ."[1] Awash in their news and our new reality—Gene's and mine—I sit stunned into my own silence.

Alex, Eliana, and I go to Chicago to receive his Hall of Fame Award from the American Society on Aging.[2] It has been a mere four months after his passing, just weeks in the grand scheme of things. It's not even that it feels like yesterday; at times it doesn't feel real at all. A widow friend of mine remembers well what she called this—her disbelief period. It is surreal, unnatural: I am here and he is not. The planning for this event had begun before Gene died—they had shared the news with him—but neither he nor the planners could have known that the sudden turn would come so swiftly, and that, unlike most of the Society's Hall of Fame inductions, Gene's would be posthumous.

Here we all are, then, gathered to celebrate him and his contribution, he who has died just five weeks after turning sixty-five, having devoted his entire career since his mid-twenties to the understanding and creative potential of people sixty-five and older. And he never got to be one. He wasn't old enough. He had accomplished so much and yet had anticipated so much more for the "second half" of his life and career. And then he was gone. The loss, for us who loved him as Gene the husband and life partner, Gene the father, Gene the family man, is barely even fathomed in full. The crowd here is not lacking in compassion—to the contrary, they are caring beyond words—yet they also bring a different love, respect, and mourning to the moment, a different platform for loss. So many of them are impassioned, as Gene was, to advance this field of science and medicine, of public policy and healthcare in their own ways. They are here to celebrate the man and his pioneering contribution—and to get on with the work to be done. I love this about them. Gene loved this about them. And: I cannot step into that space with them. They have work to do and their future is bright with the promise of gain: advancing research, integrating theory and practice, changing the world. Mine is different just now: loss. To look to the future is to assign my life with Gene to the past—*the past*—and it isn't. The same is true for Alex and Eliana. Gene's passing is not past for us. Grief calls in its own way and at its own pace for each of us.

I want to be able to pore through Gene's journals and find his entries for the part about *this*—the part about *after*, an after without him, but of course I'm on my own. I want to stand at the kitchen counter making our cups of tea, and chat with him a room away, where he lies resting on the couch in the living room, and tell him the "after" story about the time warp that grieving brings; about the wounded family body, how his absence and our loss washes through each of us and all of us as a family. I want to tell him about the weird medical thing that's come up for me. I want to say, "Gene, wait until you hear this . . ."

I want to argue with him, or argue with somebody; argue with Death. There are so many ways in which I do not get this. *Gene, I do not get why you didn't have the opportunity to write your brilliant science fiction novel that you have been incubating in your mind forever. I do not get why I would carry this book that is our life forward, without you. I do not get why you didn't have the opportunity to watch your beautiful daughter blossom from everything that we collectively gave her. I do not get how or why a love as precious as you have with your son and daughter-in-law would not have the chance to share in this deep development of character and midlife to late-life adulthood. I do not get why these four precious grandchildren will remember you in story and picture alone.*

In grief, creativity is our call to prayer. Creativity and spirituality come together as one. My mind, which can hardly focus on the mundane tasks of sorting through my mail to handle my bills in the moment, is suddenly drawn to a moment almost two months ago when I shared with Gene an unusual dream I'd had the night before. The dream and the moment of my telling it to Gene come back with vivid clarity.

I am telling him:

> I'm on a ship, a really huge ship, and we're also walking over a bridge. It's like a cruise liner and there is a trial going on. I am one of the people who is supposed to testify. The defense or prosecutors are asking for people to give sections of a story. Anyway, they look to me, and I look at my notes and I realize that the person who has already spoken, spoke about the person that I have notes on; and then there is someone else on the team of lawyers, but I can't find those notes, so I pass. I don't know if it's a lawyer exactly, because it seems like Reb David is there too. There are many of us and we are each telling parts of a story. We are on this cruise and the ship is really swaying. There are big waves in the distance, and they are coming toward us. I am really nervous and I say to you, "I know we are going down. And you say to me, "No, it's just a big wind." I say, "But look at it, Gene. We are huddling in the corner." It feels like we are underneath and we are looking out at it and you repeat, "No, it is just a big wind."

I wake up abruptly. Did we go down or did we not? I can't know, but I am mostly struck by the fact that again it is him reassuring me, or us.

And now, in his absence, I remember his part of the conversation that day. Gene had described a daydream of his own, explaining how an image in the daydream had helped him "sum up" as he put it, "what has been happening with the course of my illness." He later wrote of the unusual and illuminating daydream:

> *I have been taking one step forward and then one step backward, and it made me think of the Latin phrase Statue quo Vadis, "Where are you going? Nowhere."*[3] *So if you keep going one step forward and one step backward, you are going nowhere, and I thought, it's a limbo I can literally live with. I go nowhere, but if I go nowhere from where I am now, I'm living with it OK. It's not the greatest, but sitting down, I'm fine.*

To his bargaining, I repeated back, "Just a big wind."

"Yes, my love, it's just a big wind," Gene said. "It makes it hard for me when I'm on my feet but not while I'm sitting."

"Just a big wind" means we are existentially adrift. That is how I see it now: the Gene and Wendy soul as one that is existentially adrift—floating above anything I can recognize. We have no guide; we are on our own. In grief, creativity is not only our call to prayer. Creativity and spirituality together help us integrate experience that otherwise, in its blizzard state of grief trauma, would take everything with it, leaving us to move disoriented among the debris from the strong speed and heavy weight of the wind. Instead of chaos, the creative faculty brings congruence to events of the mind, body, and spirit.

For example, the day after Gene's memorial service, we were at lunch with my sisters and my niece, and I had a searing pain in my ear. My sister suggested that we go to Urgent Care, and before she had finished suggesting it, I was putting my coat on to go. Imagine wanting to go now to a doctor's office. When they suggested that the pain could be shingles, I tried to dismiss them. But the very next day, I followed up on their referral to a specialist, and it was in fact shingles. It was so excruciating that I could hardly think, really couldn't feel anything except the throbbing pain in my left ear and along the trigeminal nerve on the left side of my face. It was so bizarre to think that this physical nerve pain could outweigh the enormous emotional and spiritual pain I had from losing Gene. And yet it also made some strange metaphoric sense. As he had lain so completely spent on the couch nest those nights that would turn out to be his last, I had laid down by him, my left side leaning into him. I was trying to hear and understand what he needed so I could tend to him.

Now, in retrospect, half in prayer, half in conversation with him, I found myself sharing with him my hypothesis, as if we were still partners, creative detectives solving this deathbed mystery. The virus had either shut down all my immune responses, or my immune responses were already shut down and shingles virus had escaped. "*My face was up against your face, my heart up against your heart, my life force up against your life force, together we walked this terrible path of cancer/*

chemo/release of cancer cells— we fought not only for your life, but for the life of our family body which is now so run down."

As I thought about how immune systems weaken, I thought about those natural killer cells, those white blood cells that battle viruses and help prevent cancer. *Killer cells*—what a strange name for them, in a way. Cancer cells were killing everything in Gene, but in both of us, our natural killer cells were weakening. Different bodies, different ways, different times, our killer cells were wearing down.

I continued, *"How weird is this? This pain in my ear, this hurtful itching, is like a strange kind of whisper, an unearthly kind of whisper, a ghost of pain, a ghost of memory. With my ear against your heart, my desire to know what you needed is now my desire to know what I need."*

Metaphysical as it all sounds, the physical whispering is a huge pain and a distraction from functioning in this life. And I wondered how he was able to keep functioning in this life, through it all, as I was finding it so hard and my pain was so much less than his was. My system needed to just stop. The sound in my ear was really a deep resounding, like a hum from very far away, a constant hum. It was not really the sound of death, but it certainly felt like it could be. Was it coincidence that those two events—his death and the sound in my itching painful ear—happened at the same time? Was it stress related that an auditory nerve could get damaged, that a virus could wound the nerves, that as shingles healed, the ear sound diluted from pain to infection to throb to infection to itch to annoyance to a resounding remembering itching hum. This constant, maddening sensory assault accompanied my shell of a self I called "the grieving me."

You build a life. It takes years of sweat and labor—school, training, construction, psychic and physical development—and then you have to put in an equal amount, if not more work, to take it apart. And you have to do it while your friends are still building or downsizing or enjoying or retiring.

I am now a displaced person: not of the blue people, out of my identity, out of my skin. My days are spent moving books, moving papers, moving moving moving everything because everything has moved. He is not here, yet he is everywhere, and I have to find places to put his life so that we can have our life. Today I called my bereavement counselor Suzanna to ask if he was really dead—maybe he is just asleep from all of the morphine, maybe he didn't really die, maybe we made him seem like he died, maybe he will need these things, I will need these things, maybe. . ... She didn't write me off as crazy. She slowly and carefully walked me through the activated pain and the visceral cellular longing and caring for him. She understood that moving his things moved him, moved me, moved everything inside and I was there again at the moment of his moving and no, morphine is not what took him from me.

I hate everything about this process.

I wake up and move through the kitchen as if I am Gene. My presence alone in our home is now not just me, but the two of us. I have moved through my day, my home, with him here for as long as I have been here, so whatever I am doing, there has always been whatever he is doing, as well. Now, his absence is a presence.

I make my fried eggs in his small blue Le Creuset frying pan. It doesn't stick for me because I don't use the spray that he used—I use butter. Now why didn't I tell him to use butter when he was off his non-fat diet?

It was a simple thing—Gene beginning to eat fried eggs. He needed the protein; he needed to eat something through the chemotherapy that he could actually swallow. At first, it was such a treat. He needed the independence of his own cooking.

I can see Gene sitting at the table. He has slowly gone back and forth between the kitchen table and the stove. He carries one thing at a time. He is preparing his breakfast—he is making fried eggs, lonely fried eggs alone on his plate. No toast. No jam. No coffee. I am running around at a different pace, getting Eliana's breakfast, lunch, taking her to carpool to get to school on time. When I return and sit across him with my coffee, it is almost 8:10 in the morning. I know he has to leave at 9 for a meeting.

"Don't you have an appointment this morning?"

"Yes," he answers, "I am rushing." Silence. No movement.

It took me a very long time to understand what was going on for him. For such a long time, I have heard, "I am rushing" in my mind. He was rushing by trying to move at some recognizable speed that we do when we don't have to pay attention to our health. He was rushing, in his head, but his body was not moving. I was all motion. I really was rushing.

Now, I am rushing at the internal speed that he had. Illness takes time away from you that life fills with its time that moves in a cycle of speed that takes up time. We are all rushing somewhere.

Making fried eggs is a simple thing. I cook all the time. I used to feel the presence of my mother with me in the kitchen, mostly as I cooked, but now, it's the presence of my husband. My husband who hated cooking, really. A funny presence because he mostly enjoyed cooking for himself—his favorite things or at the time of his hunger or for his needs. In our domestic life, this bothered me; but in our living with chemotherapy life, it was a pleasure to watch, and an assurance of his capabilities and his capacities.

We watched it change. We watched him have no hunger or have hunger but not like the taste. We watched him feel well enough to cook but not well enough to get it to the table; well enough to eat but not well enough to move after he ate. We watched him care about the eggs; we watched him not care about the eggs. We watched the eggs, the eggs, the eggs.

Eliana and I eat fried eggs every morning now.

15

The Phoenix and the Fairy

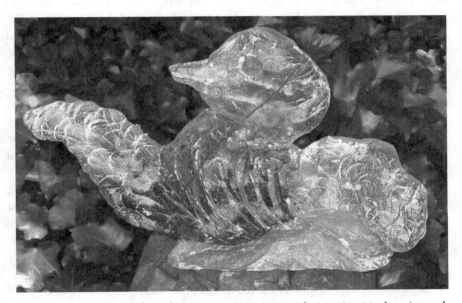

Figure 15.1 "Phoene" (2007), cast glass phoenix on rock, 9 × 12 × 4 inches. Artwork and photograph by Wendy L. Miller.

Earlier in this book I referred to this fairy tale as it came up in our conversations and eventually as Gene wrote it; now here we are at the end of our story and our tale is no longer mythical. Our fairy tale has become the narrative of our lives. How we tell our narratives, how we tell our own stories to ourselves is ultimately all we have, and in our tending to our stories, our stories bring us healing.

Self-narratives? Could that in fact be what most fairy tales are? Are they self-narratives told through the use of metaphor, creative imagery, symbol, and story? Gene and I shared a fascination with fairy tales, looking at them from the perspectives of family—women, children, changing events of transition, and aging. Why do so many tales start with the death of a parent, and usually the mother? Why do so many fairy tales face off good against evil, birth parent against stepparent, old against young, wise against ignorant, rich against poor? There are so many themes that replay throughout time, enriched by existential questions of value, timing, desire, and wisdom.

The original purpose of writing the phoenix and the fairy was not to write a book—that goal grew out of the importance of the imagery as it began to speak back to its author, Gene, the phoenix. The symbol began to grow through the years in meaning and significance, not just for Gene, but also for me. Originally, Gene started writing a fairy tale to Eliana, his young beloved toddler of a daughter, because he feared that he wasn't going to live long enough for her to remember him. He became frightened at the thought of what could happen to him, and therefore what could happen to everyone he loved, but particularly because she was so young, he feared what she would have, or not have, to hold onto as love, guidance, and dad.

We read her so many stories and fairy tales. She loved stories as all children do, and the characters and images began to come alive and be part of our family life. "One Hundred and One Dalmatians"[1] became the action dogs she loved, the party theme for her birthday, the cake, the dress code, the animal print pants and shirts that went through elementary school with her.

One night, she called out to her dad, frightened by a dream or by something in her room. He sat down on the edge of her bed to comfort her, and she cried into his chest, "Daddy, I don't want Cruella De Vil in my house. I don't like her." He held her in his arms, gently wiping away at her soft tears, trying to soothe her back into sleep. She couldn't really say what had upset her, but it didn't matter. She needed comfort and he was there to give it to her. As he began to feel that she was resting back to sleep, he quietly started to leave the room.

"Not even in a book, daddy. I don't even want her in my house in a book," her voice tiredly awakened.

Gene promised her he would take the storybook off her bookshelf, and he did. As he left the room, his heart so deeply touched by her fragile innocence, he realized how many cruel things he wanted to remove from ever frightening her. He wanted to remove everything from her house that could ever harm her. He didn't even want them in her heart. And yet he knew already that he would never be able to protect her from life itself. He wanted to remove anything and everything that could ever bring harm to his little love. He wanted her safe. He wanted her protected. He wanted her sturdy. Yet she was just a young child, naïve and innocent, all ears awaiting the knowledge of her life to become her guide.

Slowly, over time, merging her needs with his needs, he began to write the tale "The Phoenix and The Fairy." He wanted to capture something about his own life journey in which he faced challenges and setbacks, dreams of heroes and ogres, which ultimately illuminated his own fears, his own creativity, and strengths.

Gene always searched through literary authors and mentors to inspire his inner voice. W.B. Yeats' words awakened his desire for a quill pen as he read: "Come fairies, take me out of this dull world, for I would ride with you upon the wind and dance upon the mountains like a flame."[2] And the mythic voice began to speak with him. The phoenix made sense to him, it gave him a way to frame the challenges he faced, and it provided a magical way for him to describe it to his daughter. In Chapter 5, he wrote:

> *In ancient Greek mythology, the Phoenix is a mythical bird that, across intervals of times, periodically bursts into flames, falls from the sky to the earth, burning into ashes, only to emerge from the ashes renewed to soar again into flight, but destined to repeat the cycle of burning and renewal over and over again . . . (for me) en route to burning into ashes, only to seemingly miraculously be renewed to spread and lift my wings again in life.*

What other choice we do have when we are faced with challenge and adversity? We need to make sense of how to be there for our loved ones. We make our mark. We record. We imagine. We use the only medicine we have: we mix our creativity into the cauldron of our adversity. We do this naturally for ourselves. Our psyche finds ways to give us the metaphors and images that we need to both sustain us and guide us.

Gene's tale told the history of Phoene, a mortal odd bird who descended from the ancient phoenix, living, loving, and working in Washington, DC, with his son. One day, Phoene meets an enchanting and magical fairy, Faendy, and falls in love with her. The tale then progresses through all of Gene's autobiographical flights of the phoenix, his clever use of puns transposed into bird language. He imagined that he could spin for his daughter the harsh tale of facing difficulty, by filling it with her love of rainbows, magical twists of good fortune, parallel in some ways to his own night dreams yet not as threatening images, more as the clever "find your way through" images. His characters were professorial owls as doctors (the ornipod) and educators (Professor Otis), bird diseases (Baxter's disease), his son renamed as Ali, as well as the journey to the Arabian Desert to find our daughter, Ailie, a fairybirdbaby at the edge of a rainbow, weaving in the magical beginnings of her adoption story. He renamed his own book on creativity and aging *"The Aging Bird Brain—A Creative One,"* describing Fernando Nottebohm's discovery of neurogenesis in songbirds.[3] His characters faced the same sequence of challenges that cancer had brought to our family life. And in many ways, as his writing developed from his purpose of writing to his daughter into his desire to write to his whole family, his tale became its own form of a love story. He wrote:

> *So, you see, the bonds between Phoene and Faendy continued to grow. They were both fascinated with one another. For Faendy, Phoene had a fanciful side to him, but he also had his feet on the ground when he wasn't flying.*

All of this made him very interesting to her. For Phoene, Faendy was exotic and he warmed all over from the attraction he sensed Faendy felt toward him.

By this time, Gene was well past the five-year mark, and rapidly moving toward a healthy decade. He didn't always know he was going to make it as long as he did. Eliana, growing as well, replaced her love of animals with a love of fairies. My contribution was that once I understood my role as a fairy in this tale, I certainly needed the fairy's voice to make sense to me. And so I began to write my voice into his tale, describing the task and the purpose of fairies. Intuition, wisdom, watching, holding experience, fairies as travelers who can read what is happening:

You see that is why they flutter so or what you call twinkle about. It is light-ing up the movement to a different layer of the world experience. Fairies light up what needs to be seen, but their light is very gentle for they don't want to burn anyone's eyes. I know because I am a fairy.

I went on to distinguish fairies from other magical creatures, angels or bor-rowers or shape shifters, to give the fairy voice the symbolic essence of inner intuition:

Because not everyone knows who their fairy is or where or how a bird whose ancestor was the phoenix rises and falls, only to rise again. . . . Fairies are internal guides, enlightening our moral compasses. We are not the compasses themselves, but we brighten them so that they can be read and used. The compasses are always there, but so often life events and outer worldliness darken, surround, and encase them so no one is able to read the direction of the needle, and see where it is pointing. That is why everyone is always going in a million different directions; whether the direction is right or wrong isn't the issue—the issue is all that spinning. Spinning gets in fairies' air space. It gets in our way. It blurs the paths of light.

As time went on, the tale began to live through the reality of the challenges, not just in a theoretical or imagined frame. What began with the purpose of making sense to a young child who might not have the luxury of having her father throughout her life, now was becoming an act of writing to make sense to himself. Isn't this what our narratives do for each of us? In the tale, Phoene calls out:

How could this happen? He had already escaped illness. He had built a new life. It was a sickening feeling for him—not so much because he was

afraid of death—we all know that happens to everyone, no escape there—
but from the anguishing fear of not being around to be with Faendy and to
help raise their little fairybirdbaby Ailie and see the grandchildren that Ali
would one day have. Waves of darkness engulfed Phoene. Ali flew home to
be with him and to be with Faendy and his baby sister Ailie. Ali convinced
his girlbird to fly back with him too. Then he put his huge wings around
Phoene and Faendy who, of course, was holding Ailie. He hugged them
tightly, and when Ailie saw the tears in all their eyes, tears came to her eyes
as well, and a soft rainbow arced over all of them, bringing Ailie into the
light as she too became family.

The fairy tale never really had a conclusion. It ended with the time period
of his flight into and with chemotherapy. It ended with his sense of this is
where we are. The narrative of uncertainty, the narrative of continuing with the
latest hurdle

where the rainbow light appears faint on the outside, the fear and hope shift-
ing in and out of one another, yet the vision is strong as it echoes all that they
know and believe—for they know the light is there, always, forever, in sickness
and in health. Phoene and Faendy, as always, support one another through
their love and care. The family surrounds them with their love and light. The
friends sing to them and bring food to their nest. Everyone sings their special
prayers. And Phoene continues to fly, though not so high right now.

It ended without ending, the story of being present with what is:

"and she placed the world gently in the palm of my hand."[4] *(Story peo-*
ple: Selected stories & drawings of Brian Andreas)

A year later, I decided to write the fairy tale ending. At the time, I felt like it was
the right ending. It began:

With Phoene rising out of our earth sphere, riding upon the wind, like a
flame, Yeats tells us, the color of time and space changes. The light changes.
The identification of light changes. The light of identity changes. Everything
rearranges so quickly that time is unrecognizable.

Neither Phoene nor Faendy knew that grieving would turn Faendy into
ashes. She awakens with no supernatural or magical powers. She points
her wand, but no new paths appear; she spills out her dust, but there is no
sparkle or shine. She can't be the fairy OR the phoenix. She can't be the
fairy AND the phoenix. She can't be. . . .

My whole being was filled with the depth of my grief, still four years after his death. The ending of the tale was the ending of my identity, and that seemed true. I finished the tale:

> *But Faendy is not a fairy anymore. She was his fairy. Love brings out the fairy in each of us; our magic wands appear and do whatever it is that needs to be done. Love/protect/provide/shine/mirror/perceive/perform/partake. Remind/remise/remit/remittance. Because not everyone knows who their fairy is or where or how a bird whose ancestor was the phoenix rises and falls, only to rise again, then we might ask: Do we all have a fairy? Do you have a fairy? Do I have a fairy? Is there even a difference between the phoenix and the fairy? Is it possible we are both?*

More and more, I have come to understand that the purpose of this fairy tale is not to share more autobiographical information. Rather, its purpose is to observe and serve as a guiding light, not only for her, or for him, but for each of us. The task of looking at our own creativity and imagination, our own images, metaphors, and symbols—the works of our creative faculty: that is our story. That is what gives meaning to our life, to our aging, to our illnesses, and to our potential. It is this power of our creative faculty that we have for our own healing, and it is in service to us always. It is in fact what ultimately saves us. And has saved me.

Recently I read the entire fairy tale in its original form to our daughter. I wanted to find out if she remembered any parts that Gene had read to her. I wanted to know what she thought it was about. In his moments of feeling he would be disappeared from his daughter's life, he had sat down to write her a fairy tale motivated by love and fear of the deepest kind. He had desired to be there for her when he wasn't there otherwise, and here we were. Now twenty years old, she, like Alex and me, has come through her own tunnel of darkness, learning to live into her life with the loss of her father. I had my own expectations as to what she would think or feel. Of course, I was wrong. Because our narratives are not only our own stories, they are the stories of our relationships within our self and between one another. Her response becomes her narrative of what he told, regardless of the meaning he intended. He intended it to speak to her, and therefore that intention is true. He intended it to speak to us, our readers, and here we are.

Eliana told me:

> Dad wrote about our life. He was saying that even if you have a short amount of time, you should make it worthwhile, like spend as much time as you can with family, do what you want to do, and don't stress over dumb stuff. Even if you have too short a time to actually live, you shouldn't be stuck in that moment with worries. You should celebrate life with family that makes you happy. That is who he is. That is what

I imagine he would say: Accept what happened and don't let it hold you down or stop you from what you want to do.

It has been of great interest to me to hear her perspective. I had thought the tale was about hope and challenge, but for her it was about learning to accept what is in life. Acceptance. Of course, that is exactly what we have had to do, and what we all have to do, all the time: learn to accept our situation whatever we may be facing, and discover the story that is speaking to us within it.

I already have four grandchildren, three great nieces, and one great nephew to read the fairy tale to. Whatever version it grows into, "The Phoenix and the Fairy" will continue to fly through time and space, toward blue sky above clouds.

Part Six

EPILOGUE

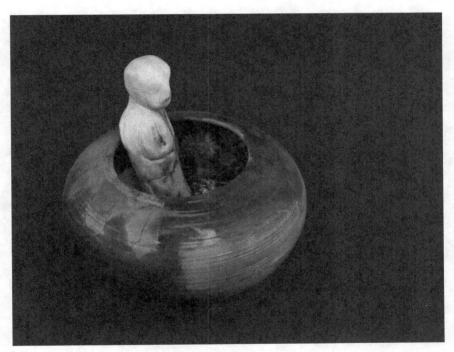

Figure VI.i "Centering in Reflection" (1999), porcelain clay figure with oxides in raku fired bowl, 8 × 7 × 8 inches. Artwork by Wendy L. Miller, photo credit: Joshua Soros.

Epilogue

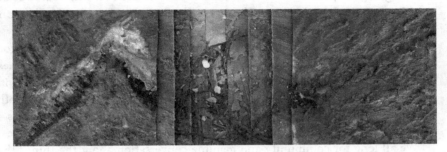

Figure VI.ii "Gray Blue Water, Wide as the Arm of the Sea" (from Rimbaud, *Illuminations XIV: Les Ponts*) (1999), mixed media of clay, paint, plaster, sand on Arches paper with egg shells, twigs, and rocks, 15 × 31 inches. Artwork by Wendy L. Miller, photo credit: Claire Blatt.

For years now, first as a quiet intuitive voice and over time as a louder, more force-ful voice, I have heard myself say: "If you don't edit and publish this book, it will be as if Gene has died twice," and I refused to let that happen. Throughout these years, there have been many other aspects of his work that have been divided up—his research, his center, his webinars, his games, his writings, his contribu-tions to the creativity and aging field—but this piece, this book, was always left to me. My commitment to our writing as Gene's legacy and his ethical commitment to both family and community was my thread from above that pulled me up out of the depths of grief and loss. It was my connection to the sky above.

In truth, it has been very difficult for me to write this book. Yet I knew that there are readers who are isolated, as Gene and I were, in their own experience, particularly the aging process, and particularly when there are medical complica-tions. So much of the isolation or struggle emerges in the course of everydayness, but the roots of it—and potential relief—lie much deeper in matters of existential identity. It can be uncomfortable for any of us to confront, much less engage in these conversations with ourselves or others, even with those we love. Whatever the reason, it is also true that there are many forms of "magical thoughts" inside all of us that say, if we don't know much about illness then it won't happen to us; that when we actually live through these "hard times," people mostly try to say the platitudes of polite positive hopeful thinking, or give advice, or change the subject, or give us that look that we can't name but somehow ends up adding to our invisibility. We can begin to feel like we have leprosy or some such thing that requires quarantine; we can feel psychically hidden and alone.

It can also be that at times we are the ones avoiding these conversations with those around us who might be in need. The stamina and willingness to be in existential conversation is often quite short. So why would I take it on in this book? Because I have been an existential seeker since I was a teen. I am attracted to meaning and purpose in all of its manifestations. It has been the source of my creativity, so, hard as it has been, I knew I had to develop my own will and writing stamina.

In so many ways, Gene and I are very ordinary; in other ways, we are far from ordinary. Maybe this is a false perception, but I think we have had both illness and health come at us from all directions. I know lots of people who work with illness, others who study it, some who live through it with their families, and others who live through it themselves. Gene and I were in all of these categories— individually, separately and together, personally, familially, and professionally.

We all long for community and genuine conversation about the things that matter most, which grow in complexity and nuance with age and especially with illness. It can be tempting, as I've said, to want to avoid all that. My hope is that this book somehow transcends that impulse we all have to avoid complexity. Whether or not we want to live through aging and illness, whether it is occurring now or later, whether it involves us or our friends, this is what is, and it happens in so many ways, at so many times, and in so many places. It doesn't really behoove us to have our heads in the sand. Whether we have named it creativity in living, or hope, or health, or illness time, or aging, the truth is that most of us are very unprepared for complex experience. We tend to keep ourselves close to the hut, separate or join ourselves, distract or immerse ourselves, or categorize into a singular perspective—be it a spiritual outlook or a medical or psychological or social or how-to or coaching voice. I hope that our combined voices in this book, together and individually, have offered each of you a voice of integration, as that voice is ultimately the voice that awakens our cells beyond their limitations, calls forth our creative faculties and our human potential, and accompanies us as an unexpected resource in unexpected places—at every age and through all life's passages.

A Note on the Future of the Arts in Healthcare

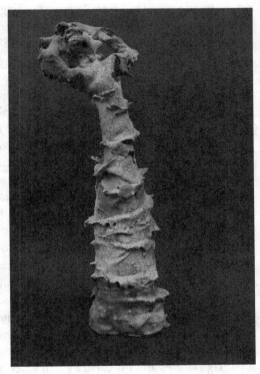

Figure VI.iii "A Soft Stance" (1986), paper-dipped porcelain and sagger fired figure, 4 × 18 × 5 inches. Artwork by Wendy L Miller, photo credit: Joshua Soros.

The field of the arts in healthcare has at this time evolved to a place where the combined skills Gene and I shared were exactly what were necessary. Gene heightened the field—gave it the authority it needed—because he knew the strength of evidence-based research, not just in science, but in creativity and within the many developmental psychological phases and processes that accompany it. He also knew how to make research accessible to the artistic types who believed they were non-research types, and he was able and willing to work with others to create educational toolkits for that process.[1]

We also both understood how creativity is related to intelligence, human potential, and all the aspects of the arts and psychotherapy to which I have committed my life. In fact, it was Gene who helped me understand that I had been collecting research my whole life: all my client stories, my images from art therapy, my images from my own studio. And here we stand today, professionally, with our fields still growing and forming themselves, yet fields that will have to return through the eye of the star with their evidence-based knowledge and understanding of science, back to a true arts-based focus at some point. Our fields will have to return to a deep and existential understanding of the power and healing potential of imagery and creativity. Gene knew that I understood this. He helped me learn why it was that I had felt so invisible, so outside of the trajectory of our field. For it is through the evidence-based language that we will arrive there, maybe in my time, maybe not, because we have been fighting to be heard from that perspective since its very inception. Creativity? Medicine? Whose language shall we use? Whose power structure, filled with degrees, certifications, resumes, exhibits, awards, and titles, will have the right to define what we know? How long will it take before we return to the wisdom, once known, that our imagination truly is our greatest medicine[2] and that creativity and medicine truly are one and the same?

Gene provided the necessary bridge of translation; he was able to cross-fertilize among the fields of medicine, psychiatry, creativity, and the full spectrum of the humanities. He lovingly promised me, before he left this planet, that my imagery alongside our voices together would bring forth this "arrival" of something new, this true creativity, in the same way that his toolkits had strengthened the voices of the artists, teachers, administrators, facilitators, and co-researchers who were part of his ground-breaking creativity and aging study.[3]

Gene's original vision for this book was going to incorporate stories from my practice. That is partially the book I have written now, but I had to do that work without him. I kept asking, how will I find a voice to convey what we understood together—the overlay of his developmental and my integrative intelligences, with my image stories and his capacity and voice of authority? Could my own work come out of its shell now, having felt before so out of sync with where my own art and expressive therapy professional worlds were headed? These worlds appeared to all be going more and more toward the research and clinical level of description, and farther and farther away from the visual, kinesthetic, imagistic, poetic, auditory knowledge. He and I both knew that I had a collection of picture narratives that could tell the essential visual complexity of the story of intuition, art, and healing.

The ten-year period of his life between writing his books, *The Creative Age* and *The Mature Mind*, and his death in late 2009 was a time when the fields of healing arts, expressive arts therapy, and creative aging needed his contribution to evidence-based research, his policy skills, and his neuroscience of the brain. Yet, to go in this scientific direction, our fields turned themselves away from the "experience" of the image to the "mechanism" of the image, so that there could be validity, scientific understanding, and potential for integrative approaches to funding, research, and publishing. His was a major voice in this happening and taking off. In so many ways, my own fields of art therapy and expressive arts therapy have been trying since their inception to do exactly what he was able to do for the field—shift the paradigm.

But Gene knew that this shift was not the whole picture; understanding mechanisms of creativity were important, but they were not sufficient. To truly understand creative faculty, we need a deep understanding of integration—an overlay for Gene and me of our developmental and integrative intelligence models—combined with learning to follow and trust our own imagistic stories and our own capacities for intuitive authority. These are what develop our creative faculties. These are what will take us to the next level. I introduced these ideas at the beginning of this book in the Introduction, but here, as a note specifically to the profession, it bears repeating. We hoped that our book, *Sky Above Clouds*, would provide the voice that could help us move to this next paradigm shift in the complex understanding of creativity, aging, and health.

This was Gene's gift to me. At a lunch we shared at a local Dupont Circle restaurant in Washington, DC, after meeting with his book agent, he articulated that this book could become the book that was needed for our professions. But without him, my own heartsong pulsed weakly through its fragile "pauses between the notes." My belief, my understanding, my joy, my partnership, my love, my pulsing knowledge flickered. I had wanted to write this book together, my life partner by my side. I had wanted to walk out into the field beyond right and wrong, beyond left and right brains, beyond. Without Gene, I stood seemingly alone; but I was not alone. Through his writings, which have been included at length in the book and in the Appendix, Gene's voice is here, and in it his wisdom and encouragement not only to me but to our field. Writing and finishing this book has been a profound gift. I just didn't know that I would have to do it without him.

Here are a few things that we need to know: we know that to move a paradigm, we need to distill ideas by playing with them in new ways, so that new edges of a field show themselves. We know that edge ideas are part of edge thinking and these ideas seem to magnetize one another so that people on the edges of their own expertise begin to find one another, and a new field creates itself. Edge thinking is made up of commonality, collaboration, complexity, creativity, and consilience. The reason these ideas or people are on the edges of their own fields is that they are willing to try out new concepts, in new ways, and they are influenced by concepts and ideas from such core commonalities.

Leading-edge thinkers understand that what has been and what has yet to be is the exact territory we need to inhabit. We need to bring forth our challenges, our opportunities, and our next steps so that we can both navigate and claim the new edges of our thinking. This is what potential means; and this is what *Sky Above Clouds* refers to in terms of creativity.

It has been the scientific, evidence-based research that has given our professions the tools to begin to actually show what was taking place, the toolkit not just for how to do the research but how to use the research. The mind–body field in its alternative health movement taught us that psychoneuroimmunology was the hybrid of study and that neuroscience was the wave of the future, teaching us; but both immunology and neurology were seemingly a huge leap of inquiry for artistic clinicians. Having the expressive arts therapy field and the creativity and aging movement begin to speak our own language, it became clearer and clearer to everyone why these results needed to be known and studied: it allowed the field to gain the reputation and equality status it deserved. It allowed the artists and creative researchers to come forth and be respected for their skills and talents, not just the statisticians, yet also the statisticians. In creativity and aging, we are moving forward, making the necessary connections in renegotiating our languages, finding our commonalities at these very edges of our fields, and we are allowing our sensory vocabularies to be both expressed and heard so that the new way truly will be led by our creative faculties.

But could it really be true that there has been so little research on "wisdom" as a cumulative product of age, experience, and creativity? We are living in an age of information, so information is exactly what people have wanted and needed. More and more information, and yet, much like the literature on technology, we are losing something as we are gaining something from this overload and over-access to information. We are losing the intuitive, gut-knowing knowledge of our hands-on insights, our capacity to be slowed down and connected internally to the type of knowing that we will definitely need as we age into ourselves. The kind of knowing that we can rest into as our seasoned, developmental, integrative wisdom is called forth to take care of our families, our professions, and everything we have generatively created throughout our lives. We will need to learn to conserve and preserve, and without knowing how to intuitively reserve energy and internal awareness, this will be a harder and harder task. We will need to do more and more of our own work, and bring the creative intuitive voice to the forefront of our fields.

Personal Acknowledgments

Having read many book acknowledgments, I now understand why authors are so grateful to their people. Like most of life, it takes a village to accomplish everything, and that is certainly true of this book, which has been in formation throughout a full decade. *Sky Above Clouds* has been shaped by a number of people, under a number of titles. I am extremely grateful to each of them: agents Gail Ross and Howard Yoon, and co-writer Teresa Barker, Gene's original "team" for *The Creative Age* and *The Mature Mind*; then, years later, narrative gerontologist Kate de Medeiros, for her remarkable retrieval; editor Bill Zeisel, who took on the task of working through an early version of the manuscript with his extraordinary organizational and word-whacking skills; and Karin Leuthy, who in the depths of all that material recognized a single few words of Gene's that would become the beautiful title for the book, then produced a clear project description that enabled me to present it to a publisher. Finally, for continued shaping of the book that eventually came to be, Teresa Barker with Kristen Rau, editor, at Readmore Communications, and Andrea Knobloch, whose vision of autobiography as parable was our guiding mantra throughout the rewriting and shaping of this book.

The written voices in this book are Gene's and mine. However, they could never have gotten to the page without the help of others who listened, collaborated, understood, and clarified our words and thoughts. Painful and uncertain as some of the raw material was, I am grateful that I was accompanied not only by Gene and Teresa but also by my own writing—my writer's voice—which allowed me to chronicle from inside experiences that might otherwise have been only a blur in retrospect.

I am grateful for the synchronicities that guided this project and drew the essential individuals to it as it progressed. First is Teresa's presence from the very beginning, through her work with Gene, then as Gene and I began our writing together, and finally four years after Gene's death, when our work with Oxford began. Her understanding of health, illness, aging, love, commitment, and all of the existential overlays to our lives infuses this narrative. Teresa taught me to trust my voice, to unpack my experiences even if I didn't know where the writing would lead me. She listened deeply to what was going on in me and, in so doing, taught me to hear my self. She has protected both our privacy and our honesty. I am so grateful to have had her beside me, to have worked with not only a fabulous collaborator but also a dear, lifelong friend.

Then there is Kate DeMedeiros, who came to me through a synchronicity in timing, trust, and writing. I am so deeply indebted to Kate. In that first year after Gene's death, I had neither heart nor mind for the project. Kate came along, with fresh eyes and ears, to help me edit a short piece of Gene's writing for a Special Section Tribute to him in the *Journal of Aging, Humanities and the Arts*. As a gerontologist, she worked with Thomas Cole to edit this tribute. Since Gene's last piece of published writing before his death was a chapter in Thomas Cole's book, *Guide to Humanistic Studies in Aging*, I knew I could trust Thomas. I was still so fragile physically and emotionally then from the loss that the best I could do was simply *find* our writing. After the essay for the tribute was finished, I asked Kate, "How did you do that?" meaning how did she make sense out of the writings that at that time were so elusive to me. I could hardly comprehend anything either Gene or I had ever thought, much less written down. My memory of her answer was, "I am very good at seeing the big picture." And she was. How grateful I am to her for taking everything out of its box or file or CD or whichever version that year had produced and reintegrating it into a working manuscript. She never added a single word of her own, but masterfully reorganized what Gene and I had in a way that I could find both my voice and our meaning again.

Sculpture is often discussed in terms of being made by those who work in an additive way or in a subtractive way. The same is true of editing. Words in three-dimensional space are the medium. Kate searched the quarry to find the pieces of stone that were gems. Bill carved away material to bring some essential aspects of the story forward. Karin, surrounded by all that material, spotted the singular few words that would name it, and in doing so gave it its place to stand. Teresa used all aspects of a sculptor, but her greatest gift was that of refining and polishing the stone. I am grateful for these fellow sculptor/editors.

The synchronicities and gratitude continued. As I searched for a publishing home for our book, I decided to do a series of readings in memory of Gene. One of those readings was requested by Gene's friend and colleague, Dr. Jim Blatt, at the George Washington University School of Medicine and Health Sciences, which led me to Dr. Christina M. Puchalski, the Director of the George Washington Institute for Spirituality and Health. I read to the medical students in her psychosocial seminar from the manuscript, and afterwards she very graciously and confidently introduced me to her publisher, Oxford University Press Senior Editor in Medicine, Andrea Seils Knobloch.

In addition to my editor, I am grateful to the Oxford University Press team: Rebecca Suzan for managing communications on the project, Emily Perry for managing production, Jerri Hurlbutt for copyediting, Newgen for their image work, and Michelle Kelly and the other members of the production, marketing, and distribution team who have created this wonderful edition of the book.

To my manuscript reviewers, Marc Agronin, Sanford Finkel, and Kristin Rau, your comments and insights have further helped us to provide our readers with clarity and meaning. A special thanks to Tarsilla Sampaio Moura, Library Services Specialist at the University of Maryland, who so painstakingly researched, fact-checked, and then helped me organize the extensive endnotes and our shared references/bibliography. We greatly appreciate her resources at the University of Maryland library, and extend thanks to my initial email helper in this pursuit, Abby Yochelson, Reference Specialist at the Library of Congress.

I am also indebted to those who contributed advance praise for the book, essentially shepherding the book and its message to a wide range of clinical, scholarly, and public policy leaders.

I am forever grateful to all of my clients, who so generously share their stories, images, and the intimacies of their lives. I am fortunate to be able to work with and develop the incredible relationships we have together. Thank you for all that you have taught me along the way.

I am filled with appreciation for my community of friends, some of whom were early readers: Lauren Leroy, Elizabeth Haase, Joan Krash, and Wende Heath. I had ongoing dialogues on so many topics and shared inquiries with Emily Randall, Rebecca Milliken, Carol Cox, Katherine Williams, Andrea Sherman, Marsha Weiner, Paula Terry, Berna Huebner, Michael Patterson, Abigail Wiebenson, Jaime Biderman, Andrea Hassiba, Joanne Rollins, Janet Crittenden, Jackie Brookman, Cara and Ed Barker, Steve Johnson, Marge Silverton, Jim Blatt, Laurie Blatt, Shira Saperstein, Maya Rovner, Mark Rovner, Sandy Finkel, Fern Finkel, Suzane Reatig, Nooni Reatig, Martha Adler, David Adler, Andy Penn, Cathy Surace, Shana Penn, Walter Reich, Gloria Capron, Ellen Pearl, Paula Rolleston, Laura Solomon, Lisa Wurtzbacher, Sue Klein, Larry Uman, Kari Uman, Sandy Katz, Kaltoum Maroufi, Judy Brody, and Johanna Wermers. Many thanks to my whole community of friends at Kehila, and in particular Rosanne Skirble, Linda Sussman, Gail Singer, Morris Ojalvo, Carla Dinowitz, Ron Milone, Judy Marx, Franca Posner, Rosana Azar, Ruth Guyer, Bonnie Friedman, and Susan Zempsky. I greatly appreciate the ongoing support for me and for Gene from the staff and board members of the National Center for Creative Aging, and for their encouragement as this book has evolved, particularly Gay Hanna, Susan Perlstein, and Greg Finch. Thanks go to Sally White and Patricia Dubroof at Iona Senior Services for so graciously organizing and creating my first book reading. Thank you to Claire Blatt for her photographs of my artwork and my portrait, and for guiding me with the help of her fiancé Daniel Felps whenever I was in a computer or image resizing panic.

Without my family, what would the point be? My sisters, Sara Miller Arnon and Julie Miller Soros, keep me laughing and remind me of the life support of love and family, through thick and thin. I am surrounded by my niece, nephews, and wonderful caring cousins, who have continued to check in on how the book is progressing. Special thanks go to my nephew, Joshua Soros, whose photographic talents made it possible to print my artwork; otherwise they never would have made it to the page. And of course to my mother, Gisele, and my father, Howard, whose memory and love accompany me in everything I do.

What better legacy of Gene's to be left with than his firm and solid belief in me as a writer, in his own manuscript, and in his children? My capacity to both survive and thrive is due to the deep presence, trust, and connection of our loving daughter Eliana, whose humor and insights keep me on my toes: thank you for your caring presence. To Gene's son Alex, daughter-in-law Kate, and our gorgeous grandchildren Ruby, Lucy, Ethan, and Bennett, I am so blessed to have you in my life. May this book provide each of you with a lifelong lens through which to keep growing in the ways you already know and will come to know Gene and who we were together.

And lastly, my gratitude for Gene's love and belief in me and in the importance of our voices together. You were like a sustainable fuel, the oil that lasted so many days beyond its capacity to create light; a fuel that allowed me to see even when you weren't here to see it with me. I know that if you were here, this book would look different; but I also know that in your final reading of it, you said, "I am going to love this book." I hope I have honored that love.

—Wendy Miller

Though Gene is not here to give his own acknowledgements, he never could have done his work without the support of the National Institute of Mental Health at the National Institutes of Health (and specifically Bert Brown, director at the time, who hired him as a 31-year-old physician), the National Institute of Aging at the National Institutes of Health, the Center for Mental Health Services of the U.S. Department of Health and Human Services, the Atlantic Philanthropies (USA) Inc., the Helen Bader Foundation, the National Endowment for the Arts (NEA), AARP, the Stella and Charles Guttman Foundation, the International Foundation for Music Research, the National Center for Creative Aging, and the Center for Aging, Health and Humanities at George Washington University, as well as his many private funders.

He was deeply appreciative of his many friends and colleagues who shared his vision for a changing aging landscape for us all. He had great appreciation for his many patients, research participants, assistants, statisticians, and colleagues, who not only significantly informed him but have continued to carry on his work in such significant ways, moving the field of creative aging to the forefront. In particular, at his Center on Aging, Health and Humanities, he would extend appreciation to Jean Johnson, Beverly Lundsford, Shari Sliwa, and those who completed the grant for the Washington DC Area Geriatric Education Center Consortium, which kept his center alive: Andrea Sherman, Elizabeth Cobbs, Kimberly

Acquaviva, and Gay Hanna. Deb Schmal stepped in many times in those early years after he died, to help find something needed from his old computers or research data files.

I struggled with how and where to put Gene's acknowledgement of his children and family in these notes. They meant the world to him. I finally realized that in fact, he says so himself throughout the whole book; the book itself is an acknowledgement of his love for them and the depth to which he felt their love for him.

—Wendy Miller

I would like to add my thanks to Wendy and to Gene for the opportunity to engage in work from the heart for so many years. Such serendipity: Gene's first book project, *The Creative Age*, landed in my hands in the final months of my mother's life, and he brought a warm presence to those days, even when under the heaviest deadline pressure. Our work on *The Mature Mind* was illuminating, and I can still hear the excitement in his voice the day he called to describe his newest creative adventure: to co-write a book with Wendy. The years that followed were rich in conversation, writing, and laughter with them both, as colleagues and friends, and it has been a special privilege to continue to work with Wendy and with Gene's material. Kristen Rau brought his editorial talents and time to this effort so generously. I am grateful, too, for the shared wisdom of close family and friends, and in a special way to my friend Kathy, whose insights informed this work and whose spirit moves forward with it. I remain grateful to my parents Maxine and George, for what they taught me about confronting health adversities and death. Finally, a special thanks to my husband Steve, my daughters Rachel and Rebecca, my son Aaron, daughter-in-law Lauren and dear granddaughter Leyna, and my beloved mother-in-law Dolly, for their unconditional love and support.

—Teresa Barker

Professional Acknowledgments

It feels important at the end of this book to have a place where I can also offer my professional acknowledgments to the many fellow thinkers whose work has been accompanying me for years. These people—some leading thinkers, some quiet writers—have so influenced me in my development. Some of you are people I have trained or studied with directly, others only in the solitary realm of reading, thinking, and writing. But all of you have unknowingly shared so much with me and have brought me to this juncture in time where my thoughts, feelings, and ideas could coalesce into this book

Early in my life it was my mother, Gisèle Baroukel Miller, who shared with me her love of art, philosophy, and French culture. Her support and understanding guided my love for learning as she and I discussed existential philosophers: Jean Paul Sartre, Simone de Beauvoir, Albert Camus, Soren Kierkegaard, Friedrich Nietzsche, and Martin Heidegger. Much later I moved on to Otto Rank, Martin Buber, Paul Tillich, Jacques Derrida, Michel Foucault, and Jacques Lacan, and most recently to the work of Emmy van Deurzen and that of Alfried Längle.

Yet my entry into psychology did not start with these sophisticated thinkers. What young college student wouldn't want to enter the field of psychology after reading works by Bruno Bettelheim, Clark Moustakas, Herbert Kohl, Virginia Axline, Theodore Rubin, Hannah Green, or Robert Coles?

How can I separate out the elements of the synergy that developed from years of inquiry into the worlds of existentialism, clinical psychology, art, feminism, art therapy, expressive arts therapy, psychoanalysis, health, healing, spirituality, narrative medicine, literature, creativity, aging, and mind–body medicine? A grand thank you in the world of art goes to to Lucy Lippard, Suzi Gablik, MC Richards, Paulus Berensohn (whose book *Finding One's Way with Clay* not only guided my clay work but found its way into titling this book), Stephen De Staebler, Seymour Locks, Karen Breschi, and Leonard Hunter and the many artists of the women's art movement.

The overlapping of feminism, philosophy, psychoanalysis, and health brought me to Luce Irigaray, Helen Cixous, Claire Lispector, Catherine Clement, Joyce

McDougal, Juliet Mitchell, Julia Kristeva, Susan Griffin, Mary Daly, Betty Friedan, Adrienne Rich, Tillie Olsen, Monique Wittig, Mary Catherine Bateson, Gina Berriault, Susan Sontag, Jean Rhys, and the Three Marias.

Evolving as a clinician in arts-based psychotherapy for thirty-five years, I am deeply appreciative of those whose work has guided my path, starting with Sigmund Freud, Carl Jung, RD Laing, DW Winnicott, Victor Frankl, Fritz Perls, Abraham Maslow, Erik Erikson, Irvin Yalom, Christopher Bollas, Thomas Ogden, Marion Woodman, James Hillman, Heinz Kohut, Claire Douglass, Virginia Satir, Elizabeth Kubler-Ross, Thomas Szasz, and Steve Shulman. In the field of psychosynthesis I am grateful to Roberto Assagioli, Piero Ferrucci, Carl Peters, Lenore Lefer, Phillip Brooks, Thomas and Anne Yeoman, Marco J. de Vries, and Molly Young Brown.

In my own fields of art therapy, expressive arts therapy, and play and sand-play therapy, without the following theoreticians, who would I be? My gratitude goes to Joan Erikson, Victor Lowenfeld, Janie Rhyne, Florence Cane, Hanna Kwiatkowska, Bernie Levy, Eleanor Ulman, Edith Kramer, Vija Lusebrink, Emmanuel Hammer, Judy Rubin, Arthur Robbins, Susan Bach, Gregg Furth, Rebecca Milliken, Tamar Hendel, Carol Cox, Barry Cohen, Mari Fleming, Elizabeth Lerner, Karen Baer, Claudia Rafael, Pat Allen, Don Jones, Rawley Silver, Katherine Williams, Peggy Heller, Cathy Moon, Bruce Moon, Cathy Malchiodi, Joseph Garai, Paolo Knill, Helen Barba (Haley Fox), Margo Fuchs, Mariagnese Cattaneo, Ellen Levine, Steven Levine, Shaun McNiff, Natalie Rogers, Jack Weller, Kate Donohue, Anin Utigaard, Laurie Goldrich, Gloria Simoneaux, Deborah Koff-Chapin, and Wende Heath, Mel Levine, Dora Kalff, Martin Kalff, Gisela de Domenico, Kay Bradway, Ruth Ammann, Gita Moreno, Estelle Weinrib, Barbara Boik, E. Anna Goodwin, Alexander Shaia, and Eliana Gill. And in creativity itself, my gratitude goes to Rollo May, Charles Johnston, Howard Gardner, Rudolf Arnheim, Suzanne Langer, Ira Progoff, Natalie Goldberg, Liz Lerman, and Twyla Tharp. I also studied guided imagery through the work of Ernest Lawrence Rossi, Carl Simonton, Annees Sheikh, Akhtar Ahsen, Michael Samuels, Mardi Horowitz, and Shakti Gawain.

The fields of psychoneuroimmunolgy and mind–body medicine came into my life as I was healing from chronic fatigue syndrome and went on to provide the language for healing with others. My thanks go to Hans Selye, Ken Pelletier, Steven Locke, Bernie Siegel, Dennis Jaffe, Arthur Klein, Herbert Benson, Larry Dossey, Arthur Frank, Carl Simonton, Rachel Naomi Remen, Michael Lerner, Jim Gordon, Larry LeShan, Norman Cousins, Jeanne Achterberg, Joan Borysenko, Candace Pert, Michael Ruff, Marc Barash, Kens Wilber, Angeles Arrien, Elizabeth Kubler-Ross, Rita Charon, Jean Shinoda Bolen, Jerome Groopman, Kat Duff, Pat Berne, Paul Van Ness, Elizabeth Lesser, Mark Epstein, Tara Brach, Pema Chödrön, Thich Nhat Hanh, and Jon Kabat-Zinn.

In the field of creativity and aging, Gene Cohen, of course, is my star teacher. Through his guidance, I continue our thanks to Thomas Cole, Kate De Medeiros, Marc Agronin, Andrea Sherman, Gay Hanna, Susan Perlstein, Michael Patterson, Berna Huebner, Maria Genet, Peter Whitehouse, Gary Glazer, John Zeisel, and Marc Freedman.

And lastly, in the category I can only imagine as calling pure love of language, my appreciation goes out to Mary Pipher, Elizabeth Tova Bailey, A.A. Milne, E.B. White, Maira Kalman, Mary Oliver, Maya Angelou, David Whyte, Anne Valley-Fox, The Three Marias, and always, Antoine de Saint-Exupéry.

Appendix

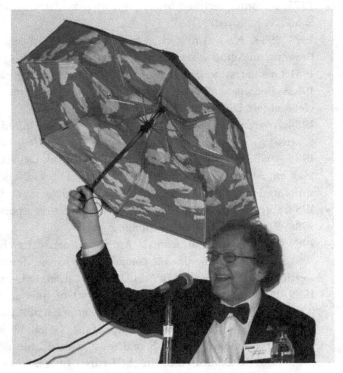

Figure A.1 Photograph of Gene D. Cohen at a professional presentation for the 2005
White House Conference on Aging, with his Sky Above Clouds umbrella.
Photograph by Wendy L. Miller.

Timeline of an Unexpected Life in the Presence of Life-Threatening Illness

I. BACKGROUNDS PRE-MEETING

Cohen
- Born September 28, 1944
- 1962: Wins first place in the MIT/MA State Science Fair Project on Aging, studying the age of the longhorn sculpin fish by using a microsaw
- 1966: Graduates from Harvard College, majoring in biology

- 1970: Graduates from Georgetown University School of Medicine
- 1971: Starts his 25-year longitudinal study on aging at Regency House, Washington, DC
- 1972: Son Alex is born
- 1972: Drafted during the Vietnam War into the Commissioned Corps of the United States Public Health Service at the National Institute of Mental Health
- 1973: Becomes certified in community psychiatry through the Washington School of Psychiatry
- 1975–1988: Named first chief of the Center on Aging and director of the Program on Aging, National Institute of Mental Health
- 1981: Graduates from The Union Institute & University with a Ph.D. in gerontology
- 1983: Becomes clinical professor in the Department of Psychiatry at Georgetown University
- 1984: Awarded the Distinguished Service Medal in United States Public Health Service
- 1986–1993: Becomes executive secretary for the Department of Health and Human Services Council on Alzheimer's Disease, and is congressionally appointed to the Federal Advisory Panel on Alzheimer's disease
- 1988: Receives the Surgeon General's Certificate of Appreciation
- 1988: Publishes *The Brain in Human Aging*
- 1989: Receives certificate from the American Board of Psychiatry and Neurology, "in recognition of significant contributions to the development of the First Certification Examination In Added Qualifications in Geriatric Psychiatry"
- 1989–1995: Becomes editor-in-chief (first) of *International Psychogeriatrics* (Official Journal of the International Psychogeriatric Association)
- 1991–1993: Appointed acting director of the National Institutes of Aging
- 1991: Misdiagnosed with ALS, realized as a misdiagnosis in 1993
- 1992–2001: Becomes editor-in-chief (first) of *American Journal of Geriatric Psychiatry* (Official Journal of the American Association for Geriatric Psychiatry)
- 1993: Concludes his 20 years in the Public Health Service at National Institutes of Health, having won numerous (30+) awards there and throughout various national and international associations; most notable to him was the Public Health Service (PHS) Distinguished Service Medal (the highest honor of the PHS)
- 1993: Forms his intergenerational board game company, Genco, International, and manufactures his first game, WWIII (Word Wars III)

Miller

- Born May 21, 1950
- 1961: Breaks her leg in a ski accident. It gets reset at Boston's Children's Hospital, where she has her first taste of art as therapy and decides this is what she wants to do when she grows up

- 1963: Wins first place in Academic Scholarship at Coburn Classical Institute
- 1972: Graduates from Simmons College, majoring in psychology
- 1978: Graduates from San Francisco State University with a MA in creative arts interdisciplinary studies
- 1978–1982 and 1984–1986: Works for the California Arts Council Artist-in-Social Institutions Program
- 1978: Creates an art program within a psychiatric aftercare program, mentored by Joan Erikson
- 1982: Becomes a certified artist-therapist with the American Artist Therapist Association (AAAT)
- 1982: Receives award of honor from the San Francisco Commission on the Status of Women for her art exhibition with psychiatric women clients, titled "Images from Our Lives"
- 1982: Has her first one-woman art show, titled "Strategies for Standing," at Southern Exposure Gallery (San Francisco)
- 1982–1983: Travels through Spain and North Africa with artist friend, interviewing women and visiting her mother's place of birth, Oran, Algeria.
- 1984–1997: Becomes adjunct instructor in various undergraduate and graduate programs, in expressive arts therapy, fine arts, sculpture, art therapy, arts and consciousness, and professional psychology, at John F Kennedy University, San Francisco State University, Southwestern College, George Washington University, Lesley College, California Institute of Integral Studies, and Vermont College of Norwich University
- 1987: Completes training at Psychosynthesis Training Institute, San Francisco
- 1992: Graduates from The Union Institute & University with a Ph.D. in clinical and health psychology
- 1992: Becomes a certified expressive therapist with the National Expressive Therapy Association (NETA)

II. MILLER AND COHEN TOGETHER

1993
- Wendy and Gene meet

1994
- Gene establishes the Washington, DC Center on Aging, a think tank focused on creative program development, problem-solving, and innovative approaches to issues of aging and intergenerational relationships
- Gene becomes professor of health care sciences and professor of psychiatry and behavioral sciences, School of Medicine and Health Sciences, George Washington University (1994–2009)

- Gene becomes director (first) of the Center on Aging, Health & Humanities at George Washington University (1994–2009).
- Gene creates his second game, Cribbage
- Daughter Eliana is born (adopted at birth)
- Wendy becomes a registered art therapist with the American Art Therapy Association (AATA)
- Wendy cofounds Create Therapy Institute (CTI), using mind–body approaches to healing through expressive arts therapies. CTI houses trainings and creative gatherings as well as her private clinical practice in arts-based psychotherapy, 1994 through the present
- Wendy helps cofound the International Expressive Arts Therapy Association (IEATA)

1996
- Wendy becomes executive co-chair of IEATA (1996–1998)
- Gene becomes president of the Gerontological Society of America (1996–1997)

1997
- Wendy becomes a registered expressive arts therapist (REAT) with the International Expressive Arts therapy Association
- Wendy becomes a licensed professional counselor (LPC) in Washington, DC
- Wendy co-runs supervision and training groups at Create Therapy Institute (1997–2001)
- Wendy publishes on imagery, art, and health, and is featured in a film about an artist recovering from lymphoma

1998
- Wendy co-juries an art exhibition at the George Washington University's Colonnade Gallery
- Gene cofounds the Creativity Discovery Corps (a component of the Center on Aging, Health & Humanities), whose mission is to identify and preserve the creative accomplishments and rich histories of underrecognized older adults, especially those who are socially isolated and homebound
- Gene is a keynote lecturer and visiting presenter both nationally and internationally for many organizations in creativity and aging (1998–2009)

2000
- Create Therapy Institute is awarded Best Practice from the first Creativity and Aging Conference (George Washington University)
- Gene publishes the first book on creativity and aging, *The Creative Age*

- Gene begins research on his Retirement Study, aimed at developing a model for comprehensive retirement planning, with particular attention to developing an adequate social portfolio

2001
- Gene begins his Creativity and Aging Study, a National Endowment for the Arts sponsored multisite national study to assess the impact on older adults of cultural programs provided by professional artists, with attention to general health, mental health, and social functioning (2001–2005)

2002
- Wendy exhibits her artwork "Mother, Daughter, Mother" in the California art show, Seven Women Across America

2003
- Gene is awarded first place in the Society for the Arts in Healthcare's international healing arts competition for his game for Alzheimer patients, "Making Memories Together" and for his Therapeutic-Reparative (TR) Bios
- Gene begins his SEA Change Program (Societal Education about Aging for Change), a new program within the Center on Aging, Health & Humanities, focused on public education of youth about aging
- Wendy's chapter for a book on creative arts therapy and adoption is published
- Wendy begins an ongoing women's art group (2004–2011)

2004
- Gene begins writing *The Mature Mind*
- Wendy presents holistic diagrams of the marriage between creativity and medicine for various art therapy groups and associations

2005
- Gene publishes *The Mature Mind*
- Gene begins his Baby Boomer Research Study
- Wendy creates an art installation for Elders Share the Arts, for the White House Conference on Aging, and is on a panel for healing environments at the Washington Craft Show, Washington, DC
- Gene and Wendy decide to write a book together

2006
- Gene manufactures his fourth game, "Making Memories Together"

2007
- Gene and Wendy present together for the Society of the Arts in Healthcare

2009
- Gene is hired to be the expert medical witness for the Brooke Astor case in New York City. He testifies in the legal battle, NYC *v.* Anthony Marshall in late August
- Wendy's Levine family reunion event occurs in Maine, with interviews for the family film, "Legacy"
- Wendy accepts the first Gene D. Cohen Research Award in Creative Aging, presented posthumously to Gene from the Gerontological Society of America (GSA) and the National Center for Creative Aging (NCCA)

2010
- Wendy accepts the Hall of Fame Award, presented posthumously to Gene from the American Society on Aging (ASA) at the Aging in America Conference
- Wendy returns part-time to her clinical practice; she also manages Washington, DC Center on Aging and Genco games
- Wendy and Alex retrieve and house all of Gene's games from their storage and distribution centers

2011
- Wendy accepts the Special Impact Award, presented posthumously to Gene from the Society for the Arts in Healthcare (SAH)
- Wendy and her sisters complete their film on their family, "Legacy: The Levine Family," which premiered at Colby College and on Voice of America

2012
- Wendy begins to edit the writings that make up this book

2013–2014
- Eliana graduates from high school and goes to Endicott College to study sports medicine and exercise science
- Wendy works with Oxford University Press to publish *Sky Above Clouds*

III. SIGNIFICANT LIFE EVENTS

Travel/Births/Marriages
- 1994: Gene and Wendy adopt their daughter Eliana at birth
- 1996: Wendy and Gene marry
- 1997: Wendy's family's clothing business, Levine's Store, closes after operating for 107 years

- 2001: Gene's son Alex marries Kate; Gene is his best man, Eliana is one of the flower girls
- 2003: First grandchild Ruby is born
- 2005: Wendy's nephew Jeremy gets married
- 2005: Second grandchild Lucy is born
- 2006: Gene, Wendy, Eliana, Alex, Kate, Ruby, and Lucy travel to the Dominican Republic
- 2007: Eliana has her Bat Mitzvah
- 2007: Twin grandsons Ethan and Bennett are born
- 2008: Wendy's niece Joslyn gets married; Eliana is one of the bride's maids
- 2008: Gene, Wendy, and Eliana travel to Costa Rica
- 2011: Wendy's nephew Ben gets married

Illnesses and Deaths
- 1991: Wendy's nana Frieda (Levine Miller) dies at age 94 of old age
- 1994: Wendy's great aunt Betty (Levine Kaplan) dies at age 92 of old age
- 1994: Wendy's mother Gisèle (Baroukel Miller) is diagnosed with cancer (multiple myeloma)
- 1996: Wendy's great uncle Pacy (Levine) dies at age 91 of a heart attack
- 1997: Gene's father Ben (Cohen) dies at age 87 of Alzheimer's disease
- 1997: Wendy's great uncle Ludy (Levine) dies at age 99 of old age
- 1997: Wendy's mother Gisèle (Baroukel Miller) dies at age 77 from complications from multiple myeloma/bacterial infection
- 2000: Wendy's cousin Harold (Wolff) dies at age 81 of Parkinson's disease.
- 2001: Wendy's brother-in-law Dan (Arnon) dies at age 63 from antiphospholipid antibody syndrome
- 2002: Wendy's father Howard (Miller) is diagnosed with chronic myeloid leukemia and begins treatment with Gleevec; he develops a toxic reaction to the drug in the hippocampus and loses his short-term memory. Wendy and Gene file an FDA complaint on the new cancer-treating "miracle" medicine.
- 2004: Gene's brother Franklin (Cohen) dies at age 64 from a brain aneurysm
- 2005: Wendy's father Howard (Miller) dies at age 85 from a hemorrhagic stroke
- 2005: Wendy's great aunt Bibby (Levine Alfond) dies at age 89 of Parkinson's disease
- 2005: Wendy's sister Sara (Miller Arnon) is diagnosed with colon cancer and begins outpatient chemotherapy
- 2006: Gene's mother Lillian (Strashun Cohen) dies at age 92 of dementia
- 2006: Wendy's sister Sara (Miller Arnon) is diagnosed with metastasis to her liver and undergoes surgery and chemotherapy
- 2006: Wendy's brother-in-law Michael (Soros) is diagnosed with acute myeloid leukemia and begins aggressive inpatient chemotherapy
- 2007: Wendy's uncle Len (Kaplan) dies at age 94 of complications from pneumonia

- 2007: Wendy's great uncle Harold (Alfond) dies at age 93 of prostate cancer
- 2008: Wendy's cousin Lenny (Cushner) dies at age 82 of a C. *difficile* infection
- 2009: Gene dies and Wendy get shingles four days later; her grieving process over the years becomes complicated grief
- 2011: Wendy's cousin Mort (Bloom) dies at age 85 of a cerebral aneurysm
- 2013: Wendy's cousin Tema (Kaplan Cushner) dies at age 88 of emphysema
- 2014: Gene's aunt Annie (Strashun Greenside) dies at age 93 of pneumonia

Trajectory of Gene's Illness

- 1996: Gene is diagnosed with metastatic prostate cancer (PSA, 360)
- 1996–2008: Gene begins hormone therapy treatment for metastatic prostate cancer (Nilandron, Lupron, bisphosphonates), which holds the cancer in remission
- 2004: Gene breaks his femur
- 2006: Gene is told, "Medically, you do not exist."
- 2007: Gene and Wendy tell Eliana about the diagnosis Gene's has lived with her whole life from the perspective of his outlier status
- 2008: Gene gets what first presents as a urinary tract infection, which is treated with many rounds of antibiotics but does not resolve
- 2009: Gene's metastatic prostate cancer returns in an active state
- 2009: Gene has bilateral hydronephrosis, followed by bilateral nephrostomies and stents
- 2009: Gene begins chemotherapy with Taxotere, changes in rounds to Cytoxan, carboplatin, and mitoxantrone
- Nov 7, 2009: Gene dies at age 65 of metastatic prostate cancer

Gene Cohen's Boomer Research Study Summary

To keep the creative juices flowing, following the publication of *The Mature Mind*, I launched a novel study on baby boomers, the first of its kind on the post–World War II baby boomer demographic, those Americans born from 1946 to 1964. Prior to this study essentially all the psychosocial research on boomers was through surveys—questionnaires. Survey research is great when you have the right question and seek a large number of responses. But its limitation is that at best you get the answers only to the questions asked. And you don't get the questions on the minds of those being queried. As a result, in the case of boomers, there have been many unasked and unanswered questions. An added value of this study is that 25% are minorities. There are 27 women and 27 men.

The new study involves the first series of longitudinal face-to-face personal interviews with baby boomers, in which the participants have an opportunity to express their own concerns instead of being limited to responding only to concerns identified by the researcher. They have a chance to express their questions, hopes, fears, dreams, dreads, expectations, passions, and more. It is a more personal and psychological view of life, designed to provide a broader, deeper, and more accurate story of a population that is redefining so much about aging in America.

One of the findings that was quickly apparent, cutting across the racial, ethnic, and socioeconomic diversity of boomers, is that they are collectively the first group in history to witness their parents or parents' generation aging healthier and being better educated, more active, and generally better off than any aging parent group before them. As a result, boomers are the first group in history, in large numbers, to have the everyday evidence and emerging science influencing their view of the continued creativity and possibility that aging can hold for them.

The significance of this finding is illustrated in the following brief case examples:

> A 60-year-old man in the study (see James, later in this summary—not his real name), recently retired, in talking about planning for his future indicated that since his father lived well until age 95, to the extent his genes reflect his father's, he needed to think carefully about what he could and should be doing for some time to come.
>
> A 53-year-old African-American woman had entered a Masters in Divinity program and indicated, "I think that when I finish this program I will finally have the confidence and know-how to accomplish something I will really be satisfied with. I look ay my father at 77, and he started a new business in his mid-70s, investing in a van and starting

a chauffer service that gives him a lot of satisfaction and sense of independence, not to speak of extra money."

ON THE LIMITS OF THE VIEW OF SUCCESSFUL AGING

The definition of "successful aging," as defined by Rowe and Kahn, is that of "aging with minimal decline." While this definition was in many ways what the optimal application of a problem focus aimed at reducing deficits would accomplish, it is not a concept that addresses the potential for growth. What has become apparent in this boomer study is that for most of the boomers, while the idea of having minimal decline is in one sense appealing, in another sense there is the feeling that if minimal decline is as good as it gets, it is not good enough—that what aging promises according to the successful aging model is not new opportunity or growth, and this is not appealing.

As a 61-year-old subject put it, "I have had a series of bests in my life, I expect more and different bests to continue for some time to come."

Boomers expect that opportunity can and should be ahead of them. It would be like rain on their parade for older boomers to think this is as good as it gets.

ON BRAIN FITNESS AND STAYING SHARP AMONG BOOMERS

Virtually all the subjects in the study view mental fitness as very important to them. There is a high interest in staying involved in challenging full-time or part-time work, mixing the latter with challenging volunteer activities. Lifelong learning is highly valued, the majority of subjects taking or planning to take formal continuing education classes or to develop mastery in some new area, ranging from learning Spanish, to taking up comedy, to learning how to restore an automobile. Collectively, the boomers describe a clear increased involvement in physical fitness and mental fitness activities (e.g., crossword puzzles, sudoku, extensive reading, and the like).

LESSONS FROM THE BOOMER STUDY: PLANNING OF ACTIVE ADULT COMMUNITIES

At a meeting hosted by one of the premier developers of active adult communities targeting boomers, one of the most apparent gaps in their planning process was that in the midst of all their strengths—quality of residence, appeal of location, opportunity for physical fitness, social opportunity, entertainment opportunity—what was lacking was comparable attention to lifelong learning and mental challenge, where instead, a strong social and entertainment focus was viewed as addressing this area of boomer interest and concern. Lessons from this study perhaps influenced the strategic planning of these communities at a critical point in their development.

REVEALING SNAPSHOTS OF INDIVIDUAL BOOMERS

On Boomers' Orientation Toward Challenge and Change

"Those of us who were socially conscious during the 1960s became aware that your country can be profoundly wrong. This heightened our orientation toward questioning things in society, as well as our comfort level with pushing for change."

On Retirement

One view is that "retirement is more a financial position than a planned transition. The finances have to be right before the transition can be planned." Another finding is that a number of the boomers retired not with enthusiasm and advance planning but because of changes in the workplace that they found unacceptable, whether from poor or unfriendly management or a lack of significant new opportunity. Hence, these individuals had not been seeking retirement and therefore had not been planning for it. They developed instead some sense of urgency to retire from a no longer fulfilling work environment, without their options carefully thought out.

On Civic Engagement

Compared to the principle investigator's prior "retirement study" with an older cohort, the boomers in this study tend to be looking at civic engagement more through the nature of part-time work than volunteerism, though both working and volunteering are important to them. The issue in the volunteer sector is the lack of an infrastructure that has the capacity to match individuals with specific skills with programs in need of those skills. Equally fundamental is the lack of an infrastructure with the capability of simply identifying interesting civic engagement programs or opportunities apart from those that are highly visible but limited in number, like the Experience Corps.

On African-American Boomers

"My parents had all they could do to have the opportunity to learn how to read and write. They told me and my siblings, 'Get an education; nobody can take that away from you.' My generation is telling their children, 'You can do anything.' Hence, over a period of three generations, our sense of being constrained has progressively diminished and our feeling of freedom to dream has been rising— soaring with our children."

On Creative Strategies

A study of this nature captures many creative strategies on the part of individuals. Consider the following illustration. Boomers have more divorced parents than prior generations, and are therefore more challenged with staying close to both parents when the latter are separated. If married, the parents can be visited at the same time. One participant described how it was very important to find activities that enabled her relationship to continue to grow with each of her divorced parents. She described how both of her parents had developed an interest in art, and she began getting involved in art herself. Now yearly she spends a week with each parent separately in creative arts workshops, where she and each of her parents individually have an opportunity to grow, while her relationship with each parent also is growing. *This is an important example of the role of the arts in lifelong learning and lifelong relationship maintenance and growth.*

A further example of a creative strategy was given by a boomer working out with her brothers a long-distance lifelong learning program for their visually impaired mother living out-of-state. The siblings take turns calling their mother and reading a novel to her on the phone, which, like a book club, the family as a whole discusses with their mother.

WHEN THE FOCUS ON TIME CHANGES FOR BOOMERS

The issue of time has emerged as an especially poignant phenomenon with unique attributes for boomers. This started to become apparent when I interviewed James (not his real name), who was 60 years old and where he worked was eligible for retirement. He came into our session wanting to talk about his starting to think about retirement. As the discussion unfolded, we talked about others in his social circle as well as in his extended family who had retired, and what their experiences had been. In the process, he mentioned that both his parents were still alive, and doing well at 95. Then, as he said this, he paused, with a very pensive look on his face, and with a sense of awe stated that he had just realized in talking about his parents that they were as many years older than him as the number of years he had worked—35. He then, with more feeling in his voice, pointed out as much to himself as to me that if he retired now, he could have as many years to deal with retirement as his entire working career. He then wondered if he was ready for that, if he was he up to it, if that was what he really wanted to do.

Many discussions related to James' followed, and what became apparent was the perceived very significant amount of time that boomers approaching retirement age had to live. Realizing this, they began to seriously think about how to spend that time. Moreover, they viewed this time fundamentally differently than how many had viewed time ahead of them upon entering middle age. Upon turning 40, many thought about the coming years as time left until they died. That "until they died" aspect colored their experience of that time, and contributed to feelings of uneasiness or angst. But with the aging boomers, though demographically closer to death, their orientation to the years ahead was strongly about living. There was no anxiety about that time—concerns, yes, but generally not angst. The issue again is in how well they can live those years, what they can do, what will be worthwhile and meaningful, what won't bore them, and what will provide them opportunities for challenge and growth. They more typically had a sense of positive anticipation, excitement, and a looking forward to change and more freedom with how to use their time. They were almost like runners in a marathon who, after traversing many miles, were experiencing an energizing *second wind*. There was more of a sense of control they could take of that time than control time could take of them. It was akin to how Andy Warhol viewed time: "They say that time changes things, but you actually have to change them yourself."

What also affected their sense of what that time could be like in later life was what James experienced. The boomers are the first cohort group in history, in large numbers, to have a good close-up and personal glimpse that aging can be OK, that we can in fact age well, even creatively. To observe in one's own family a different view of aging reduces psychological defenses that lead to a denial of aging; denial was characteristic of virtually all aging cohorts prior to the boomers. The boomers see what can be with aging. This leads to the feeling that what can be, *should be!* This, in turn, leads to the conviction that this *should be for me*— that things should change to make this happen, and that *you* (society) better make it happen! Such is a context for social change, a new view of aging, a new set of expectations of what aging can and should offer, and a new set of positive personal experiences that redefine the experience of aging. It all points to what had been uncharted for so long about aging is now being defined and experienced in new ways. It all points to the realization that in the second half of life, today—*the times they are a changin'!*

This more positive collective attitude, emerging as it does from historic denial, fear, and negativity about aging, has produced a shift in expectations toward a conviction that what can be, should be. With that conscious engagement comes new attention to the steps required to create the context for optimal aging in our personal lives, our communities, and our country.

Why is this attitudinal shift significant as a health factor? Because awareness of the linkage between creativity, aging, health, and healing is a powerful motivating force for an individual's preventive health behaviors and use of a more holistic response to illness. And in this instance, what is powerful in the life of one is powerful for all. There is a growing interest and demand in making fundamental changes in the way we promote health and provide care for this nation's aging population. It is a fundamental focus of my work, and it has becomes fundamental in how I attempt to navigate my own everyday personal and family life with my own aging and illness.

Gene Cohen's Op-Ed Essay: "What Is a Lucid Moment?"

I was retained as the expert medical witness for the New York County District Attorney's office in the Brook Astor Case. I am a geriatric psychiatrist with a doctorate in gerontology, having done extensive research and clinical work in the area of Alzheimer's disease (AD). I was asked for my opinion as to whether Brooke Astor had the cognitive capacity to understand the changes made to her will after she was diagnosed with Alzheimer's disease. My opinion was that she lacked this capacity.

One of the key issues that emerged from the defense was that during the signing of the two codicils that changed Mrs. Astor's will, she exhibited lucid moments. A lucid moment is a very poorly understood and very often misunderstood concept around which courts, lawyers, physicians, families, and individuals need to be better educated. A lucid moment is an elusive concept.

In considering the nature of a lucid moment, there are two fundamental questions: What constitutes being lucid, and what is a moment?

Regarding what is lucid, there is much misunderstanding and considerable variation in what experts and the public perceive about being lucid. For example, many family members seeing their loved one appearing alert, view this as being lucid. But in medicine, being alert simply means being awake; one can be very alert and very confused at the same time. For others, seeing a smile on a loved one's face following a given comment may also elicit a perception of lucidity, whereas, behind the smile may be a complete misinterpretation of the comment. Also qualitative and quantitative distinctions so often fail to be made. A qualitative perception of lucidity may be the product of viewing only a fragment of lucidity, though experienced quantitatively by the viewer as constituting overall lucidity at that moment. Even healthcare professionals and attorneys can fall into this perceptual trap. To really understand a will, its changes, and the ramifications of those changes—to possess what is technically referred to as testamentary capacity—one needs to be able to see more than fragments but the whole picture. If you want to take in an entire landscape, you don't want to look through a pinhole in a single section of window with several sections; you want to view what can seen within the entire window frame and all its sections.

In my more than 40 years of working with patients with Alzheimer's disease and other dementias, I have reached the following conclusions about the capacity for lucidity. They are based on the three major stages of AD—mild, moderate, and severe. For healthy persons, their lucidity allows them to see the forest. For persons in the mild stage of AD, they can no longer see the forest, just some trees. For persons in the moderate stage of AD, they can no longer see the trees, just some branches. For persons in the severe stage of AD, they can no longer see branches, just a blur. At the time Brooke Astor's will was changed, an international expert on AD who had evaluated Mrs. Astor considered her to be moving toward the severe stage of Alzheimer's disease.

What about the moment part of a lucid moment? A moment typically refers to something that is fleeting. In relation to time as well, too often qualitative and quantitative distinctions disappear when one is trying to determine if a lucid moment occurred. If a comment is made that seems in the moment to make some sense, somehow the experience of that fleeting moment is transformed into an extended interval of lucid capacity for the duration of the encounter—even if that encounter is lengthy. To comprehend the complexities of a will and its changes requires an extended period of comprehension, not just a glimpse that can notice a branch without taking in the forest. More than a moment of lucidity is required.

One's sense of a lucid moment is often transformed or magnified through uninformed assumptions or a wishful moment on the part of the viewer, desperately searching for more than what actually meets their eye. When I hear professionals emphasizing the importance of a lucid moment, I flash back to a scene in the movie version of Nicholas Meyer's novel, "The Seven-Percent-Solution," about the fictional meeting of Sherlock Holmes and Sigmund Freud. In that scene, the famous Dr. Freud is sharing an observation with the legendary Holmes. As first Holmes is patient, but then with some exasperation asserts, "I say Herr doctor, you look but do not see." Many look but do not see—or see what they want to see—in contemplating that elusive lucid moment.

Gene D. Cohen, M.D., Ph.D.
Director, Center on Aging, Health & Humanities
George Washington University,
and a Past President of the Gerontological Society of America

Gene D. Cohen Bibliography

Papers and editorials published in peer-reviewed journals and professional/scientific newsletters

Cohen, G.D., Conwell, M., Ozarin, L.D., & Ochberg, F.M. (1974). PSROs, problems and potentials for psychiatry. *American Journal of Psychiatry, 131*, 1378–1381.

Goldstein, H., & Cohen, G.D. (1975). CMHCs and PSROs: The emerging interface. *Administration in Mental Health*, Winter, 12–18.

Kopolow, L., & Cohen, G.D. (1975). Milieu therapy: Towards a definition for reimbursement. *American Journal of Psychiatry, 133*, 1060–1063.

Cohen, G.D. (1976). Mental health services and the elderly: Needs and options. *American Journal of Psychiatry, 133*, 65–68.

Cohen, G.D. (1977). Approach to the geriatric patient. *Medical Clinics of North America, 61*, 855–866.

Cohen, G.D. (1978). Comment: Organic brain syndrome. *Gerontologist, 19*, 313–314.

Cohen, G.D. (1979). Research on aging: A piece of the puzzle. *Gerontologist, 19*, 503–508.

Cohen, G.D. (1979/1980). An alternative setting for community-based gero-psychiatric care. *International Journal of Mental Health, 8*(Fall/Winter), 173–184.

Cohen, G.D., O'Brien, J. Gillilan, J., Walsh, T.L., & Anthony, R. (1980). Geriatric psychiatry training: A brief clinical rotation. *American Journal of Psychiatry, 137*, 297–300.

Cohen, G.D. (1981). Perspectives on psychotherapy with the elderly. *American Journal of Psychiatry, 138*, 347–350.

Cohen, G.D. (1981). Prospects for mental health and aging: At a crisis and crossroad. *Gerontology and Geriatrics Education, 1*, 277–231.

Cohen, G.D. (1982). The older person, the older patient, and the mental health system. *Hospital and Community Psychiatry, 33*, 101–104.

Finkel, S.I., & Cohen, G.D. (1982). Guest editorial: The mental health of the aging. *Gerontologist, 22*, 227–228.

Cohen, G.D. (1983). Psychogeriatric program in a public housing setting. *Psychiatric Quarterly, 55*(Summer/Fall), 173–181.

Cohen, G.D. (1983). Translating research into education: Programs and practice. *Gerontology and Geriatrics Education, 3*, 171–176.

Cohen, G.D. (1984). Counseling psychology and aging. *Counseling Psychologist, 12*(Fall), 97–99.

Cohen, G.D. (1984). Psychotherapy of the elderly. *Psychosomatics, 25*, 455–463.

Cohen, G.D. (1984). The mental health professional and the Alzheimer patient. *Hospital and Community Psychiatry, 35*, 115–116.

Crook, T., & Cohen, G.D. (1984). Future directions for research on alcohol and the elderly. *Alcohol Health and Research World, 8*(3), 24–29.

Goldman, H.H., Cohen, G.D., & Davis, M. (1985). Expanded Medicare coverage for Alzheimer's disease and related disorders. *Hospital and Community Psychiatry, 36*, 939–942.

Crook, T., Bartus, R.T., Ferris, S.H., Whitehouse, P., Cohen, G.D., & Gershon, S. (1986). Age-associated memory impairment: Proposed diagnostic criteria and measures of clinical change—report of a National Institute of Mental Health work group. *Developmental Neuropsychology, 2*, 261–276.

Nickens, H.W., Crook, T., & Cohen, G.D. (1986). Psychotropic drugs. *Generations, 10*(Spring), 33–37.

Cohen, G.D. (1989). Biopsychiatry of Alzheimer's disease. *Annual Review of Gerontology and Geriatrics, 9*, 216–231.

Cohen, G.D. (1989). The movement toward subspecialty status for geriatric psychiatry in the United States. *International Psychogeriatrics, 1*, 201–205.

Cohen, G.D. (1989). The interface of mental and physical health phenomena in later life: New directions in geriatric psychiatry. *Gerontology & Geriatrics Education, 9*, 27–38.

Lebowitz, B.D., & Cohen, G.D. (1989). Education and training in geriatric psychiatry. *Advances in Psychosomatic Medicine, 19*, 167–178.

Cohen, G.D. (1990). Alzheimer's disease: Clinical update. *Hospital and Community Psychiatry, 41*(5), 496–497.

Cohen, G.D. (1990). The prevalence of psychiatric problems in older adults. *Psychiatric Annals, 20*, 433–438.

Finkel, S.I., Cohen, G.D., Bergener, M., & Hasegawa, K. (1991). Psychogeriatrics and medical informatics. *International Psychogeriatrics, 3*, 7–9.

Bergener, M., Cohen, G.D., Finkel, S.I., & Hasegawa, K. (1992). Psychogeriatrics—an interdisciplinary specialty. *International Psychogeriatrics, 4*(1), 7–8.

Cohen, G.D. (1992). What is the value of psychiatric home visits to the elderly? *Harvard Mental Health Letter, 9*(6), 8.

Hasegawa, K., Bergener, M., Cohen, G.D., & Finkel, S.I. (1992). Late-life suicide. *International Psychogeriatrics, 4*(2), 163.

Cohen, G.D. (1993). African American issues in geriatric psychiatry: A perspective on research opportunities. *Journal of Geriatric Psychiatry and Neurology, 6*(4), 195–199.

Cohen, G.D. (1993). A tale of two Decembers: The journal of December 1992 & the case of December 1843. *American Journal of Geriatric Psychiatry, 1*(1), 1–2.

Cohen, G.D. (1993). Comprehensive assessment of older adults: Capturing strengths, not just weaknesses. *Generations*, Winter/Spring, 47–50.

Cohen, G.D. (1993). How old is too old? *American Journal of Geriatric Psychiatry, 1*(2), 91–93.

Cohen, G.D., Bergener, M., Finkel, S.I., & Hasegawa, K. (1993). May you live amidst interesting dichotomies—from manifest behavior to molecular biology. *International Psychogeriatrics, 5*(1), 3–4.

Cohen, G.D., & Cahan, V. (1993). Older women's health: Avoiding a tragedy of mythic proportions. *Archives of Family Medicine, 2*(4), 361–363.

Cohen, G.D., & Havlik, R.J. (1993). Epidemiology of aging comes of age. *Annals of Epidemiology, 3*(4), 448–450.

Cohen, G.D. (1994). Alzheimer's disease: Puzzle and paradox, pain and pathway. *Gerontologist, 34*, 845–846.

Cohen, G.D. (1994). Creativity and aging: Relevance to research, practice, and policy. *American Journal of Geriatric Psychiatry, 2*(4), 277–281.

Cohen, G.D. (1994). Health care at an advanced age: Myths and misinformation. *Annals of Internal Medicine, 121*(2), 146–147.

Cohen, G.D. (1994). Health care reform and older adults. *Gerontologist, 34*, 584–585.

Cohen, G.D. (1994). Journalistic elder abuse: It's time to get rid of fictions, get down to facts. *Gerontologist, 34*(3), 399–401.

Cohen, G.D. (1994). The geriatric landscape—toward a health and humanities research agenda in aging. *American Journal of Geriatric Psychiatry, 2*(3), 185–187.

Cohen, G.D. (1994). Toward new models of dementia care. *Alzheimer Disease and Associated Disorders, 8*(Supplement 1), S2–S4.

Cohen, G.D. (1995). Health care costs associated with aging: What is your HCA IQ—your "health costs associated with aging" intelligence quotient? *American Journal of Geriatric Psychiatry, 3*, 185–190.

Cohen, G.D. (1995). Humor and aging: Methuselah and Thalia as close friends. *American Journal of Geriatric Psychiatry, 3*, 93–95.

Cohen, G.D. (1995). Intergenerationalism: A new "ism" with positive mental health and social policy potential. *American Journal of Geriatric Psychiatry, 3*, 1–5.

Cohen, G.D. (1995). Management of Alzheimer's disease. *Advances in Internal Medicine, 40*, 31–67.

Cohen, G.D. (1995). Mental health promotion in later life: The case for the social portfolio. *American Journal of Geriatric Psychiatry, 3,* 277–279.

Cohen, G.D. (1996). Can research on aging deliver on its promises? *Perspectives on Aging,* 25(1), 4–8.

Cohen, G.D. (1996). Consistency of care: What will be its fate under managed care?. *American Journal of Geriatric Psychiatry, 4*(4), 277–280.

Cohen, G.D. (1996). Put the reimbursement with the rhetoric: Medicare, managed care, and mental health. *American Journal of Geriatric Psychiatry, 4*(2), 93–95.

Cohen, G.D. (1996). The special case of mental health in later life: The obvious has been overlooked. *American Journal of Geriatric Psychiatry, 4*(1), 17–23.

Cohen, G.D. (1996). Time, managed care, and mental health. *American Journal of Geriatric Psychiatry, 4*(3), 185–187.

Cohen-Mansfield, J., Reisberg, B., Bonnema, J., Berg, L., Dastoor, D.P., Pfeffer, R.I., & Cohen, G.D. (1996). Staging methods for the assessment of dementia: Perspectives. *Journal of Clinical Psychiatry, 57*(5), 190–198.

Butler, R.N., Cohen, G., Lewis, M.I., Simmons-Clemmons, W., & Sunderland, T. (1997). Late life depression: How to make a difficult diagnosis. *Geriatrics, 52*(March), 37–50.

Butler, R.N., Cohen, G., Lewis, M.I., Simmons-Clemmons, W., & Sunderland, T. (1997). Late life depression: Treatment strategies for primary care practice. *Geriatrics, 52*(April), 51–64.

Cohen, G.D. (1997). Citizen Kane as senior citizen: A mental health perspective. *American Journal of Geriatric Psychiatry, 5*(2), 93–96.

Cohen, G.D. (1997). Dorothy and the wizard: Intergenerational issues in mental health and aging. *American Journal of Geriatric Psychiatry, 5*(4), 277–278.

Cohen, G.D. (1997). Progress in Alzheimer's disease: Pause and perspective. *American Journal of Geriatric Psychiatry, 5*(3), 185–187.

Cohen, G.D. (1997). Sky above clouds: Mental health in later life. *American Journal of Geriatric Psychiatry, 5*(1), 1–3.

Cohen, G.D. (1998). Aging to sleep, perchance to dream. *American Journal of Geriatric Psychiatry,* 6(2), 93–96.

Cohen, G.D. (1998). Anxiety in Alzheimer's disease: Confusion and denial. *American Journal of Geriatric Psychiatry, 6*(1), 1–4.

Cohen, G.D. (1998). Anxiety in Alzheimer's disease: Theoretical and clinical perspectives. *Journal of Geriatric Psychiatry, 31*(2), 103–115.

Cohen, G.D. (1998). Creativity and aging: Ramifications for research, practice, and policy. *Geriatrics, 53*(Supplement), S4–S8.

Cohen, G.D. (1998). Do health science concepts influence care? The case for a new landscape of aging. *American Journal of Geriatric Psychiatry, 6*(4), 273–276.

Cohen, G.D. (1998). The magic bullets are blanks: Purported shortcuts to improving the aging mind. *American Journal of Geriatric Psychiatry, 6*(3), 185–195.

Finkel, S.I., Costa e Silva, J., Cohen, G.D., Miller, S., & Sartorius, N. (1998). Behavioral and psychological symptoms of dementia: A consensus statement on current knowledge and implications for research and treatment. *American Journal of Geriatric Psychiatry, 6*(2), 97–100.

Cohen, G.D. (1999). Aging and peaking. *American Journal of Geriatric Psychiatry, 7*(4), 275–278.

Cohen, G.D. (1999). Human potential phases in the second half of life: Mental health theory development. *American Journal of Geriatric Psychiatry, 7*(1), 1–7.

Cohen, G.D. (1999). Marriage and divorce in later life. *American Journal of Geriatric Psychiatry,* 7(3), 185–187.

Cohen, G.D. (1999). The aging brain vs. the aging body. *American Journal of Geriatric Psychiatry,* 7(2), 93–95.

Cohen, C.I., Cohen, G.D., Blank, K., et al. (2000). Schizophrenia and older adults. An overview: directions for research and policy. *American Journal of Geriatric Psychiatry,* 8(1), 19–28.

Cohen, G.D. (2000). Aging at a turning point In the 21st century. *American Journal of Geriatric Psychiatry, 8*(1), 1–3.

Cohen, G.D. (2000). Creativity and aging. *Grantmakers in the Arts Reader, 11*(2), 1, 16–19.

Cohen, G.D. (2000). If you were an old woman who lived in a shoe, what would you do? *American Journal of Geriatric Psychiatry, 8*(2), 93–95.

Cohen, G.D. (2000). Loneliness in later life. *American Journal of Geriatric Psychiatry, 8*(4), 273–275.

Cohen, G.D. (2000). The future of being old in America: A mental health perspective. *American Journal of Geriatric Psychiatry, 8*(3), 185–187.

Cohen, G.D. (2000). Two new intergenerational interventions for Alzheimer's disease patients and families. *American Journal of Alzheimer's Disease, 15*(3), 1–6.

Finkel, S.I., Burns, A., & Cohen, G.D. (2000). Overview, behavioral and psychological symptoms of dementia (BPSD): A clinical and research update. *International Psychogeriatrics, 12*(Supplement 1), 13–18.

Blank, K., Cohen, C.I., Cohen, G.D., Gaitz, C., et al. (2001). Failure to adequately detect suicidal intent in elderly patients in the primary care setting. *Clinical Geriatrics, 9*(1):26–36.

Cohen, G.D. (2001). Creativity with aging: Four phases of potential in the second half of life. *Geriatrics, 56*(4), 51–57.

Cohen, G.D. (2001). Criteria for success in interventions for Alzheimer's disease. *American Journal of Geriatric Psychiatry, 9*(2), 95–98.

Cohen, G.D. (2001). Exeunt Omnes everybody leaves. *American Journal of Geriatric Psychiatry, 9*(3), 187–190.

Cohen, G.D. (2001). Robert N. Butler, MD, charismatic leader and advocate. *Contemporary Gerontology, 7*(4), 113–115.

Cohen, G.D. (2001). The course of unfulfilled dreams and unfinished business with aging. *American Journal of Geriatric Psychiatry, 9*(1), 1–5.

Cohen, G.D. (2002). Alzheimer's disease: Managing behavioral problems in patients with progressive dementia. *Geriatrics, 57*(2), 53–54.

Cohen, G.D. (2002). Creative interventions for Alzheimer's disease. *Geriatrics, 57*(3), 62–66.

Cohen, G.D. (2002). Depression in later life: An historic account demonstrates the importance of making the diagnosis. *Geriatrics, 57*(12), 38–39.

Cohen, G.D. (2002). Promoting mental health, treating mental illness: Broadening the focus on intervention. *Geriatrics, 57*(1), 47–48.

Cohen, G.D. (2002). Retirement: Advising older adults who are contemplating this change. *Geriatrics, 57*(8), 37–38.

Cohen, G.D. (2002). The art of caring in health care: Lost, relocated, rediscovered. *Gerontologist, 42*(6), 863–867.

Cohen, G.D. (2003). Enhancing connections between the young and the old in and age of technology by impacting the young with positive images of aging: Mental health implications. *International Psychogeriatrics, 15*(Supplement 2), 9.

Cohen, G.D. (2003). Intergenerational interventions for people with Alzheimer's disease. *Dimensions, 10*(2), 6.

Cohen, G.D., Blank, K., Cohen, C.I., Gaitz, C., Liptzin, B., Maletta, G., Meyers, B., & Sakauye, K. (2003). Mental health problems in assisted living patients: The physician's role in treatment and staff education. *Geriatrics, 58*(2), 44, 54–56.

Cohen, G.D. (2004). Development and personal growth in middle age and older adulthood. *Dimensions, 11*(1), 1, 6.

Cohen, G.D. (2004). The golden awakening. *Visions, 9*, 4–5.

Cohen, G.D. (2005). National study documents benefits of creativity programs for older adults. *The Older Learner, 13*(2), 1, 6.

Cohen, G.D. (2006). Research on creativity and aging: The positive impact of the arts on health and illness. *Generations, 30*(1), 7–15.

Cohen, G.D. (2006). Smarts and aging: The learning potential of the brain in later life. *The Older Learner, 13*(4), 1, 6–7.

Cohen, G.D. (2006). The mature mind: The positive power of the aging brain. *Adult Development & Aging News, 34*(1), 4–6.

Cohen, G.D., Perlstein, S., Chapline, J., Kelly, J., Firth, K., & Simmens, S. (2006). The impact of professionally conducted cultural programs on the physical health, mental health, and social functioning of older adults. *Gerontologist, 46*(6), 726–734.

Cohen, G.D. (2007). A key component of the aging brain: The human capacity for spirituality. *Aging & Spirituality, 19*(3), 1.

Cohen, G.D., Perlstein, S., Chapline, J., Kelly, J., Firth, K., & Simmens, S. (2007). The impact of professionally conducted cultural programs on the physical health, mental health, and social functioning of older adults—2-year results. *Journal of Aging, Humanities and the Arts, 1*(1-2), 5–22.

Cohen, G.D. (2008). A new perspective on sustaining and increasing learning capacity with age. *Dimensions*, Summer, 1–3.

Cohen, G.D. (2008). Answering half-asked questions from doomsayers of aging. *Aging Today, XXIX*(5), 1–4.

Cohen, G.D. (2008). The creativity fitness movement. *Aging Today, XXIX*(6), 7.

Cohen, G.D. (2009). New theories and research findings on the positive influence of music and art on health with ageing. *Arts & Health, 1*(1), 48–63.

Cohen, G.D. (2009). Historical lessons to watch your assumptions about aging: Relevance to the role of *International Psychogeriatrics. International Psychogeriatrics, 21*(3), 425–429.

Cohen, G.D., Firth, K.M., Biddle, S., Lewis, M.J.L., & Simmens S. (2009). The first therapeutic game specifically designed and evaluated for Alzheimer's disease. *American Journal of Alzheimer's Disease and Other Dementias, 23*(6), 540–551.

Chapters and reviews published in books

Cohen, G.D. (1980). Prospects for mental health and aging. In J.E. Birren & R.B. Sloane (Eds.), *Handbook of mental health and aging* (pp. 971–993). New York: Prentice-Hall.

Cohen, G.D. (1981). Senile dementia of the Alzheimer type (SDAT): The nature of the disorder. In T. Crook & S. Gershon (Eds.), *Strategies for the development of an effective treatment for senile dementia* (pp. 1–5). New Canaan, CT: Mark Powley Associates.

Miller, N.E., & Cohen, G.D. (1981). Clinical aspects of Alzheimer's disease and senile dementia: Synopsis and future perspectives in assessment, treatment, and service delivery. In N.E. Miller & G.D. Cohen (Eds.), *Clinical aspects of Alzheimer's disease and senile dementia* (pp. 17–35). New York: Raven Press.

Cohen, G.D. (1982). Geriatric psychiatry. In D. Oken & M. Kakovics (Eds.), *A clinical manual of psychiatry* (pp. 131–138). New York: Elsevier/North Holland.

Cohen, G.D. (1983). Alzheimer's disease—the human concept. In R. Katzman (Ed.), *Biological aspects of Alzheimer's disease* (pp. 3–6). Cold Spring Harbor, NY: Banbury Reports.

Cohen, G.D. (1983). Senile dementia and Alzheimer's disease: Historical views and evolution of concepts. In B. Reisberg (Ed.), *Alzheimer's disease* (pp. 29–33). New York: The Free Press.

Cohen, G.D. (1984). Treatment of Alzheimer's disease and related disorders: Research, practice, and policy. In W.E. Kelley (Ed.), *Alzheimer's disease and related disorders: Research and management* (pp. 3–17). Springfield, IL: Charles C. Thomas.

Crook, T., & Cohen, G.D. (1984). Future directions for alcohol research in the elderly. In J.T. Hartford & T. Samorajski (Eds.), *Alcoholism in the elderly* (pp. 277–282). New York: Raven Press.

Cohen, G.D. (1985). Mental health aspects of nursing home care. In E.L. Schneider et al. (Eds.), *The teaching nursing home* (pp. 157–164). New York: Raven Press.

Cohen, G.D. (1985). Psychotherapy with an eighty-year old patient. In R.A. Nemiroff & C.A. Colaruso (Eds.), *The race against time* (pp. 195–204). New York: Plenum Press.

Cohen, G.D. (1985). The future of psychotherapy and the elderly. In C.M. Gaitz & T. Samorajski (Eds.), *Aging 2000: Our health care destiny* (pp. 497–507). New York: Springer-Verlag.

Cohen, G.D. (1985). Toward an interface of mental and physical health phenomena in geriatrics: Clinical findings and questions. In C.M. Gaitz & T. Samorajski (Eds.), *Aging 2000: Our health care destiny* (pp. 283–299). New York: Springer-Verlag.

Cohen, G.D. (1987). Alzheimer's disease. In G.L. Maddox (Ed.), *The encyclopedia of aging* (pp. 27–30). New York: Springer.

Cohen, G.D. (1988). Disease models of aging: Brain and behavior considerations. In J.E. Birren & V.L. Bengtson (Eds.), *Emergent theories in aging* (pp. 83–89). New York: Springer.

Cohen, G.D. (1988). One psychiatrist's view. In L. Jarvik & C. Winograd (Eds.), *Treatments for the Alzheimer's patient—the long haul* (pp. 96–104). New York: Springer.

Cohen, G.D. (1989). Psychodynamic perspectives in the clinical approach to brain disease in the elderly. In D.K. Conn, A. Grek, & J. Sadavoy (Eds.), *Psychiatric consequences of brain disease in the elderly* (pp. 85–99). New York: Plenum Press.

Cohen, G.D. (1989). The geriatric patient. In T.B. Karasu (Ed.), *Treatments of psychiatric disorders*, Vol. 2 (pp. 800–803). Washington, DC: American Psychiatric Association.

Cohen, G.D. (1990). Lessons from longitudinal studies on mentally ill and mentally healthy elderly: A 17 year perspective. In M. Bergener & S.I. Finkel (Eds.), *Clinical and scientific psychogeriatrics*, Vol. 1 (pp. 135–148). New York: Springer.

Cohen, G.D. (1990). Normal changes and patterns of psychiatric disease in aging. In *The Merck manual of geriatrics* (pp. 995–1004). Rahway, NJ: Merck Sharp & Dohme Research Laboratories.

Cohen, G.D. (1991). Anxiety and general medical disorders. In C. Salzman & B.D. Lebowitz (Eds.), *Anxiety in the elderly* (pp. 47–62). New York: Springer.

Cohen, G.D. (1991). Directions and developments in research on aging. In J.L. Albarède & P. Vellas (Eds.), *L'Année Gérontologique facts and research in gerontology* (pp. 295–300). Paris: Serdi.

Cohen, G.D. (1992). Aging. In *McGraw-Hill encyclopedia of science & technology*, 7th ed., Vol. I (pp. 173–174). New York: McGraw Hill.

Cohen, G.D. (1992). Alzheimer's disease: Current policy initiatives. In R.H. Binstock, S.G. Post, & P. Whitehouse (Eds.), *Dementia: Moral and policy issues*. Baltimore: Johns Hopkins University Press.

Cohen, G.D. (1992). Development of subspecialization for geriatric psychiatry in the United States. In M. Bergener, K. Hasegawa, S.I. Finkel, & T. Nishimura (Eds.), *Aging and mental disorders: International perspectives* (pp. 407–412). New York: Springer.

Cohen, G.D. (1992). The future of mental health and aging. In J.E. Birren, R.B. Sloane, & G.D. Cohen (Eds.), *Handbook of mental health and aging* (pp. 893–914). New York: Academic Press.

Lebowitz, B.D., & Cohen, G.D. (1992). Introduction: Older Americans and their illness. In C. Salzman (Ed.), *Clinical geriatric psychopharmacology* (pp. 3–14). Baltimore: Williams & Williams.

Cohen, G.D. (1994). Linkages between public and private sectors. In J. Copeland, M. Abou-Saleh, & D. Blazer (Eds.), *The psychiatry of old age: An international textbook* (pp. 157.1–157.4). Chichester, UK: John Wiley & Sons.

Cohen, G.D. (1995). Normal changes and patterns of psychiatric disease in aging. In W.B. Abrams, M.H. Beers, & R. Berkow (Eds.), *The Merck manual of geriatrics*, 2nd ed. (pp 1215–1225). Rahway, NJ: Merck Sharp & Dohme Research Laboratories.

Cohen, G.D. (1996). Commentary: The role of values in influencing ethical, legal, and policy decisions. In M. Smyer, K.W. Schaie, & M.B. Kapp (Eds.), *Older adults' decision-making and the law* (pp. 175–181). New York: Springer.

Cohen, G.D. (1996). Neuropsychiatric aspects of aging. In J.C. Bennett & F. Plum (Eds.), *Cecil textbook of medicine,* 20th ed. (pp. 17–21). Philadelphia: W.B. Saunders.

Cohen, G.D. (1997). Gaps and failures in attending to mental health and aging in long-term care. In R.L. Rubinstein & M. Powell Lawton (Eds.). *Depression in long-term and residential care* (pp. 211–233). New York: Springer.

Cohen, G.D. (1998). Health, modifiability, and human potential with aging. In T.T. Yoshikawa, E.L Cobbs, & K. Brummel-Smith (Eds.), *Ambulatory geriatric care,* 2nd ed. St. Louis: Mosby.

Lebowitz, B.D., Pearson, J., & Cohen, G.D. (1998). Older Americans and their illnesses. In C. Salzman (Ed.)., *Clinical geriatric psychopharmacology,* 3rd ed. (pp. 3–20).

Cohen, G.D. (1999). Creativity and healthy aging. In K. Dychtwald (Ed.), *Healthy aging* (pp. 145–153). Gaithersburg, MD: Aspen Publishers.

Cohen, G.D. (1999). Mental health and the future of elders. In M.L. Wykle & A.B. Ford (Eds.), *Serving minority elders in the 21st century* (pp 131–146). New York: Springer.

Cohen, G.D. (2000). A brief history of geriatric psychiatry in the United States, 1944_1994. In R.W. Menninger & J.C. Nemiah (eds.), *American psychiatry after World War II, 1944–1994* (pp. 481–501). Washington, DC: American Psychiatric Press.

Cohen, G.D. (2000). Aging and mental health. In M.H. Beers & R. Berkow (Eds.), *The Merck manual of geriatrics,* 3rd ed. (pp. 307–310). Whitehouse Station, NJ: Merck Research Laboratories.

Cohen, G.D. (2003). The social portfolio: The role of activity in mental wellness as people age. In J.L. Ronch & J.A. Goldfield (Eds.), *Mental wellness in aging* (pp. 113–122). Baltimore: Health Professions Press.

Cohen, G.D. (2006). The geriatric patient. In M.A. Agronin & G.J. Maletta (Eds.), *Principles and practice of geriatric psychiatry* (pp. 3–16). Philadelphia: Lippincott, Williams & Wilkins.

Edited books and special journal issues guest edited

Cohen, G.D. (Guest Editor). (1979/1980). Community mental health programs for the elderly. *International Journal of Mental Health* (Fall/Winter--Double Issue).

Crook, T., & Cohen, G.D. (Eds.). (1981). *Physicians' handbook on psychotherapeutic drug use in the aged.* New Canaan, CT: Mark Powley Associates.

Miller, N.E., & Cohen, G.D. (Eds.). (1981). *Clinical aspects of Alzheimer's disease and senile dementia.* New York: Raven Press.

Cohen, G.D. (Guest Editor). (1982). Special issue on mental health and aging. *Hospital and Community Psychiatry.*

Crook, T., & Cohen, G.D. (Eds.). (1983). *Physicians' guide to the diagnosis and treatment of depression in the elderly.* New Canaan, CT: Mark Powley Associates.

Miller, N.E., & Cohen, G.D. (Eds.). (1987). *Schizophrenia and aging.* New York: Guilford Press.

Birren, J.E., Sloane, R.B., & Cohen, G.D. (Eds.). (1992). *Handbook of mental health and aging* (2nd ed.). New York: Academic Press.

Individually authored books

Cohen, G.D. (1988). *The brain in human aging.* New York: Springer. (Also published in Spanish and Portuguese)

Cohen, G.D. (2000). *The creative age: Awakening human potential in the second half of life.* New York: Avon Books/Harper Collins [hardcover].

Cohen, G.D. (2001). *The creative age: Awakening human potential in the second half of life.* New York: Quill/Harper Collins [paperback]. (Also published in Japanese)

Cohen, G.D. (2004). *Uniting the heart and mind: Human development in the second half of life.* San Francisco: American Society on Aging Mind Alert Publication.

Cohen, G.D. (2005). *The mature mind: The positive power of the aging brain.* New York: Basic Books [hardcover]

Cohen, G.D. (2006). *The mature mind: The positive power of the aging brain.* New York: Basic Books [paperback]. (Translated into six other languages in six other countries)

Posthumous publications

Cohen, G.D. (2010). Creativity and aging. In T.R. Cole, R. Kastenbaum, & R.E. Ray (Eds.), *A guide to humanistic studies in aging.* Baltimore: Johns Hopkins University Press.

Cohen, G.D. (2010). Creativity in later life. In the *Encyclopedia of the sociology of the life course.* Farmington Hills, MI: Gale Publishers.

Cohen, G.D., & Miller, W. (2010). In T.R. Cole & K. de Medeiros (Eds.), Special Section: A Tribute to Gene D. Cohen. *Journal of Aging, Humanities, and the Arts, 4*(4), 235–311.

Notes

Epigraph

1. See http://www.creativeaging.org/dr-gene-d-cohen-research-award-creativity-and-aging and http://ce.columbia.edu/narrative-medicine/news/dr-rita-charon-will-receive-2014-gene-d-cohen-award for a better understanding of Rita Charon, recipient of the Gene D. Cohen Research Award in Creativity and Aging, sponsored by both the Gerontological Society of America (GSA) and the National Center for Creative Aging (NCCA) since 2009. The epigraph comes from her November 6, 2014, lecture at the GSA's annual scientific meeting "Making Connections from Cells to Societies," November 5–9, 2014, in Washington, DC, where Charon received the award.

Foreword

1. See http://www.nytimes.com/2009/11/12/us/12cohen.html and http://www.washingtonpost.com/wp- dyn/content/article/2009/11/10/AR2009111018634.html and http://gwtoday.gwu.edu/memoriam-gene-cohen for Gene Cohen's expanded obituaries.
2. See http://smhs.gwu.edu/gwish/about/dr-puchalski for a better understanding of Christina Puchalski, founder and director of the George Washington Institute for Spirituality and Health (GWISH), and professor of medicine and health sciences at George Washington University School of Medicine.

Preface

1. See Cohen (2000) for further explanation of aging stereotypes as "weird, wicked, wick," in *If you were an old woman who lived in a shoe, what would you do? American Journal of Geriatric Psychiatry*, 8(2), 93.
2. See Hasrick, Messinger, Novak, Rose, and Georgia O'Keeffe Museum (1997) for further information on O'Keeffe's "Sky Above Clouds" paintings, in *The Georgia O'Keeffe Museum* (pp. 44-45). New York: Harry N. Abrams, Inc., in association with the Georgia O'Keefe Museum.

Introduction

1. See Thomas (1957) for a better look at Carol's reference, "do not go gentle into the night," in *The Collected Poems of Dylan Thomas* (p. 128). New York: New Directions.
2. See http://cahh.gwu.edu/founders-tribute for a better understanding of George Washington University's Center on Aging, Health and Humanities.

3. See www.dccenteronaging.org for a better understanding of the Washington DC Center on Aging, a non-profit organization created by Gene Cohen that continues to launch innovative projects focusing on intergenerational communication and older persons as a national resource.

4. See www.genco-games.com for a better understanding of Genco games, from the game company GENCO, created by Gene Cohen, that specializes in board games that are at the same time educational, intergenerational, and artistic. In addition, the games contain built-in mental exercises for aging; vocabulary, for example, is a mental skill that research shows can improve with practice at least into one's 80s.

5. The boomer generation refers to those born between the years 1946 and 1964. The phrase "sandwich generation" refers to people who care for their aging parents while supporting their own children. The phrase "sideways generation" refers to people who were caring for parents and children and facing health crises within their own generation of siblings and friends.

6. See www.artsandhealthalliance.org for a better understanding of the Society for the Arts in Healthcare (SAH), a professional organization dedicated to advancing arts as integral to healthcare and supporting research into the beneficial effects of the arts in healthcare. Both Cohen and Miller were SAH members. Their 2007 presentation at the conference was titled "Developmental Intelligence & Integrative Intelligence—Impact on Creativity, Healing & Cultural Responsibility."

7. See Kierkegaard and Hannay (1996) for a better understanding of how we view living our life, in *Papers and journals: A selection* (p. 63). New York: Penguin Books.

8. See Frankl (1959) for a better understanding of the need for meaning, in *Man's search for meaning: An introduction to logotherapy* (p. 107). Boston: Beacon Press.

Chapter 1

1. See Cousins (1979) for a better understanding of the reluctance to write due to anecdotal value, in *Anatomy of an illness as perceived by the patient: Reflections on healing and regeneration* (p. 27). New York: W.W. Norton & Company.

2. See Cohen (2000) for a full story and history of his ALS misdiagnosis, in *The creative age: Awakening human potential in the second half of life* (pp. 177–181). New York: Avon Books.

3. See Rodin (1986) for a closer look at her research on sense of control with older adults, in Aging and health: Effects of the sense of control. *Science, 233*(4770), 20–42.

4. See Rodin (1989) for a closer look at her research on interventions, in Sense of control: Potentials for intervention. *Annals of the American Academy of Policy and Social Science, 503*, 29–42.

5. Natural killer cells are a type of lymphocyte (white blood cell) critical to the innate immune system which play a role in the host rejection of tumors and virally infected cells. See Lutgendorf, Vitaliano, Tripp-Reimer, Harvey, and Lubaroff (1999) for more information on natural killer cells, in Sense of coherence moderates the relationship between life stress and natural killer cell activity in older adults in *Psychology and Aging, 14*(4), 552–563.

6. Psychoneuroimmonology (PNI) is the study of the various kinds of interactions among our psychological systems, our nervous system, and our immune systems. PNI uses an interdisciplinary approach to this study and has transformed our understanding of health and wellness. See Kiecolt-Glazer, McGuire, Robles, and Glazer (2002) for a better understanding of psychoneuroimmunology, in Emotions, morbidity, and mortality: New perspectives from psychoneuroimmunology. in *Annual Review of Psychology, 53*, 83–107.

7. See Pert, Dreher, and Ruff (1998) for further information on psychoneuroimmunology, in The psychosomatic network: Foundations of mind-body medicine. *Alternative Therapies*, 4(4), 30–41.

8. See http://www.smithcenter.org/ for a better understanding of Smith Center for Healing and the Arts, which is a non-profit health, education, and arts organization in Washington, DC, whose mission is to develop and promote healing practices that explore physical, emotional, and mental resources that lead to life-affirming changes for people affected by cancer. As well, Miller was part of an original brainstorming group of artists, educators, and healthcare professionals brought together by Barbara Smith Coleman for the Smith Center for Healing and the Arts, a sister program to Commonweal.

9. See http://www.commonweal.org/health-healing/ for a better understanding of Commonweal and their Cancer Help Program, which is featured by Bill Moyers in his award-winning series *Healing and the Mind*. It is also among the foremost residential support programs for people with cancer. In addition, their Institute for the Study of Health and Illness pioneered their healer's art curriculum that is now in 70 medical schools internationally, and the Collaborative on Health and the Environment is the premier global network for environmental health science dialogue.

10. See Huxley (1976) to see how experience is not what happens to a person, in *Texts & pretexts: An anthology with commentaries* (p. 5). Westport, CT: Greenwood Press.

11. See Thoreau (1892) for more discussion of castles in the air, in *Walden, in two volumes* (Vol. 11x, p. 499). Boston: Houghton, Mifflin.

12. See King (1968) for a closer look at hope as the vitality that keeps life moving, in *Trumpet of conscience* (p. 76). New York: Harper and Row.

13. See Havel (1993) for a closer look at how hope is not the mere conviction that something will turn out well, in Never hope against hope. *Esquire*, 68.

Chapter 2

1. See Gene in www.genco-games.com for more history and a full set of cribbage rules and game orders for *The Essential Cribbage Board*.

2. See http://www.cancer.gov/cancertopics/factsheet/detection/PSA for a better understanding of the PSA test and prostate cancer.

3. See http://en.wikipedia.org/wiki/American_International_Toy_Fair for more information on the Toy Fair. It was the 93nd North American International Toy Fair (1996) at the Javits Center in New York City where Cohen first introduced his games *Word Wars III* and *Cribbage*.

4. See Cohen (2005) for a better understanding of postformal thought and to find his extensive bibliography on the literature of postformal thought and aging, in *The mature mind: The positive power of the aging brain* (p. 197). New York: Basic Books. Jean Piaget's work on the four stages of intellectual development, his model of cognitive development, although it stopped at young adulthood with the formal operational stage, was a process-oriented model of development. Many developmentalists describe a fifth stage as postformal thought, which helps us to understand emotions as this thought process integrates the subjective and the objective, our feelings (heart) and our thoughts (mind). In addition, postformal thinking emerges with aging and with the complexity of wisdom, providing us with an ability to understand and compare relationships or systems which may compete with one another; to think less logically and less universally, more relatively and pragmatically; and to appreciate the tension between one's own thinking and that of other people.

5. See Cohen (2005) for a better understanding of the amygdalae with aging, in *The mature mind: The positive power of the aging brain* (pp. 14–18). New York: Basic Books.

6. See Cohen (2005) for a closer look at developmental intelligence as wisdom, in *The mature mind: The positive power of the aging brain* (pp. 34–39, 95). New York: Basic Books.

7. See http://www.cancer.org/treatment/treatmentsandsideeffects/guidetocancerdrugs/docetaxel for a better understanding of Taxotere, a chemotherapeutic medicine that is also called docetaxel and Docefrez. It is a cancer medication used for prostate cancer that interferes with the growth and spread of cancer cells in the body.

8. See http://en.wikipedia.org/wiki/Nephrostomy for a better explanation of the procedure of nephrostomy tubes, which refer to an opening created between the kidney and the skin, allowing for urinary diversion from the upper part of the urinary system.

9. See Johnston (1984) for more information on the term capacitance, in *The creative imperative: A four-dimensional theory of human growth and planetary evolution* (p. 58). Berkeley, CA: Celestial Arts.

10. See http://plato.stanford.edu/entries/paradox-zeno/ for a better look at the difference between Zeno's and Socrates' Age, providing background information for Cohen's constructed reference to Zeno's fifth paradox.

11. See http://examinedexistence.com/the-four-states-of-competence-explained/ for a deeper understanding of unconscious competence, a phrase taught to Miller by her Union Institute Ph.D. advisor, Penny MacElveen-Hoehn, for trusting inner knowledge to make connections. Academically, it comes from a learning model developed in the 1970s by Noel Burch describing the processes one develops learning new skills. Additionally, see Miller's elaboration on unconscious competence, in Miller and Milliken (2002). Pushing the experiential edge in therapy, training and supervision: A case study of Create Therapy Institute's experiential supervision program. *Poiesis: A Journal of the Arts and Communication, 4*, 87–88.

12. See http://talltimo.blogspot.com/2009/03/cribbage-rhymes.html for an informal reference on cribbage rhymes.

Chapter 3

1. See Kleinman (1988) for a better distinction between illness and disease, in *The illness narratives: Suffering, healing, and the human condition* (pp. 3–8). New York: Basic Books.

2. See Frank (1991) for more information on how a critical illness offers us the experience of being taken to the threshold of life, in *At the will of the body: Reflections on illness* (p. 1). Boston: Houghton Mifflin.

3. See the McGraw-Hill/Glencoe Companies biology textbook (2009) for a description of forest fires in Eliana's ninth-grade biology class, in *Biology* (p. 62). Columbus, OH: McGraw–Hill.

4. See http://www.webmd.com/heart-disease/electrocardiogram for a better understanding of electrocardiography (EKG or ECG), a test that checks the electrical activity of each of the chambers in the heart to look for the source of possible problems.

5. Create Therapy Institute was cofounded by Wendy Miller and Rebecca Milliken. The institute offers mind–body approaches to health through therapy, training, and the expressive arts and is currently located in Kensington, MD (301-652-7183).

6. Gene had been treated successfully through hormone therapy from the time of his initial metastatic diagnosis in 1996. He took Nilandron, also known generically as nilutamide, daily, had shots of Lupron, and took the bisphosphonate Zometa to prevent further bone damage. This form of treatment is called an androgen blockade, depriving the cancer cells of testosterone so they can become dormant. When the cancer cells became no longer hormone sensitive, the therapies stopped working, and his metastatic cancer returned. Only then was he treated with monthly rounds of chemotherapy.

7. See http://chemocare.com/chemotherapy/drug-info/cytoxan.aspx#.VO90zChqnaI for a better understanding of Cytoxan, also known generically as cyclophosphamide, or Neostar, the anti-cancer chemotherapy drug that works to slow or stop cell growth.

Chapter 4

1. See Carroll (1962) for a further elaboration of Alice in the well, in Chapter 1: Down the rabbit hole, in *Alice's adventures in wonderland and through the looking glass* (pp. 24–25). Baltimore: Penguin Books.
2. See Schopenhauer (1974) for a better understanding of all things following one another, in *On the fourfold of the principle of sufficient reason* (p. 32). New York: Cosimo Classics.
3. See Wells (1927) for a better understanding of time as a fourth dimension, in Time Machine, in *The short stories of H.G. Wells* (p. 11). London: Ernest Benn.
4. See Cicero and King (1950) for how the Roman orator and statesman Cicero describes the sword of Damocles, in Book V, item 61, in *Cicero: XVIII Tusculan disputations* (p. 487). Cambridge, MA: Harvard University Press.
5. See Cohen (2009) in the Appendix for more information on his qualitative interview findings from his boomer research study summary (unpublished).
6. See Cohen (2000) for a closer look at his George Burns story, in *The creative age: Awakening human potential in the second half of life* (pp. 175, 190). New York: Avon Books.
7. See Williams and Rosenthal (1966) for the concept of age that adds as it takes away, in The Catholic bells, in *The William Carlos Williams reader* (p. 38). New York: New Directions.
8. See Pandora's Box (n.d.) in the *Oxford English Dictionary* for further information on Pandora. Retrieved from http://www.oed.com.proxy-um.researchport.umd.edu. In addition, see Hesiod and Sinclair (1979) for Hesiod's poem on Pandora, in *Works and days* (p. 11). New York: Arno Press, which shows that in Greek mythology, Pandora was sent to Earth to be with Prometheus' brother, Epimetheus. When she arrived, she found another gift from the gods—a jar into which each god had put something. Pandora was warned not to open it, but she was overcome by curiosity. As she lifted the lid to peek inside, all the evils in the world flew out, including disease. She quickly replaced the lid, but it was too late because troubles had already covered the world. The only thing left in the jar was hope.
9. See the 1939 musical film *Wizard of Oz* for a better reference to the hourglass, in the production by Metro-Goldwyn-Mayer based on Baum (1900) *The wonderful wizard of Oz*.

Chapter 5

1. See Hamilton (1937) for translations of this passage from Aeschylus, in *Three Greek plays: Prometheus bound, Agamemnon, the Trojan women* (p. 161). New York: W.W. Norton & Co. But these words, as quoted, are closest to those used by Robert F. Kennedy, in his famous eulogy to Martin Luther King, Jr., the evening of April 4, 1968, in Indianapolis, Indiana; retrieved from http://www.pbs.org/wgbh/americanexperience/features/primary-resources/kennedys-death-mlk/
2. See http://www.tcm.com/mediaroom/video/336525/Wait-Until-Dark-Original-Trailer-.html for Audrey Hepburn in *Wait Until Dark*.
3. See http://www.hallmarkmoviesandmysteries.com/perry-mason for *Perry Mason* on TV.
4. See Jung (1966) for more information on enantiodromia, in *Two essays on analytical psychology*, Bollingen Series XX, *The collected works of C.G. Jung*, Vol. 7 (p. 73). Princeton, NJ: Princeton University Press. Enantiodromia is a term which Jung wrote about extensively on the psychology of the unconscious to describe the regulatory function of opposites. Miller uses the term *enantiodromia* as a visceral description of the pulls

within consciousness. She uses the terms more mythopoetically than psychologically to describe the pulls and tensions of illness experiences.

5. See http://en.wikipedia.org/wiki/Bisphosphonate for a better understanding of bisphosphonates, a class of drugs that prevent the loss of bone mass.

6. See http://www.nih.gov/about/ for more information on the National Institutes of Health (NIH), a part of the U.S. Department of Health and Human Services, which is the nation's medical research agency. After Cohen graduated in 1970 from the Georgetown University School of Medicine and started his residency in psychiatry there, he was drafted into the U.S. Public Health Service (1973) during the Viet Nam War and assigned to work at the National Institute of Mental Health (NIMH) at NIH. Then, in 1975, NIMH director Bert Brown appointed Gene as the first director of the Center for Studies of the Mental Health of Aging, the first federal research program on mental health and aging established in any country. It predated the creation of the National Institute on Aging, under the helm of Robert Butler, by 6 months.

7. See Lerner (1994) for a better understanding of cancer alternative treatments and choices, in *Choices in healing: Integrating the best of conventional and complementary approaches to cancer.* Cambridge, MA: MIT Press.

8. See Ginsburg and Milken (1998) for a better understanding of Gene's low-fat diet, in *The taste for living cookbook: Mike Milken's favorite recipes for fighting cancer.* Boston: Allen & Osborne.

9. See Broek (1972) for more information about the phoenix, in *The myth of the phoenix, according to classical and early Christian traditions.* Leiden: E.J. Brill.

10. See van Gelder (1977) for more information on the nature of fairies, in *The real world of fairies: A first-person account.* Wheaton, IL: Quest Books.

11. See http://www.commonweal.org for a closer look at Commonweal. Michael Lerner is president of Commonweal, a healing center in Bolinas, California, and of Smith Center for Healing and the Arts, in Washington, DC. He is cofounder (with Rachel Naomi Remen) of the Commonweal Cancer Help Program, as well as the collaborative on health and the environment, healthcare without harm, and the new school at Commonweal. And see http://www.commonweal.org/program/commonweal-cancer-help-program/ for more information on the reference to the goal of Commonweal's Cancer Help Program.

12. See Remen (1996) for more information on health and healing, in *Kitchen table wisdom: Stories that heal.* New York: Riverhead Books.

13. Multiple myeloma is described by the Mayo Clinic as a cancer that forms in a type of white blood cell called a plasma cell, which are the cells that help fight infections by making antibodies to recognize and attack germs. In addition, multiple myeloma causes cancer cells to accumulate in the bone marrow, where they push out healthy blood cells, not making helpful antibodies but producing abnormal proteins that cause problems. Definition retrieved from: http://www.mayoclinic.org/diseases-conditions/multiple-myeloma/basics/definition/con-20026607.

14. See Miller (1992) for a closer look at a dissertation on patients with chronic fatigue syndrome, in *The experience of nine women living with chronic fatigue syndrome, as demonstrated through mental imagery, drawings, and verbal description.* University Microfilms International (9219128); can be retrieved at 800-521-0600 (Ann Arbor, MI). Chronic fatigue syndrome (CFS) has been called by a variety of names, including epidemic myalgia, myalgic encephalomyelitis, chronic viral syndrome, chronic mononucleosis, chronic fatigue immune dysfunction syndrome, and post-viral fatigue syndrome. The syndrome is characterized by extreme fatigue, sore throats, headaches, low-grade fever, body muscle aches, neurological problems, impairment in memory and concentration, and swollen or tender lymph nodes. Causes of CFS include some kind of post-viral disruptions of immune functions, as well as chemical and/or environmental exposures. Also see Miller (1992) for a portrait of the illness in the Phase Diagram, in *My healing journey through chronic fatigue. Yoga Journal,* Nov/Dec, pp. 62–67, 123–125.

15. Miller's reference to her study and training in psychosynthesis took place in San Francisco, CA, during the years 1984–1987, with psychosynthesis clinicians Carl Peters, Rachel Naomi Remen, Phillip Brooks, and Lenore Lefer. In addition, psychosynthesis is an approach to humanistic and transpersonal psychology, developed by the Italian psychiatrist Roberto Assagioli. The focus is on the work of integration of the personality around the core self, using imagery exercises and the study of the will. See Assagioli (1965) for a better understanding of his psychosythesis theory, in *Psychosynthesis: A manual of principles and techniques*. New York: Hobbs, Dorman & Co. See Assagioli (1973) for a closer look on the development of the will, in *The act of will*. Middlesex, England & New York: Penguin Books.

16. See Williams and Rosenthal (1966) for the concept of age that adds as it takes away, in "The Catholic Bells," in *The William Carlos Williams reader* (p. 38). New York: New Directions.

17. See Hanna and Perlstein (2008) for more information on Cohen's quote about potential and creativity. In addition, this quote from his PowerPoint talks and webinars has been reproduced by the National Center for Creative Aging (NCCA) for their conferences on creativity and aging and can be retrieved from *Creativity Matters: Arts and Aging in America*, September monograph published by the Americans for the Arts.

18. See Cohen (2000) for an elaboration on creativity as an intellectual process, in *The creative age: Awakening human potential in the second half of life* (p. 176). New York: Avon Books.

19. See Cohen (2000) for a closer look at creativity and the way that it alters our thinking, in *The creative age: Awakening human potential in the second half of life* (pp. 12–13). New York: Avon Books.

20. See Cox and Heller (2006) (eds.) for a closer look at orchids growing in skinny spaces, in *Portrait of the artist as poet* (p. 121). Chicago: Magnolia Street Publishers.

21. *Creative faculty* is a term we have defined to encompass creative ability, creative spirit, creative mastery, and the wellspring of resources from which these all arise.

22. See http://nypost.com/2014/04/20/how-a-brain-injury-turned-a-college-dropout-into-a-genius/ and April 22, 2014, http://www.fox4news.com/story/25305307/head-injusry-turns-man-into-math-whiz for a clearer understanding of the story of Jason Padgett.

23. Penny MacElveen-Hoehn was Miller's core advisor during her Ph.D. studies at The Union Institute where MacElveen-Hoehn was a professor for 28 years, facilitating many learners to earn their doctorates. In addition, she was at the University of Washington for 21 years, as assistant professor in the Department of Psychosocial Nursing as well as a nurse researcher fellow in the Department of Parent and Child Nursing, where her research was on the correlation between social networks and positive patient outcomes. Also, she was one of the cofounders of Hospice of Seattle.

Chapter 6

1. See Miller (1992) for a better understanding of the background and development of the Phase Diagram, in *The experience of nine women living with chronic fatigue syndrome, as demonstrated through mental imagery, drawings, and verbal description* [PhD dissertation] (pp. 211–225). Ann Arbor, MI: University Microfilms International #9219128. Additionally, see Miller (1997) for more information on the Phase Diagram, in *Imagery, art and health: Excerpts form a series of presentations on art as complementary medicine. C.R.E.A.T.E.: Journal of the Creative and Expressive Arts Therapy Exchange, 6,* 41–46.

2. See Cohen (2005) for more information on the inner push and the phases, in *The mature mind: The positive power of the aging brain*. New York: Basic Books.

3. See Cohen (2000) for more information on his creativity equation, in *The creative age: Awakening human potential in the second half of life* (pp. 34–38). New York: Avon Books.

4. See Erikson (1997) for more information on the ninth stage of psychological development, in *The life cycle completed: Extended version with new chapters on the ninth stage of development by Joan Erikson.* New York and London: W.W. Norton & Co.

5. See Cohen (2000) for a closer look at wisdom as a developmental product, reviving our lives, and better understanding of formal thought, in *The creative age: Awakening human potential in the second half of life* (p. 77). New York: Avon Books.

Chapter 7

1. See Ross (1976) for *The seven-per-cent solution: Sherlock Holmes meets Sigmund Freud* [motion picture]. United States: Universal Pictures. Also, see http://www.tcm.com/this-month/article/111437%7C0/The-Seven-Per-Cent-Solution.html for some quotes taken from the 1976 screenplay of *The Seven Percent Solution* and other quotes by Holmes and Freud, from Nicolas Meyer's 1974 novel, *The seven-per-cent solution: Being a reprint from the reminiscences of John H. Watson, M.D.* New York: EP Dutton. The "seven percent solution" refers to a 7% solution of cocaine used by Sherlock Holmes.

2. See Boorstin (2001) for a closer look at how the greatest obstacle to discovery is not ignorance but illusion of knowledge, in *The discoverers: A history of man's search to know his world and himself* (Chapter 11, p. 134). London: Phoenix.

3. See Ming and Song (2005) for a better understanding of Ramon and Cajal on neurogenesis, in Adult neurogenesis in the mammalian central nervous system. *Annual Review of Neuroscience, 28,* 223–225. In addition, see http://webvision.med.utah.edu/book/part-x-primary-visual-cortex/regeneration-in-the-visual-system-of-adult-mammals/ for more information on Ramon y Cajal. *Neurogenesis* means the birth of neurons and refers to the process by which new nerve cells are generated from neural stem cells and from progenitor cells.

4. See Kiester, Jr. and Kiester (2002) for information on Fernando Nottebohm, in Birdbrain breakthrough: Startling evidence that the human brain can grow new nerves began with unlikely studies of birdsong. *Smithsonian Magazine,* June, p. 2 Also, see Nottebohm (2002) for a closer look on his work in neurogenesis, in Neurogenesis in embryos and in adult neural stem cells. *Journal of Neuroscience, 22*(3), 624–642.

5. See Kempermann, Kuhn, and Gage (1998) for a better understanding of neurogenesis, in Experience-induced neurogenesis in the senescent dentate gyrus. *Journal of Neuroscience, 18*(9), 3206–3212.

6. See http://www.neoamericanist.org/paper/woody-allen-and-golden-age-kitsch for more information on Woody Allen and his train description in Gene's dreams. Allen's description also can be found in Clarkson, S. (2011–2012). Woody Allen and the golden age of kitsch. *NeoAmericanist, 5*(2; Fall/Winter) [original publication].

7. *Authority of the unconscious* is a term that Miller has defined to discuss many elements and voices of our creative faculty and the knowledge that accompanies it. Certainly these ideas of the unconscious and its power or authority have been discussed in many schools of psychology, including those of Freud, Jung, Assagioli, and others.

8. See Goethe (1797) for more on the poem "The Sorcerer's Apprentice," in which a sorcerer's apprentice becomes tired of getting water using a pail so he uses a spell on a broom to do the work for him, but because he is not trained in magic, he does not know how to stop the brooms and the floor become increasingly filled with water.

9. *Creative faculty* is a term we have defined to encompass creative ability, creative spirit, creative mastery, and the wellspring of resources from which these all arise.

10. See White, Wilbur, and Panzer, (1995) for a closer look at the Perils of Pauline, in *The perils of Pauline, 1914: The hidden voice.* Phoenix, AZ: Grapevine.

11. See Spengler and Donner (1978) for a better understanding of Cohen's dream reference to the movie where Superman's girlfriend, Lois Lane, died in *Superman* [Motion picture]. United States: Warner Bros.

12. See http://www.thegreatharryhoudini.com/ for a closer look at Houdini.

13. See http://www.theartstory.org for a reference to a De Chirico surrealist painting in Cohen's dream.

14. See Huggins, R. (1958–1964) for more information on the television show "77 Sunset Strip," in *77 Sunset Strip* [Television series]. (Hollywood, CA: American Broadcasting Company).

15. See Knill, Barba, and Fuchs (1995) for better understanding of the concepts of inter-modal expressive arts process, the theory of crystallization, and the arrival of the third, developed by expressive arts therapist Paulo Knill, in *Minstrels of soul: Intermodal expressive therapy* (pp. 33–38, 123–124, and 131–138; Palmerston Press). The phrase "intermodal in expressive arts therapy" refers to the use of various modalities—image, sound, movement, words, action—combined with various art disciplines—visual art, music, dance, literature, and theater. It could also be called an integrated use of the arts in psychotherapy. Crystallization theory refers to the basic human drive to move toward clarity in feeling and thought. When material is crystallized, our experience seems right to us. The arts and imagination as sensory and communication modalities help us come to meaning phenomenologically, and in this way our language of imagination coalesces as crystallization. Arrival of the third refers to emergence of the imaginal realm, Examples would be a gift or presence in an encounter in art making or between parts of self, or in the encounter between therapist and client. Serving this encounter requires an openness to uncertainty, as this arrival is usually an unexpected surprise, becoming what Knill calls the transmediated. Expressive arts theory is based on serving this transmediated process because practicing the arts exercises this attitude of respect for the arrival of this emergent third.

16. See Bollas (1989) for a closer look at the concept of not knowing and the unthought known, in *Forces of destiny: Psychoanalysis and human idiom* (p. 63). London: Free Association Books. Christopher Bollas is an object relations theorist who has written extensively on the "unthought known" and "unknowing," which represents experiences we have which are known to us, but we are unable to think about them.

17. See Winnicott (1989) for a better understanding of the concept of transitional phenom-enon, in *Playing and reality* (p. 2). New York: Routledge. D.W. Winnicott is an object relations theorist who has written extensively on transitional space and transitional phe-nomenon based on attachment theories of child development.

18. See Assagioli (1965) for more information on the development and integration of the personality within the self, in *Psychosynthesis: A manual of principles and tech-niques*. New York: Hobbs, Dorman & Co. Also, see Assagioli (1973) for more infor-mation on the development of the will, in *The act of will*. Middlesex, England & New York: Penguin Books.

19. See Frank (1991) for a better understanding of illness writing, in *At the will of the body: Reflections on illness*. Boston: Houghton Mifflin. Also, see Kleinman (1988), in *The illness narratives: Suffering, healing, and the human condition*. New York: Basic Books. See Charon (2006) for a closer look at her narratives of illness, in *Narrative medicine: Honoring the stories of illness*. New York: Oxford University Press, as well as Remen (1996) for more on health and wellness, in *Kitchen table wisdom: Stories that heal*. New York: Riverhead Books.

20. See Johnston (1984) for a better understanding of formative theory, in *The Creative imper-ative: A four-dimensional theory of human growth and planetary evolution* (p. 11). Berkeley, CA: Celestial Arts.

21. See http://www.cancer.org/treatment/treatmentsandsideeffects/guidetocancerdrugs/docetaxel for a better understanding of Taxotere, a chemotherapeutic medicine that is also called docetaxel and Docefrez. It is a cancer medication used for prostate cancer that interferes with the growth and spread of cancer cells in the body.

Chapter 8

1. See Rosenberg (2010) for a better understanding of Brooke Astor and the case, in Regrettably unfair: Brooke Astor and the other elderly in New York. *Pace Law Review, 30*(3), 1004–1060. Robert Morgenthau was the longest serving district attorney for New York County in Manhattan, serving from 1975 to 2009. He is the second longest-serving district attorney in U.S. history. Serving nine terms in office, homicides in Manhattan were reduced by over 90% and his staff conducted approximately 3.5 million criminal prosecutions.
2. See http://www.ehow.com/how_5312998_make-diamonds-coal.html, Robinson (n.d.), for more information on how to make diamonds into coal.
3. See Freedman (1994) for the book mentioned in the Astor trial, titled *Clock drawing: A neuropsychological analysis* (New York: Oxford University Press).
4. See the Appendix for Cohen's complete editorial, "What is a Lucid Moment?"
5. The pericardium is a thin double-layered sac which encloses the heart. Normally, fluid is contained within these layers, but due to hardening of the pericardium from chemotherapy, it became difficult for Cohen's heart to stretch properly when it beat, therefore making it hard to breathe. Retrieved from http://www.nlm.nih.gov/medlineplus/ency/imagepages/18081.htm

Chapter 9

1. See Grimm, Grimm, Colum, and Scharl (1972) for the older German fairy tale called "Snow White," written by the Brothers Grimm and published in 1812; tale 53 in *The complete Grimm's fairy tales* (pp. 249–258). New York: Pantheon.
2. See Miller (2016) for the essay on her mother's death, "Do you think that is the face of a dying woman?" in Cox and Harrison (Eds.) (in press). *Saying goodbye to our mothers for the last time: A collection of essays*, Lisa Hagan Books.
3. See McCartney (1967) for the Beatles song "When I'm 64," on *Sgt. Pepper's Lonely Hearts Club Band* [CD] (London: EMI Studios). Also, note that the song is about growing old together. Paul McCarthy was only 16 when he wrote the song but his father was 64 that year.
4. See Hampson (2009) for more information on Cohen, in Gene Cohen: The guru of grey matter. *The Globe and the Mail*, from http://www.theglobeandmail.com/life/the-guru-of-grey-matter/article4212154/
5. See Gould (2002) http://cancerguide.org/median_not_msg.html for more information on statistics and illness, in The median isn't the message, in *CancerGuide,*.
6. See Lerner (1990) for more information on the price paid for honesty about his illness in terms of lecture requests, in *Wrestling with the angel: A memoir of my triumph over illness.* New York: Norton.
7. See Graves (1995) for a better understanding of the Greek mythology of Tiresias and Athena, in *The Greek myths*, Vol. 2 (p. 10). Baltimore: Penguin Books.
8. See http://www.nih.gov/about/almanac/organization/NCCIH.htm for information about the National Center for Complementary and Alternative Medicine (NCCAM), which was established in October 1991 as the Office of Alternative Medicine (OAM), and reestablished as NCCAM in October 1998 to explore complementary and alternative healing practices in the context of rigorous science; train complementary and alternative medicine researchers; and disseminate authoritative information to the public and professionals. Miller makes reference to many writers, doctors, and practitioners of the 1980/90s mind–body health movement, which helped to change the healthcare landscape.

9. See Miller (1992) for more information on chronic fatigue syndrome, in pages 23-42 of *The experience of nine women living with chronic fatigue syndrome, as demonstrated through mental imagery, drawings, and verbal description* [PhD dissertation] (pp. 23–42). Ann Arbor, MI: University Microfilms International, #9219128.

Chapter 10

1. See Schnabel (1958) for a better understanding of pauses between the notes, in Kundtz, D. (1998). *Stopping: How to be still when you have to keep going* (p. 42; Berkeley, CA: Conari Press). In addition, Artur Schnabel's quote was first quoted on page 4 of the *Chicago Daily News*, June 11, 1958.
2. See Hemingway (1995) for a better understanding of his reflections, in *The Old Man and the Sea* (p. 103). New York: Scribner.
3. *Lossness* is a term Miller has made up to refer to the phenomenological state in which the experience of loss, seemingly invisibly, seeps into many other aspects of a person's life.
4. See Joyce (1997) for Molly Brown's soliloquy, in *Ulysses*. London: Picador.
5. "Twilight zone" is a reference to the 1959 television series created by Rod Steiger called *The Twilight Zone*. It was a series of stories filled with drama, science fiction, tension, and suspense, always with an unexpected twist. Retrieved from http://en.wikipedia.org/wiki/The_Twilight_Zone
6. Denial can be known as a defense mechanism used to protect one's ego from things that are difficult to cope with. The concept implies that a person is not able to face an aspect of reality or recognize that something has happened.
7. See Abood, Chase, Pappalardo-Robinson, Rounds, Budd, and Cook (2002) for a closer look at Tinker Bell's light, in *Return to Never Land* [Motion picture] (United States: Buena Vista Pictures).
8. See LeShan (1989) for more information on working with cancer patients, in *Cancer as a turning point: A handbook for people with cancer, their families, and health professionals*. New York: Dutton. In addition, Miller's personal conversation comes from a 1990 Washington, DC lecture.

Chapter 11

1. See http://en.wikipedia.org/wiki/Bisphosphonate for a better understanding of bisphosphonates, a class of drugs that prevent the loss of bone mass.
2. See Allen (1979) for a better look at his saying, in My speech to the graduates, *The New York Times*, August 10, p. 25
3. See McCartney (1965) for the Beatles song in Cohen's story: "Yesterday," on *Help!* [CD] (London: EMI Studios).
4. See Hermanns and Einstein (1983) for a better look at Einstein's saying, in *Einstein and the poet: In search of the cosmic man* (p. 58). Brookline Village, MA: Branden Press.
5. See note in Chapter 2 on post-formal thought. Gene referred to post-formal thought and aging in all of his writing; it can be found in the 2005 publication of *The mature mind: The positive power of the aging brain* (New York: Basic Books), with his extensive bibliography on the literature of post-formal thought and aging (p. 197), and in his 2000 publication *The creative age: Awakening human potential in the second half of life* (p. 77). New York: Avon Books.
6. See Sperry (1952) for a better understanding of the right/left brain differences in fantasy and analytic skills, in Neurology and the mind-brain problem. *American Scientist, 40*(2), 291–312.

7. See Cabeza (2002) for a better understanding of the HAROLD model, in Hemispheric asymmetry reduction in older adults: the HAROLD model. *Psychology and Aging, 17*(1), pp. 85–100. Additional information on Cabeza can be found in Cabeza, Daselaar, Dolcos, Prince, Budde, and Nyberg (2004). Task-independent and task-specific age effects on brain activity during working memory, visual attention, and episodic retrieval. *Cerebral Cortex, 14*(4), 364–375.

8. See Maguire, Frith and Morris (1999) for the studies Cohen discusses, in The functional neuroanatomy of comprehension and memory: The importance of prior knowledge. *Brain, 122*(10), 1839–1850 Additionally, see Maguire, Burgess, Donnett, Frackowiak, Frith, and O'Keefe (1998). Knowing where and getting there: A human navigation network. *Science, 280*(5365), 921–924; and Maguire and Frith (2003). Aging affects the engagement of the hippocampus during autobiographical memory retrieval. *Brain, 126*(7), 1511–1523.

9. See Cohen (2005) for a look at the phrase "like chocolate to the brain," in *The mature mind: The positive power of the aging brain* (p. 77). New York: Basic Books, as well as further elaboration on developmental intelligence (pp. 34–39).

10. See Atalay (2004) for plates of Leonardo Da Vinci's Mona Lisa, in *Math and the Mona Lisa: The art and science of Leonardo da Vinci*. Washington, DC: Smithsonian Books.

11. See Drohojowska-Philp and O'Keeffe (2005) for O'Keefe's "Sky Above Clouds" paintings, in *Full bloom: The art and life of Georgia O'Keeffe*. New York: W.W. Norton & Company.

12. *See* www.donotgogently.com for a closer look at *Do Not Go Gently: The power of imagination in aging*. Narrated by Walter Cronkite [DVD 2007 NEWIST/CESA 7].

13. See Cohen (2005) for a better understanding of Pearce, in *The mature mind: The positive power of the aging brain* (pp. 88–89). New York: Basic Books.

14. See Delaney, Delaney, and Hearth (1993) on living into one's hundreds, in *Having our say: The Delany sisters' first 100 years*. New York: Kodansha International.

15. See Cohen (2016), "When My Mother's Inner Light Began to Flicker," essay on his mother's death, in Cox and Harrison (eds.) (2016), *Saying goodbye to our mothers for the last time: A collection of essays*. New York: Lisa Hagan Books.

16. See Gardner (1983) for a better understanding of multiple intelligences, in *Frames of mind: The theory of multiple intelligences* (New York: Basic Books), and for an elaboration with school children, in Miller (2006) in Why art in education matters. *Lowell Ledger, 15*(2), 7.

17. See http://www.wendylmiller.com/media/written%20works/individual/Ripening%20Seeds.pdf for a better understanding of integrative intelligence: the star. Also see Miller (2004) in Ripening seeds: The star of identity through imagery interplay. *International Expressive Arts Therapy Newsletter, 1*, 17–20.

18. See Miller (1992) for a closer look at the development of the star model, in The experience of nine women living with chronic fatigue syndrome, as demonstrated through mental imagery, drawings, and verbal description [PhD dissertation] (pp. 58–63; 234–238). Ann Arbor, MI: University Microfilms International # 9219128; can be retrieved at 800-521-0600.

19. See Remen (1986) for more information on how health is the movement toward wholeness, in Healing and wholeness: Living well and dying well. *Institute of Noetic Sciences Newsletter, 14*(1), 3–7.

20. Information about Elmer Green's research on reverie as the state of healing comes from Miller's attendance at a 1993 conference, The Heart of Healing, at The Menninger Clinic in Topeka, Kansas. Additionally, for Miller's elaboration on reverie, see Miller and Milliken (2002). Pushing the experiential edge in therapy, training and supervision: A case study of Create Therapy Institute's experiential supervision program. *Poiesis: A journal of the arts and communication, 4*, 87–88.

Chapter 12

1. See Strunk and White (1959) for a better understanding of Cohen's use of elements of style for doctor/patient communication, in *Elements of style* (New York: Macmillan), as well as Strunk, White, and Kalman (2005). *The elements of style* (New York: Penguin Press).
2. See Faber and Mazlish (1982) for an insightful analysis on talking and listening, in *How to talk so kids will listen & listen so kids will talk* (New York: Avon).
3. This comment is from her November 6, 2014, lecture at the Gerontological Society of America's annual scientific meeting, "Making Connections from Cells to Societies," November 5–9, 2014, in Washington, DC, where Charon received the Gene D. Cohen Research Award in Creativity and Aging.
4. See De Medeiros (2014) for an elaboration on telling the right story, in *Narrative gerontology in research and practice* (p. 51). New York: Springer.
5. See Charon (2006) for more understanding on doctor–patient communication, in *Narrative medicine: Honoring the stories of illness* (p. 177). New York: Oxford University Press.
6. See http://www.ishiprograms.org/ for further elaboration on the healer's art and other resources at the Institute for the Study of Health and Illness.
7. See Remen (1996) for further information on medical lineage, in *Kitchen table wisdom: Stories that heal* (p. 164). New York: Riverhead Books.
8. See Agronin (2011) for further information on lessons from fire, in *How we age: A doctor's journey into the heart of growing old* (p. 254). Cambridge, MA: De Capo Press.
9. See Gould (2002) http://cancerguide.org/median_not_msg.html for more information on statistics and illness, in *The median isn't the message*, in *CancerGuide*.

Chapter 13

1. See http://www.bettyfordcenter.org/index.php for a better understanding of Cohen's morphine reference to The Betty Ford Center, a non-profit rehab center. In addition, see http://www.hospicepatients.org/terminal-agitation.html for further information on Ativan, morphine, and Haldol, in Terminal agitation: A major distressful symptom in the dying.
2. See Folkenflik (2007) for more information on journalist Art Buchwald, in Columnist Art Buchwald leaves us laughing, *National Public Radio: NPR*, from http://www.npr.org/templates/story/story.php?storyId=5249437
3. See Holland (2007) for a closer look at Pavarotti, Cohen's choice for music on his last night, from http://www.nytimes.com/2007/09/06/arts/music/06pavarotti.html?pagewanted=all&_r=0
4. See Heschel and Rothschild (1959) for the first paragraph quote and prayer, in *Between God and man: An interpretation of Judaism* (p. 208). New York: The Free Press.
5. See Heschel (1976) for second paragraph quote and prayer in *Man is not alone: A philosophy of religion* (p. 16). New York: Farrar, Straus & Giroux. See all three paragraphs of Heschel quotes together in *The New Kehila Makhzor* (2003) (p. 34). Rockville. MD: Kehila Chadasha & Am Kolel Judaic Resource and Renewal Center.

Chapter 14

1. See http://www.nytimes.com/2009/11/12/us/12cohen.html and http://www.washingtonpost.com/wp-dyn/content/article/2009/11/10/AR2009111018634.html and http://gwtoday.gwu.edu/memoriam-gene-cohen for Gene Cohen's expanded obituaries.

2. In 2010, Miller accepted the Hall of Fame Award presented posthumously to Cohen by the American Society on Aging, Aging in America Conference, Chicago, Illinois.
3. See Knowles (2006) for a better understanding of Cohen's story of the Latin phrase "Statue quo vadis," in Quo vadis. *The Oxford Dictionary of Phrase and Fable*, from http://www.encyclopedia.com/doc/1O214-quovadis.html

Chapter 15

1. See Smith and Walt Disney Company (1995) for more on Cruella De Vil, in *Disney's 101 Dalmatians* (California: Mouse Works).
2. See Yeats (1934) for a better look at the quotation, in *The land of heart's desire* (p. 10). New York: French.
3. See Kiester, Jr. and Kiester (2002) for information on Fernando Nottebohm, in Birdbrain breakthrough: Startling evidence that the human brain can grow new nerves began with unlikely studies of birdsong. *Smithsonian Magazine*, June, p. 2.
4. See Andreas (1997) for a better look at the quotation, in *Story people: Selected stories & drawings of Brian Andreas*. Decorah, IA: StoryPeople.

A Note on the Future of the Arts in Healthcare

1. See Boyer (2007) for a better look at the arts and aging toolkit, in *Creativity matters: The arts and aging toolkit*. New York: National Guild of Community Schools of the Arts.
2. See Achterberg (1985) for more information on imagination and medicine, in *Imagery in healing: Shamanism and modern medicine* (p. 72). Boston: New Science Library.
3. See Cohen, Perlstein, Chapline, Kelly, Firth, and Simmens (2006) for an elaboration on the creativity and aging study, in The impact of professionally conducted cultural programs on the physical health, mental health, and social functioning of older adults. *Gerontologist*, 46(6), 726–734.

Further References

Abood, C., Chase, C., Pappalardo-Robinson, M., Rounds, D. (Producers), & Budd, R., Cook, D. (Directors). (2002). *Return to Never Land* [Motion picture]. United States: Buena Vista Pictures.

Achterberg, J. (1985). *Imagery in healing: Shamanism and modern medicine. Boston.* MA: New Science Library.

Agronin, M. E. (2011). *How we age: A doctor's journey into the heart of growing old.* Cambridge, MA: Da Capo Press.

Allen, W. (1979, August 10). My speech to the graduates. *The New York Times,* p. A25.

American Experience. (n.d.). Primary resources: RFK on the death of MLK. Retrieved from http://www.pbs.org/wgbh/americanexperience/features/primary-resources/kennedys-death-mlk/

Andreas, B. (1997). *Story people: Selected stories & drawings of Brian Andreas.* Decorah, IA: StoryPeople.

Assagioli, R. (1965). *Psychosynthesis: A manual of principles and techniques.* New York: Viking Press.

Assagioli, R. (1973). *The act of will.* New York: Viking Press.

Atalay, B. (2004). *Math and the Mona Lisa: The art and science of Leonardo da Vinci.* Washington, DC: Smithsonian Books.

Biggs, A., Glencoe/McGraw-Hill., & National Geographic Society (U.S.). (2009). *Biology.* New York: McGraw-Hill/Glencoe.

Bollas, C. (1989). *Forces of destiny: Psychoanalysis and human idiom.* London: Free Association Books.

Boorstin, D. J. (2001). *The discoverers: A history of man's search to know his world and himself.* London: Phoenix.

Broek, R. (1972). *The myth of the Phoenix, according to classical and early Christian traditions.* Leiden: E.J. Brill.

Cabeza, R. (2002). Hemispheric asymmetry reduction in older adults: The HAROLD model. *Psychology and Aging, 17*(1), 85–100. Retrieved from http://dx.doi.org/10.1037/0882-7974.17.1.85

Cabeza, R., Anderson, N.D., Locantore, J.K., & McIntosh, A.R. (2002). Aging gracefully: Compensatory brain activity in high-performing older adults. *Neuroimage, 17*(3), 1394–1402.

Cabeza, R., Daselaar, S.M., Dolcos, F., Prince, S.E., Budde, M., & Nyberg, L. (2004). Task-independent and task-specific age effects on brain activity during working memory, visual attention and episodic retrieval. *Cerebral Cortex, 14*(4), 364–75.

Cahalan, S. (2014, April 20). From mullet to math genius after a concussion. *New York Post.* Retrieved from http://nypost.com/2014/04/20/how-a-brain-injury-turned-a-college-dropout-into-a-genius/

Carroll, L., & Tenniel J. (1962). *Alice's adventures in wonderland and through the looking glass*. Baltimore: Penguin Books.

Charon, R. (2006). *Narrative medicine: Honoring the stories of illness*. New York: Oxford University Press.

Cicero, M.T., & King. J.E. (1950). *Cicero: XVIII Tusculan disputations*. Cambridge, MA: Harvard University Press.

Cohen, G.D. (1998). Sky above clouds: Mental health in later life. *American Journal of Geriatric Psychiatry, 5*(1), 1–3.

Cohen, G.D. (2000). If you were an old woman who lived in a shoe, what would you do? *American Journal of Geriatric Psychiatry, 8*(2), 93–95.

Cohen, G.D. (2000). *The creative age: Awakening human potential in the second half of life*. New York: Avon Books.

Cohen, G.D. (2005). *The mature mind: The positive power of the aging brain*. New York: Basic Books.

Cohen, G.D. (2009). Historical lessons to watch your assumptions about aging: Relevance to the role of *International Psychogeriatrics*. *International Psychogeriatrics, 21*(03), 425–429.

Cohen, G.D. (2009). New theories and research findings on the positive influence of music and art on health with aging. *Arts & Health, 1*(1), 48–62.

Cohen, G.D. (2011). The geriatric patient. In M.E. Agronin & G.J. Maletta (Eds.), *Principles and practice of geriatric psychiatry* (pp. 15–30). Philadelphia: Lippincott Williams & Wilkins.

Cohen, G.D., Perlstein, S., Chapline, J., Kelly, J., Firth, K.M., & Simmens, S. (2006). The impact of professionally conducted cultural programs on the physical health, mental health, and social functioning of older adults. *Gerontologist, 46*(6), 726–734.

Cole, T.R., & de Medeiros, K. (Eds.). (2010). Special section: A tribute to Gene D. Cohen. *Journal of Aging, Humanities, and the Arts, 4*(4), 235–311.

Cousins, N. (1979). *Anatomy of an illness as perceived by the patient: Reflections on healing and regeneration*. New York: W.W. Norton & Company.

Cox, C.T., & Harrison, W.A. (Eds.). (in press). *Saying goodbye to our mothers for the last time: A collection of essays*. New York: Lisa Hagan Books.

Cox, C.T., & Heller, P.O. (Eds.). (2006). *Portrait of the artist as poet*. Chicago: Magnolia Street Publishers.

de Chirico, G. (1910). *Metaphysical town square* [Painting]. Retrieved from http://www.theartstory.org.

Delany, S.L., Delany, A.E., & Hearth, A.H. (1993). *Having our say: The Delany sisters' first 100 years*. New York: Kodansha International.

De Medeiros, K. (2014). *Narrative gerontology in research and practice*. New York: Springer Publishing.

Disney, W., Smith, D., & Walt Disney Company. (1986). *The 101 Dalmatians*. New York: Gallery Books.

Erikson, E. (1997). *The life cycle completed: Extended version by Joan Erikson*. New York: W.W. Norton.

Faber, A., & Mazlish, E. (1982). *How to talk so kids will listen & listen so kids will talk*. New York: Avon.

Folkenflik, D. (2007, January 18). Columnist Art Buchwald leaves us laughing. *National Public Radio*. Retrieved from http://www.npr.org/templates/story/story.php?storyId=5249437

Freedman, M. (1994). *Clock drawing: A neuropsychological analysis*. New York: Oxford University Press.

Frank, A. (1991). *At the will of the body: Reflections on illness*. Boston: Houghton Mifflin Co.

Frank, A.W. (2013). *The wounded storyteller: Body, illness, and ethics*. Chicago: University of Chicago Press.

Frankl, V.E. (1959). *Man's search for meaning: An introduction to logotherapy*. Boston: Beacon.

Gardner, H. (1983). *Frames of mind: The theory of multiple intelligences*. New York: Basic Books.

Ginsberg, B., & Milken, M. (1998). *The taste for living cookbook: Mike Milken's favorite recipes for fighting cancer*. Santa Monica, CA: CaP CURE.

Godoy, M. (Producer/Director). (2007). *Do not go gently* [Motion picture]. United States: American Public Television.

Gould, S.J. (2002, May 31). The median isn't the message. *CancerGuide.* Retrieved from http://cancerguide.org/median_not_msg.html.

Graves, R. (1955). *The Greek myths.* Baltimore: Penguin Books

Grimm, J., Grimm, W., Colum, P., & Scharl, J. (1972). *The complete Grimm's fairy tales.* New York: Pantheon.

Hamilton, E., Aeschylus, & Euripides. (1937). *Three Greek plays: Prometheus bound, Agamemnon, the Trojan women.* New York: W.W. Norton & Co.

Hampson, S. (2009, June 14). Gene Cohen: The guru of grey matter. *The Globe and the Mail.* Retrieved from http://www.theglobeandmail.com/life/the-guru-of-grey-matter/article4212154/

Hassrick, P.H., Messinger, L.M., Novak, B., Rose, B., & Georgia O'Keeffe Museum. (1997). *The Georgia O'Keeffe Museum.* New York: Harry N. Abrams, Inc. in association with the Georgia O'Keefe Museum.

Havel, V. (1993, October). Never hope against hope. *Esquire*, 68.

Hemingway, E. (1995). *The old man and the sea.* New York: Scribner.

Heraclitus, & Robinson, T.M. (1987). *Fragments.* Toronto: University of Toronto Press.

Hermanns, W., & Einstein, A. (1983). *Einstein and the poet: In search of the cosmic man.* Brookline Village, MA: Branden Press.

Heschel, A.J. (1976). *Man is not alone: A philosophy of religion.* New York: Farrar, Straus & Giroux.

Heschel, A.J., & Rothschild, F.A. (1959). *Between God and man: An interpretation of Judaism.* New York: The Free Press.

Hesiod, & Sinclair, T.A. (1979). *Works and days.* New York: Arno Press.

Holland, B. (2007, September 6). Luciano Pavarotti is dead at 71. *The New York Times.* Retrieved from http://www.nytimes.com/2007/09/06/arts/music/06pavarotti.html?pagewanted=all&_r=0

Huggins, R. (Creator). (1958–1964). *77 Sunset Strip* [Television series]. Hollywood, CA: American Broadcasting Company.

Huxley, A. (1976). *Texts & pretexts: An anthology with commentaries.* Westport, CT: Greenwood Press.

Johnston, C.M. (1984). *The creative imperative: A four-dimensional theory of human growth and planetary evolution.* Berkeley, CA: Celestial Arts.

Joyce, J., & Rose, D. (1997). *Ulysses.* London: Picador.

Jung, C.G. (1966). *Two essays on analytical psychology.* Princeton, NJ: Princeton University Press.

Kempermann, G., Kuhn, H.G., & Gage, F.H. (1998). Experience-induced neurogenesis in the senescent dentate gyrus. *Journal of Neuroscience, 18*(9), 3206–3212.

Kiecolt-Glaser, J.K., McGuire, L., Robles, T.F., & Glaser, R. (2002, January 01). Emotions, morbidity, and mortality: New perspectives from psychoneuroimmunology. *Annual Review of Psychology, 53,* 83–107.

Kierkegaard, S., & Hannay, A. (1996). *Papers and journals: A selection.* New York: Penguin Books.

Kiester, E., & Kiester, W. (2002, June 1). Birdbrain breakthrough: Startling evidence that the human brain can grow new nerves began with unlikely studies of birdsong. *Smithsonian Magazine.* Retrieved from http://www.smithsonianmag.com/science-nature/birdbrain-breakthrough-64765165/?no-ist=&page=2.

King, M.L., Jr. (1968). *The trumpet of conscience.* New York: Harper & Row.

Kleinman, A. (1988). *The illness narratives: Suffering, healing, and the human condition.* New York: Basic Books.

Knill, P.J., Barba, H.N., & Fuchs, M. (1995). *Minstrels of soul: Intermodal expressive therapy.* Toronto: Palmerston Press.

Knowles, E. (2006). Quo vadis. *The Oxford Dictionary of Phrase and Fable.* Retrieved from http://www.encyclopedia.com/doc/1O214-quovadis.html

Kobasa, S.C. (1979). Stressful life events, personality and health: An inquiry into hardiness. *Journal of Personality and Social Psychology, 37,* 1–11

Kobasa, S.C., Maddi, S.R., & Kahn, S. (1982). Hardiness and Health: a prospective study. *Journal of Personality and Social Psychology, 42*(1), 168–177.

Kundera, M. (1984). *The unbearable lightness of being.* New York: Harper & Row.

Kundtz, D. (1998). *Stopping: How to be still when you have to keep going.* Berkeley, CA: Conari Press.

Lerner, M. (1990). *Wrestling with the angel: A memoir of my triumph over illness.* New York: Norton.

Lerner, M. (1994). *Choices in healing: Integrating the best of conventional and complementary approaches to cancer.* Cambridge, MA: MIT Press.

LeShan, L.L. (1989). *Cancer as a turning point: A handbook for people with cancer, their families, and health professionals.* New York: Dutton.

Lutgendorf, S.K., Vitaliano, P.P., Tripp-Reimer, T., Harvey, J.H., & Lubaroff, D.M. (1999). Sense of coherence moderates the relationship between life stress and natural killer cell activity in healthy older adults. *Psychology and Aging, 14*(4), 552–563.

Maguire, E.A., Burgess, N., Donnett, J.G., Frackowiak, R.S., Frith, C.D., & O'Keefe, J. (1998). Knowing where and getting there: A human navigation network. *Science, 280*(5365), 921–924.

Maguire, E.A., & Frith, C.D. (2003). Aging affects the engagement of the hippocampus during autobiographical memory retrieval. *Brain: A Journal of Neurology, 126*(7), 1511–1523.

Maguire, E.A., Frith, C.D., & Morris, R.G.M. (1999). The functional neuroanatomy of comprehension and memory: The importance of prior knowledge. *Brain, 122*(10), 1839–1850.

Maugham, W.S. (2001). *The summing up.* London: Vintage.

McCartney, P. (1965). Yesterday [Recorded by the Beatles]. On *Help!* [CD]. London: EMI Studios.

Meyer, N. (Ed.). (1974). *The seven-per-cent solution: Being a reprint from the reminiscences of John H. Watson, MD.* New York: Dutton.

Miller, D.P. (1992). My healing journey through chronic fatigue. *Yoga Journal, 11/12*(62–67), 123–125.

Miller, W. (1988). Living with illness. *Pathways,* Spring, 31, 33.

Miller, W. (1991). Art as a therapeutic element in the healing process with chronic fatigue syndrome: Grant recipients. *The Rose Window: Newsletter of Healing Through Arts, 3–4*

Miller, W. (1992). *The experience of nine women living with chronic fatigue syndrome, as demonstrated through mental imagery, drawings, and verbal description* (Doctoral dissertation). University Microfilms International (9219128).

Miller, W. (1996). Imagery, art and health: Excerpts from a series of presentations on art as complementary medicine (pp. 1–15). Strategic Implications International.

Miller, W. (1997). Imagery, art and health: Excerpts from a series of presentations on art as complementary medicine. *C.R.E.A.T.E., Journal of the Creative and Expressive Arts Therapy Exchange, 6,* 41–46.

Miller, W. (2003). Metaphors of identity and motifs of expression: Clinical observations on international adoption and the use of the sand tray process in art therapy with internationally adopted children. In D. Betts (Ed.), *Creative arts therapies approaches in adoption and foster care: Complementary strategies for working with individuals and families.* New York: Charles C. Thomas.

Miller, W. (2003). Still searching for the ground of memory. *Poiesis: A Journal of the Arts and Communication, 5,* 127–139.

Miller, W. (2004). Ripening seeds: The star of identity through imagery interplay. *International Expressive Arts Therapy Newsletter, 1,* 17–20. Retrieved from http://www.wendylmiller. com/media/written%20works/individual/Ripening%20Seeds.pdf.

Miller, W. (2006). Wendy Miller. In C.T. Cox & P.O. Heller (Eds.), *Portrait of the artist as poet* (pp. 120–125). Chicago: Magnolia Street Publishers.

Miller, W. (2006). Why art in education matters. *Lowell Ledger, 15*(2), 7.

Miller, W., & Cohen, G.D. (2010). On creativity, illness and aging. *Journal of Aging, Humanities, and the Arts, 4*(4), 302–311.

Miller, W., & Milliken, R. (2002). Pushing the experiential edge in therapy, training, and supervision: A case study of Create Therapy Institute's experiential supervision program. *Poiesis: A Journal of the Arts and Communication, 4*, 79–89.

Ming, G.L., & Song, H. (2005). Adult neurogenesis in the mammalian central nervous system. *Annual Review of Neurosciences, 28*, 223–250.

Mitoxantrone. (2012, April 20). Retrieved from http://www.cancer.org/treatment/treatment-sandsideeffects/guidetocancerdrugs/mitoxantrone

Nottebohm, F. (2002). Why are some neurons replaced in adult brain? *Journal of Neuroscience, 22*(3), 624–8.

Nottebohm, F., Stokes, T.M., & Leonard, C.M. (1976). Central control of song in the canary, *Serinus canarius*. *Journal of Comparative Neurology, 165*(4), 457–486.

Ornish, D., Gerdi, W., Fair, W.R., Ruth, M., Pettengill, E.B., Raisin, C.J., & Barbard, R.J. (2005). Intensive lifestyle changes may affect the progression of prostate cancer. *Journal of Urology, 174*(3), 1065–1070.

Padgett, J., & Seaberg, M.A. (2014). *Struck by genius: How a brain injury made me a mathematical marvel*. Boston: Houghton Mifflin Harcourt.

Pert, C.B., Dreher, H.E., & Ruff, M.R. (1998). The psychosomatic network: Foundations of mind-body medicine. *Alternative Therapies in Health and Medicine, 4*(4), 30–41.

Phoenix. (n.d.). In *Oxford English Dictionary* online. Retrieved from http://www.oed.com.proxy-um.researchport.umd.edu.

Remen, R.N. (1980). *The human patient*. Garden City, NY: Anchor Press.

Remen, R.N. (1986). Healing and wholeness: Living well and dying well. *Institute of Noetic Sciences Newsletter, 14*(1), 3–7.

Remen, R.N. (1996). *Kitchen table wisdom: Stories that heal*. New York: Riverhead Books.

Remen, R.N. (2000). *My grandfather's blessings: Stories of strength, refuge, and belonging*. New York: Riverhead Books.

Remen, R.N. (2001). Recapturing the soul of medicine: Physicians need to reclaim meaning in their working lives. *Western Journal of Medicine, 174*(1), 4.

Rimbaud, A., & Ashbery, J. (2011). *Illuminations*. New York: W.W. Norton.

Robinson, A. (n.d.). How to make diamonds from coal [eHow]. Retrieved from http://www.ehow.com/how_5312998_make-diamonds-coal.html

Rodin, J. (1986). Aging and health: Effects of the sense of control. *Science, 233*(4770), 1271–1276.

Rodin, J. (1989). Sense of control: Potentials for intervention. *Annals of the American Academy of Policy and Social Science, 503*, 29–42.

Rosenberg, J.A. (2010). Regrettably unfair: Brooke Astor and the other elderly in New York. *Pace Law Review, 30*(3), 1004–1060.

Ross, H. (Producer/Director). (1976). *The seven-per-cent solution: Sherlock Holmes meets Sigmund Freud* [Motion picture]. United States: Universal Pictures.

Schnabel, A. (1963). *My life and music*. New York: St. Martin's Press.

Schopenhauer, A. (1974). *On the fourfold of the principle of sufficient reason*. New York: Cosimo Classics.

Shneyer (Ed.). (2003). *The New Kehila Makhzor*. Rockville: MD: Kehila Chadasha, Am Kolel Judaic Resource and Renewal Center.

Smith, D., & Walt Disney Company. (1995). *Disney's 101 Dalmatians*. California: Mouse Works.

Spengler, P. (Producer), & Donner, R. (Director). (1978). *Superman* [Motion picture]. United States: Warner Bros.

Sperry, R.W. (1952). Neurology and the mind-brain problem. *American Scientist, 4*(2), 291–312.

Sperry, R.W. (1982). Some effects of disconnecting the cerebral hemispheres. *Bioscience Reports, 2*(5), 265–276.

Sperry, R.W., Gazzaniga, M.S., & Bogen, J.E. (1969). Interhemispheric relationships: The neocortical commissures; syndromes of hemisphere disconnection. *Handbook of Clinical Neurology, 4*, 273–290.

Strategic Implications International (Producer). (1996). *Healing through art: The story of an artist's experience with lymphoma (Darcy Lynn)* [Video]. (Available form Cogent Interactive Communications, 1921 Galloway Rd., Suite 360, Vienna, Virginia, 22182).

Strunk, W., & White, E.B. (1959). *The elements of style.* New York: Macmillan.

Strunk, W., White, E.B., & Kalman, M. (2005). *The elements of style.* New York: Penguin Press.

Terminal agitation: A major distressful symptom in the dying. (n.d.). Retrieved from http://www.hospicepatients.org/terminal-agitation.html

Thomas, D. (1957). *The collected poems of Dylan Thomas.* New York: New Directions Books.

Thoreau, H.D., & Krutch, J.W. (Ed.). (1971). *Thoreau: Walden and other writings.* New York: Bantam Books.

van Gelder, D. (1999). *The real world of fairies: A first-person account.* Wheaton, IL: Quest.

Wells, H.G. (1927). *The short stories of H.G. Wells.* London: Ernest Benn Limited.

White, P., Wilbur, C., Panzer, P., Grapevine Video (Firm), & Eclectic Film Company. (1995). *The perils of Pauline, 1914: The hidden voice.* Phoenix, AZ: Grapevine Video.

Williams, W.C., & Rosenthal, M.L. (1966). *The William Carlos Williams reader.* New York: New Directions.

Yeats, W.B. (1934). *The land of heart's desire.* New York: French.

About the Authors

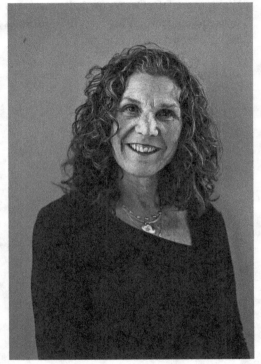

photo credit: Claire Blatt

Wendy L. Miller, PhD

Wendy Miller Ph.D., LPC-BCPC, ATR-BC, LCPAT, REAT, is a writer, sculptor, expressive arts therapist, and educator. She has taught at JFK University, San Francisco State University, Southwestern College, Lesley College, California Institute of Integral Studies, and George Washington University. She is the cofounder of Create Therapy Institute, which offers clinical services in arts-based psychotherapy and trainings in experiential approaches to learning. She is a founding member and first elected (past) executive co-chair of the International Expressive Arts Therapy Association, where she continues to be on their Advisory

Council. She is also on the Advisory Board of MaineGeneral's Healthy Living Resource Center and Blossom Arts Board of Advisors.

Miller's skills take her into the worlds of fine art, writing, psychology, expressive arts therapy, and mind–body medicine. She has published on medical illness and the arts as complementary medicine, the use of sand tray therapy with internationally adopted children, experiential approaches to supervision in expressive arts therapy, and the cultural responsibility of the arts in therapy. Her current work is evolving as she continues the legacy of her late husband's work and his Washington, DC, Center on Aging, where she is guiding it into projects on intergenerational communication. She continues to research the relationships among the arts, creativity, and health.

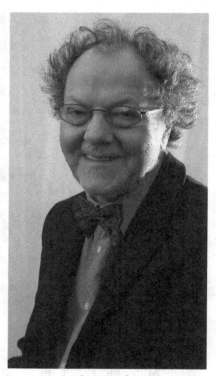

photo credit: Joshua Soros

Gene D. Cohen, MD, PhD

Gene D. Cohen, M.D., Ph.D., is considered one of the founding fathers of the field of geriatric psychiatry. He was the first director of the Center on Aging, Health & Humanities (established in 1994) at George Washington University, where he held the positions of professor of health care sciences and professor of psychiatry. He is a past-president of the Gerontological Society of America. During 1991–1993, he served as acting director of the National Institute on Aging (NIA) at the National Institutes of Health (NIH). Before coming to NIA, Dr. Cohen served as the first chief of the Center on Aging of the National Institute of Mental Health—the first federal center on mental health and aging established in any country. In addition, he also coordinated the Department of Health and Human Services' planning and programs on Alzheimer's disease, through the efforts of the Department's Council and Panel on Alzheimer's disease. For his recent research on Alzheimer's disease, he was awarded first place in the Blair Sadler International Healing Arts Competition from the Society for the Arts in Health Care. He was founding director of the Washington, D.C. Center on Aging and past president of the Gerontological Society of America. He appeared on *Nightline, The MacNeil/Lehrer Report*, and the *CBS Nightly News*, and appeared in a series of public service messages on aging with George Burns and Steve Allen. He invented four inter-generational board games, one that was selected by an international art jury for a three-year museum tour.

He is the author of more than 150 publications in the field of aging, including *The Brain in Human Aging*, published by Springer, in their Series on Life Style and Issues in Aging, in 1988, and the first book on creativity and aging, published in 2000 by Avon, *The Creative Age: Awakening Human Potential in the Second of Life*. PBS did a one-hour TV program on *The Creative Age*, and the book is published in six languages. In 2005, Basic Books published *The Mature Mind: The Positive Power of the Aging Brain*.

Teresa H. Barker, Co-writer

A career journalist and book collaborator, Teresa Barker has co-written more than a dozen books in the fields of parenting and child development, adult psychology, creativity and aging, personal growth, healing, and spirituality. She collaborated with Gene Cohen on *The Creative Age* and *The Mature Mind*. She also is co-writer of *The New York Times* bestsellers *Raising Cain: Protecting the Emotional Life of Boys* (Michael G. Thompson and Dan Kindlon) and *The Spiritual Child: The New Science of Parenting for Health and Lifelong Thriving* (Lisa Miller). Other recent titles include *The Big Disconnect: Protecting Childhood and Family Relationships in the Digital Age* (Catherine Steiner-Adair), and *Self-Reg: How to Help Your Child (and You) Break the Stress Cycle and Successfully Engage with Life* (Stuart Shanker).

Additional information about the authors and the book

www.sky-above-clouds.com
www.Facebook.com/skyaboveclouds
www.Instagram.com/sky_above_clouds
https://global.oup.com/academic/product/sky-above-clouds-9780199371419
http://dccenteronaging.org/

Index

References to figures are denoted by an italicized *f*